CANCER ETIOLOGY, DIAGNOSIS AND TREATMENTS

PENILE CANCER

CHALLENGES AND CONTROVERSIES

CANCER ETIOLOGY, DIAGNOSIS AND TREATMENTS

Additional books and e-books in this series can be found on Nova's website under the Series tab.

MEN'S ISSUES

Additional books and e-books in this series can be found on Nova's website under the Series tab.

Cancer Etiology, Diagnosis and Treatments

Penile Cancer

Challenges and Controversies

Francisco E. Martins
and
Miroslav L. Djordjevic
Editors

Nova Medicine & Health
New York

Additional color graphics may be available in the e-book version of this book.

Library of Congress Cataloging-in-Publication Data

ISBN: 978-1-53615-950-9
Library of Congress Control Number: 2019946125

Published by Nova Science Publishers, Inc. † New York

CONTENTS

PREFACE

This book on penile cancer is the end-result of the contribution of an international panel of worldwide renowned experts on the field, who so kindly have lent their time, patience and efforts to make this book a worthy backlog of up-to-date information on challenges and controversies of a still uncommon malignant disease in western, industrialized countries such as penile cancer.

"Penile Cancer: Challenges and Controversies" is divided into five sections. Section A includes 4 chapters featuring Introduction, Epidemiology, Pathology, and Diagnosis and Staging of Penile Cancer. Relevant issues pertaining to epidemiology, pathological characteristics of the most common type of penile cancer and other less common types and subtypes of penile malignancy. The final part of this section will cover the capabilities of the modern imaging tools employed in the clinical diagnosis and staging of penile cancer which are the cornerstones of staging, risk stratification and treatment planning as prognosis depends heavily on accurate inguinal node staging. Section B covers an in-depth discussion of the current surgical treatment approaches to penile cancer where surgical resection can yield remarkably high cure rates if employed in the early stages of the disease, especially in patients with clinically negative groins. In more advanced stages, cure rates decrease dramatically and a multimodal therapeutic approach by a multidisciplinary team is the path to follow for rescue and salvage of these unfortunate patients. This nonsurgical multimodal management and contemporary recommendations for follow-up is the scope of Section C. Sections D and E deal with critical issues linked to quality of life of the penile cancer survivor. Historically, mutilating and disfiguring partial or total penile amputation was the rule and the only therapeutic option penile cancer patients were offered which was associated with devastating impact on sexual and urinary functions, as well as psychosocial traits of manhood. Penile-preserving strategies have become standard treatment in localized, low-to-intermediate risk disease. Recently, restoration of penile anatomy and function has taken bolder steps in an attempt to legitimize penile transplantation in penile cancer survivors who underwent amputation and remain disease-free. Section F tackles some still unresolved challenges and controversies surrounding penile cancer disease, like "is prevention and early diagnosis routinely possible?", changes in management decision-making according to clinical stage of the disease, how to best manage patients with clinically negative groins, impact of minimally invasive technology on inguinal lymphadenectomy, the exact risks and benefits of surgery involving penile preservation as well as "what is the best timing for penile preservation approaches and who should perform these operations"? A number of these challenges and controversies result, on one hand, from the rarity of the disease in the developed countries where most of the scientific and financial resources are allocated. And, on the other hand, the relative lack of interest and incentives from the pharmaceutical industry in penile cancer. And lastly, Section F also attempts to uncover what's in the horizon to improve our current strategies in terms of, first and foremost, prevention, but also diagnostic and staging accuracy, delineation of a molecular profile for patients with clear impact on epidemiology, and ultimately introduction of newer and more efficacious systemic treatments capable of implementing cure with minimal morbidity and thus converting penile cancer into a medically curable disease. This desideratum will need a global collaboration including dedicated scientific, industry and political partnerships. Unfortunately, we still foresee a long journey looming ahead to reach this destination.

Francisco E. Martins, MD
Miroslav L. Djordjevic, MD, PhD

SECTION A. INTRODUCTION, EPIDEMIOLOGY, PATHOLOGY, DIAGNOSIS AND STAGING OF PENILE CANCER

In: Penile Cancer: Challenges and Controversies
Editors: F. E. Martins and M. L. Djordjevic
ISBN: 978-1-53615-950-9

Chapter 1

INTRODUCTION

Francisco E. Martins[1,*], MD and Miroslav L. Djordjevic[2], MD, PhD
[1]Department of Urology, University of Lisbon, School of Medicine, CHULN, Lisbon, Portugal
[2]University of Belgrade, School of Medicine, Children's Hospital, and Belgrade Center for Genital Reconstructive Surgery, Belgrade, Serbia

Penile cancer is an uncommon neoplasm in developed and industrialized western nations occurring in approximately 1 per 100,000 males in the USA and Europe. However, its occurrence can reach between 10% and 22% in developing countries, particularly in some regions of Africa, Asia and South America. The rarity of the disease, its variable clinical manifestation, delay in seeking medical attention due to frequent embarrassment, shame and sense of guilt felt by the patients, as well as potential misdiagnosis by the initial physician constitute negative factors that often delay diagnosis and, consequently, successful treatment outcomes. Because of this delay, clinical evaluation often results in erroneous staging with dismal implications on prognosis. If performed early, clinical evaluation alone can often characterize the disease with a high level of accuracy and this can be significantly complemented by modern imaging diagnostic modalities currently available such as magnetic resonance imaging (MRI), ultrasound-guided fine-needle aspiration cytology (US-guided FNAC), dynamic sentinel lymph node biopsy (DSLNB) based on lymphoscintigraphic imaging patterns as well as other novel imaging techniques, namely positron emission tomography/computed tomography (PET-CT) and nanoparticle enhanced MRI allowing for detailed depiction of penile anatomy, assessment of lymph nodes, confirmation of metastatic involvement in

* Corresponding Author's E-mail: faemartins@gmail.com.

suspicious inguinal nodes (or even to predict its occult spread) in order to achieve a most accurate clinical status of a patient with penile cancer.

Significant advances have occurred in the various facets of penile cancer treatment, subsequent cancer survivorship and quality of life. Traditional penile mutilating resections have given way to currently standard minimally invasive treatment modalities for localized disease with no negative impact on recurrence and prognosis. In case of recurrence, this is easily and promptly salvageable with wider resection and non-surgical treatments without compromising successful outcomes and prognosis.

Novel systemic chemotherapeutic and immunomodulating agents are currently under investigation and the preliminary results are promising.

This book, authored by a panel of dedicated experts in the various aspects of penile cancer, comprehensively discusses the standard management of penile cancer simultaneously highlighting the ongoing challenges and controversies that still surrounds this malignant disease.

In: Penile Cancer: Challenges and Controversies ISBN: 978-1-53615-950-9
Editors: F. E. Martins and M. L. Djordjevic

Chapter 2

EPIDEMIOLOGY, ETIOLOGY, NATURAL HISTORY AND RISK FACTORS

Ryan W. Speir**, Adam Calaway and Timothy A. Masterson
Indiana University School of Medicine,
Department of Urology, Indianapolis, Indiana, US

ABSTRACT

The purpose of this review is to present an updated summary of the incidence and geographic distribution of this disease, the associated risk factors for its development, as well as an overview of the natural progression of disease by stage, patterns of spread, and associated survival for penile cancer patients. Covered herein are several main themes. Penile cancer incidence, stratified by geographic and economic factors, as trended over time, is discussed. This is followed by an extensive review of risk factors, including circumcision status, physical, chemical and infectious exposures, and lifestyle/social factors. Finally, this review is concluded with the natural history of penile cancer along with the patterns of spread and associated survival outcomes. Recent literature, combined with a significant contribution from historical studies suggest that while penile cancer is uncommon, it remains a significant source of morbidity in the developing world. Many risk factors have been identified, some of which are modifiable. Early identification and treatment significantly improve survival outcomes. The key message is that education and public health initiatives in developing countries should be aimed at improving healthcare infrastructure and identifying locally relevant risk factors with the subsequent development of mitigation programs.

Keywords: penile cancer, epidemiology, etiology, natural history, risk factors, incidence, prevalence

---

* Corresponding Author's E-mail: rwspeir@gmail.com.

Introduction

Penile cancer is an uncommon malignancy worldwide, accounting for less than 1% of solid tumors among men in the United States and around 300 deaths per year [1]. Associated with devastating physical and psychological effects for patients, it can affect men of all ages and across all nationalities [2]. While histologic subtypes of primary penile malignancies can vary, squamous cell carcinoma predominates in the vast majority of cases. The epidemiological and socioeconomic factors associated with the development of penile squamous cell carcinoma have been well characterized. Within this chapter, we present an updated summary of the incidence and geographic distribution of this disease, the associated risk factors for its development, as well as an overview of the natural progression of disease by stage, patterns of spread, and associated survival for penile cancer patients.

Epidemiology

Incidence

There is marked discrepancy worldwide in the overall rates of penile cancer. Penile cancer is rare in North America, Europe and other industrialized countries being diagnosed in <1/100000 men. It accounts for 0.4-0.6% of all cancers and 0.1% of cancer related deaths in the US and Europe [3]. In the US, about 2,320 new cases are expected in 2018 with about 380 deaths from penile cancer [1]. In contrast, penile cancer is more common in Asia, Africa and South America, where it can account for up to 6% of all cancers in men [4]. This tends to be related to a high rate of economic disparity and low rate of neonatal circumcision, as has been shown in assessing rates of penile cancer in relation to religious practices. In fact, Israeli Jews have the lowest overall rate of penile cancer amongst all religious groups at 0.1/100,000, likely related to their circumcision practice [5].

Penile cancer typically affects older men with peak incidence between the ages of 50-70 years although it can be seen in much younger men and tends to occur earlier among those with HIV and HPV infections [2]. Additionally, the incidence of penile cancer varies by race. In evaluating men with penile cancer in the United States, white and black men have similar incidence (0.81 vs 0.82 per 100,000) while Hispanic men have a >2-fold increased risk (1.72/100,000) and lower in Asian/Pacific Islanders (0.45/100,000) at every age group. Hispanic men aged 80 years or older have the highest incidence of any-race/any-age group [6].

Geographic/Economic Distribution

In the United States, there is geographic variability with regards to the incidence of new penile cancer diagnoses. Compared to western states, penile cancer is significantly more prevalent in the south, northeast and Midwest [7]. This has been reportedly related to both economic disparity within the US as well as racial distributions and religious practices.

Penile cancer risk is 43% higher in men from countries with 20% or more of the population living at the poverty level compared with men living in regions of <10% poverty [7]. Additionally, penile cancer rates are higher in countries where <75% of men completed high school education [8]. Brazil has the highest incidence with 2.8-6.8/100,000 and penile squamous cell carcinoma is the 4th most common tumor in men in this country, accounting for 2.1% of male malignancies nation-wide [9]. Even within this country, tremendous economic disparity exists resulting in dispirit incidence rates. In the northeast region, where it is less economically developed, the rate is 5.7%, while in the southeast region, the rate is 1.2% [10].

Trends over Time

Overall, rates in industrialized nations over time seem to be relatively stable, although a closer evaluation shows a decrease in rates in the US between 1970 and 1990 from 0.84/100,000 to 0.58/100,000. A review of the SEER data base between 1998 and 2003, however, showed rates returning to 1970 level at 0.81. Similarly, in the UK, rates since the mid 1990's seem to be increasing, with incidence rates ranging from 1.1 to 1.33/100,000. This is perhaps associated with higher rates of HPV and other STDs in association with lower circumcision rates [11].

This is in contrast to the rates of penile cancer in developing nations. In Uganda, for example, the nation with the second highest rate of penile cancer behind Brazil, the rate has decreased. While it remains high at 3-4/100,000, it has decreased since 1960. This is attributed in part by improved urbanization and piped water supply leading to improved penile hygiene [12]. Additionally, there has been a significant effort to perform pre-pubertal circumcisions and the effect of this on the incidence of a cancer which tends to occur in the 5-6th decade of life will be realized over the coming decades.

RISK FACTORS (TABLE 1)

Lack of Circumcision

The protective effect of circumcision against the development of penile cancer was first suggested in the 1930's. An epidemiologic cohort study evaluated 1,103 cases of penile cancer diagnosed in the United States. Analysis of patient demographics revealed that no Jewish men were included in this cohort which drastically contrasted the 33 expected penile cancer cases in Jewish men (Jewish men made up 3% of the population at that time). Circumcision, a universal religious practice for Jewish men, was offered as an explanation for this epidemiologic finding [13]. This observation was confirmed by a smaller study of 120 cases of penile cancer diagnosed in New York City. No patient with penile cancer was Jewish despite the fact that 1/3 of all other cancers in the hospital occurred in Jewish patients [14].

The timing of circumcision is also an important factor in penile cancer risk. Cases of penile cancer in men who had a neonatal circumcision are extremely rare; however, circumcision later in life does not confer the same beneficial effect. In a cohort of 50,000 male penile cancer patients, only 10 were circumcised as a newborn leading to a ratio of uncircumcised to neonatal circumcised men with cancer of 5000:1 [15]. A population-based case-control study from Washington State and British Columbia demonstrated that uncircumcised men has a 3.2x higher risk for penile cancer than men who had a neonatal circumcision. Moreover, men who were circumcised after the neonatal period had a 3x higher risk of penile cancer than men who had a neonatal circumcision [16]. The beneficial effect of neonatal circumcision was confirmed in numerous other studies [10, 17, 18].

Table 1. Risk factors associated with increased incidence of penile SCC

Lack of Circumcision
Phimosis and Poor Hygiene
Lichen Sclerosus and Inflammatory Conditions
Obesity
Social Factors (marital status, income, education, insurance status, etc.)
Premalignant Lesions and Immune Compromise
Smoking and Marijuana Use
UVA phototherapy
HPV (strains 16, 18, 31, 45, 56 and 65)

Human papilloma virus (HPV) is another risk factor of penile cancer as discussed in a following section. After numerous randomized controlled trials in Africa provided compelling evidence to suggest circumcision was protective against Human Immunodeficiency Virus (HIV) infection, it was hypothesized that circumcision may also be protective against HPV acquisition and transmission [19-21]. The first study investigating this hypothesis was a continuation of two parallel trials in Uganda evaluating circumcision and HIV infection rates. In a subgroup analysis evaluating HPV infection at baseline and during follow-up, prevalence of high-risk HPV genotypes was 18% in those who underwent circumcision and 27.9% in those who did not (adjusted risk ratio 0.65, 95% CI 0.46-0.90).[22] These findings were supported by data from two other male circumcision studies conducted in Sub-Saharan Africa documenting similar results [23, 24]. Finally, a randomized trial in Uganda demonstrated that male circumcision reduced HPV transmission to female partners. HIV-negative men were randomized to either immediate or delayed circumcision. HPV prevalence was similar in the spouses of the intervention and control groups at baseline. After two years, HPV prevalence (27.8 vs 38.7%) and incidence (20.7 vs 26.9 per 100-person years) in the spouse was lower in the intervention group than the control group, respectively. Clearance of genotype-specific HPV was also higher in wives of men in the intervention group (66.2 vs 59.2%) [25].

Phimosis and Poor Hygiene

The protective effect of circumcision on penile cancer risk is likely due to the decreased risk of phimosis in uncircumcised males. A population-based case-control study reported that uncircumcised men with penile cancer were 5x more likely to report a history of phimosis than controls. Phimosis in uncircumcised males was strongly associated with the development of invasive penile cancer [Odds Ratio (OR): 11.4]. This association was negated in uncircumcised men without phimosis [26]. A second case-control study of 100 matched pairs of men from Los Angeles County confirmed that phimosis was a strongly associated with invasive penile carcinoma (OR: 16). This association persisted in a restricted group of uncircumcised patients thus suggesting that the protective effect of circumcision on penile cancer risk is due in large part to the reduced risk of phimosis [27]. The relationship between phimosis and penile cancer was further observed in numerous European countries in which circumcision is not routinely performed after birth [28]. Poor hygiene, especially in uncircumcised males, may increase the risk of phimosis and thus the risk of penile cancer. In Paraguay, the incidence of penile cancer is 4-times higher than the rate in the United States. In a cohort of 103 Paraguayan men with penile cancer, phimosis was a common finding in men who had moderate or poor hygiene habits thus suggesting that better hygiene could minimize phimosis and subsequent risk for penile cancer [29].

Lichen Sclerosis and Inflammatory Conditions

Chronic inflammation is the proposed pathophysiologic mechanism for carcinogenesis of penile cancer in men with phimosis. Thus, many studies have investigated the association between chronic inflammatory disorders and penile cancer. Chronic balanitis has been shown to be associated with risk of penile cancer in a recent meta-analysis of 4 studies (OR: 3.82, 95% Confidence Interval 1.61-9.06) [15, 26, 30,

31]. Penile lichen sclerosis, also known as balanitis xerotica obliterans (BXO), is associated with penile cancer and often seen in conjunction with penile cancer on pathology specimens. A single-institution retrospective cohort study of 522 patients reported that 2.3% of patients treated surgically for lichen sclerosis had squamous cell carcinoma of the penis as well [32]. Conversely, in a cohort of 223 men surgically treated for squamous cell carcinoma of the penis, 23.3% of men had synchronous lichen sclerosis. When comparing patients with and without synchronous lichen sclerosis, there was no difference in oncological outcomes suggesting that presence of lichen sclerosis is not associated with adverse outcomes [33]. Moreover, an observational study over a 10-year period in Italy reviewed 130 patients with pathologically confirmed genital lichen sclerosis to assess for concurrent premalignant or malignant histopathological features. Overall, 11 and 7 men had premalignant or malignant features, respectively, suggesting that patients with lichen sclerosis should be observed closely for the development of malignant lesions [34].

Obesity

Obesity is a well-known risk factor for many malignancies; however, the association between obesity and penile cancer is unclear. A case-control study comparing penile cancer patients with Behavioral Risk Factor Surveillance System (BRFSS) cancer-free controls indicated that higher body mass index (BMI) was associated with a higher risk of invasive penile cancer and higher stage of disease at presentation. For every 5-unit increase in BMI, the odds of having invasive penile cancer increased 2-fold (OR 2.0, 95% Confidence Interval 1.72-2.33) and the odds of higher stage disease at presentation increased by 49% (OR 1.49, 95% Confidence Interval 1.16-1.91) [35]. The same group confirmed these results in a matched case-control study using different population databases [36]. These associations contradict a single-center cohort study of 433 men with penile cancer treated over a 6-year period in Europe. No relationship was seen between BMI and American Joint Committee on Cancer stage at diagnosis (OR 1.01, 95% Confidence Interval 0.9-1.05). Disease-specific survival stratified by BMI categories was similar amongst all groups suggesting that BMI at penile cancer treatment did not affect disease prognosis [37].

Social Factors

Social determinants of health (marital status, income, education, insurance status, etc.) are well-established risk factors for cancer incidence and mortality. A population-based registry from Sweden compared 1,676 men with penile cancer to 9,872 controls.

Lower educational level was associated with an increased risk of invasive penile cancer and a more advanced stage at diagnosis. These trends also were seen in divorced, never-married and men living in single family households. Importantly, these socioeconomic factors did not influence cancer-specific mortality [8]. Studies using population databases from the United States demonstrate similar results. Using the Surveillance, Epidemiology and End Results (SEER) database, unmarried men had a 1.5-fold higher risk of having locally advanced disease at the time of surgery than married men on multivariate logistic regression analysis. Again, marital status did not have an effect on disease-specific mortality in this cohort [38]. More recently, the National Cancer Database was used to identified socioeconomic risk factors of advanced pathological stage (pT2 or higher) at diagnosis. Uninsured (OR 1.79), lower education (OR 1.13), African American (1.17) and Hispanic (1.66) race and geographic location (non-metropolitan) were significant factors on multivariable analysis [39].

Premalignant Lesions and Immune Compromise

Premalignant lesions of the penis are thought to be benign lesions with the potential for malignant transformation. The risk of malignant transformation is dependent upon the site of diagnosis and type of lesion. Premalignant lesions are often dichotomized into HPV and non-HPV associated lesions. Lichen sclerosis, as previously discussed, is a non-HPV associated premalignant lesion [33]. Cutaneous penile horns are rare exophytic lesions associated with chronic inflammation. Roughly 30% of these tumors have concurrent malignant penile lesions at the base of the lesion [40].

There are numerous HPV-associated premalignant lesions. Penile intraepithelial neoplasia (PIN) is commonly associated with aggressive strains of HPV (16 and 18). More aggressive PIN lesions (PIN II and III) pathologically resemble carcinoma in situ of the glans (erythroplasia of Queyrat) or penile shaft (Bowen's disease) [41]. Buschke-Löwenstein tumors, or giant condyloma acuminata, are large warty exophytic growths that require aggressive surgical resection. The majority of these tumors are thought to be associated with HPV 11. Malignant progression may be seen in upwards of 30% of cases [42, 43].

Human Immunodeficiency Virus (HIV) infection increases the risk of penile cancer. In a population-based cohort study, the relative risk of penile cancer was 3.9-fold higher in patients with HIV/AIDS than what would have been expected in the general population [44]. The pathophysiology of this association is likely due to the high rates of HPV co-infection and poor clearance rates of HPV in men with HIV/AIDS. In an evaluation of male circumcision trials in Uganda, 776 HIV-negative and 223 HIV-positive males were tested for HPV co-infection. HIV-positive males had higher incidence rates (66.5 vs 32.9 per 100 person-years) and lower clearance rates (114.7 vs

170.2 per 100 person-years) of high-risk HPV strains [45]. Furthermore, a retrospective cohort of men diagnosed with penile cancer at a single institution in South Africa over an 8-year period documented that men with HIV were younger and more likely to be infected with HPV than men with penile cancer who did not have HIV [46].

Smoking and Marijuana

Numerous studies have investigated the association between tobacco and penile cancer. A study of 503 patients diagnosed with penile cancer and age-matched controls demonstrated a significant association between smoking or chewing tobacco in patients with penile carcinoma. The use of snuff was also more common in men with penile cancer. Smoking was associated with a 44% higher risk of penile cancer. A strong dose-response relationship was demonstrated as men who smoked >10 cigarettes a day (OR 2.14), >5 years in duration (OR 1.43) and who had smoked > 30-pack years (OR 1.86) all had significantly increased risks of developing penile cancer [47]. The strong association and dose-response relationship between smoking and squamous cell carcinoma of the penis was confirmed in a case-control study of 100 matched pairs. Ever smokers had a 2.4 higher risk of penile cancer and the risk was greatest (OR: 5.9) in men who smoked >20 cigarettes/day [27]. To date, there has only been one study published which assessed marijuana use and risk of penile cancer. In a case-control study of 110 cases and 355 population controls matched by age and date of diagnosis, ever use of marijuana was not associated with penile cancer risk and no dose-relationship was observed [16].

UVA Phototherapy

UVA phototherapy is a potential treatment for patients with psoriasis. The first report of UVA phototherapy and penile cancer was published in 1979. This patient had previously undergone UVA therapy and later developed multiple areas of Bowen's disease and squamous cell carcinoma of the penis and pubic area [48]. The 'PUVA follow-up study' was a prospective cohort of patients that were followed long-term to investigate the treatment related side effects of UVA and UVB phototherapy. The initial publication using this cohort observed that men treated with UVA had an increased risk of penile tumors (Standard Morbidity Ratio 95.7, 95% Confidence Interval 43.9-181.8) compared to the expected incidence in the United States population [49]. A follow-up study on this same cohort of patients published 12-years later confirmed that the risk of invasive scrotal and penile squamous cell carcinoma was 81.7-fold higher in men previously treated with UVA compared to the general population [50]. Finally, a systematic review investigated the carcinogenic risk of PUVA and PUVB for the treatment of chronic plaque psoriasis. Results clearly demonstrated that previous treatment was associated with an increased risk of non-melanoma skin cancers. Other notable findings included that squamous cell carcinoma can develop even with very low exposures and the risk of cancer increases with increasing dose. Second, there appeared to be an elevated risk of squamous cell carcinoma in areas of skin that were not-exposed directly to UVA phototherapy [51].

HPV

Human papilloma virus is the most common sexually transmitted disease in the United States. The Center of Disease Control and Prevention (CDC) estimated that 14.1 million new cases of HPV were diagnosed and 79.1 million people were living with the virus in 2008 [52]. There are many known strains of HPV and the clinical manifestations and association with squamous cell carcinoma varies by strain. Classically, HPV strains 6 and 11 are associated with cutaneous genital warts which have not been proven to be associated with an increased risk of cancer. More virulent strains such as 16, 18, 31, 33, 45, 56, and 65 have been associated with the risk of developing squamous cell carcinoma of numerous organs including the cervix, anus, head/neck and penis. Previously, estimations suggested that HPV was associated with anywhere from 36-48% of penile cancer cases [53-55]. A collaborative study between the CDC and 7 population-based cancer registries in the United States reported that HPV DNA was detected in 63.3% of penile cancer cases. Using this data, the group further estimated the number of cancers potentially preventable through vaccination. The previous standard quadrivalent vaccine against HPV strains 6, 11, 16 and 18 was estimated to potentially prevent 47.9% of all penile cancers. The newer 9-valent vaccine also targeting strains 31, 33, 45, 52 and 58 may prevent an additional 15.3% of all penile cancers [56].

Although the benefits of vaccination against HPV are unquestionable, the lack of population knowledge and poor vaccination rates, especially in adolescent and young adult males, is startling and a significant public health issue. Contemporary perceptions of HPV and penile cancer was assessed using the Health Information National Trends Survey (HINTS) which a cross-sectional telephone survey performed by the National Cancer Institute. In 3376 respondents, only 64.4% had ever heard of HPV and under 30% were aware that HPV could cause penile cancer. Men, when compared to women, were much less likely to have ever heard of HPV (OR: 0.32, 95% Confidence Interval 0.24-0.43) [57]. Furthermore, National Immunization Surveys conducted by the CDC between 2008-2016 were used to determine how many males completed the 3-shot HPV vaccination schedule. Only 29.5% of males aged 13-15 and 31.5% of males aged 13-17 received all three shots [58]. Improving vaccination rates in female and males has the potential to reduce the incidence, morbidity and mortality of HPV related cancers and should remain a public health priority over the next decade.

Natural History

Evolution of Invasion (CIS --- Ta/1 ---- T2/3 ----N+/M+)

To fully understand the invasive characteristics and patterns in penile cancer, a thorough understanding of the penile anatomy is a prerequisite. The penis is composed of three cylindrical chambers surrounded by an enveloping fascia and its overlying skin. Since most cancers of the penis arise from the squamous epithelium of the epidermis and dermis, it is most relevant to understand the natural pattern of infiltration into deeper tissues and metastatic progression to loco-regional sites. In the penis, the erectile bodies are surrounded by Buck fascia, Dartos fascia and skin. It is between Buck and Dartos fascia in which the mobility of the overlying skin of the penile shaft arises due to loose connective tissue attachments. This remains in stark contrast to the skin of the glans penis, which remains fixed in place due to direct attachments of the epidermis and dermis to a thin layer of tunica albuginea. Buck fascia fuses with the tunica albuginea both distally at the corona of the glans and proximally at the level deep to the bulbospongiosus and ischiocavernosus muscles in the perineum, enveloping the corpus spongiosum along its length. Within the tunica albuginea lies the erectile tissue of the corpora cavernosum and the cavernosal artery. The corpora cavernosum are not distinct cylinders and instead communicate freely through an incomplete septum [59].

The most common site for penile cancer is the glans, which accounts for 48% of the diagnoses followed by the prepuce in 21%, both glans and prepuce in 9%, the coronal sulcus in 6% and the shaft in <2% [60]. The initial lesion can range from subtle induration to a papule or even ulcerative lesion. The most common signs of penile cancer at presentation are a painless lump (25%), ulcer (13%), rash (6%), bleeding (4%) or balanitis (4%). From the glans, the neoplastic growth gradually extends to involve the entire glans and shaft of the penis. If left unchecked, the lesion will often erode through the prepuce and will present with a foul odor and discharge with or without bleeding.

Patterns of Spread

While Buck's fascia will temporarily act as a barrier for spread, once this barrier is penetrated, it allows tumor to seed within the lymphatic channels in a sequential manner. Typically, tumor cells disseminate through first-echelon regional inguinal lymph nodes and then on to second-echelon deep pelvic nodes [61]. Inguinal adenopathy is demonstrated in 30-60% of penile cancer cases at time of diagnosis although malignant infiltration of the lymph nodes is only present in about half of these cases, with the other 50% of cases presumably due to inflammatory causes [62]. The lymphatic channels are interconnected and cross the midline throughout the penis at both the level of the shaft and the base. Accordingly, the lymphatic drainage of the penis occurs to the inguinal lymph nodes in each groin with no predictable laterality of drainage patterns, and cross-over occurring in 60-85% of cases [63].

When nodal metastases develop, Penile SCC will spread in a stepwise fashion to the superficial and deep inguinal lymph nodes, which are categorized according to their location above or below the fascia lata. These lymphatic channels continue to course superiorly along the medial aspect of the femoral vein, sending efferent vessels beneath the inguinal ligament through the femoral canal and draining into the node of Cloquet and pelvic lymph nodes (external iliac, internal iliac, and obturator). The drainage of penile SCC is consistent without any known evidence of "skip" lesions occurring [64]. If left untreated the natural history of inguinal lymphadenopathy is that of enlargement, ulceration both superficially through the skin and deep into the femoral vessels with resulting hemorrhage [65]. Distant metastases are an uncommon finding in penile cancer until late in the course with only 1-10% of patients presenting with metastases at time of diagnosis [66]. Most commonly, penile cancer metastasizing to the visceral organs such as the lung, liver, bone or brain represents a late manifestation of disease and uniformly is associated with prior lymph node metastases.

Survival Outcomes by Spread

Overall, penile cancer has a 5-year survival rate of approximately 50%, in spite of the fact that 62% of penile cancer is diagnosed at a localized stage [7]. There is a significant delay in patients seeking care for penile lesions. It has been reported that 45.7% of patients waited more than 3 months before evaluation of a self-identified penile lesion [67]. This delay resulted in significant risks for a larger lesions size, more advanced stage of the primary tumor (>pT1b), a higher positive rate of regional lymph nodes and a lower rate of penile sparing procedures. A delay in presentation of greater than 6 months led to a significant risk for lower survival at the second-year endpoint compared to un-delayed patients.

Early diagnosis is of utmost importance, as a delay in the management of both the primary tumor and regional lymph nodes can negatively impact recurrence and survival. In the setting of clinically negative lymph nodes, the surgical detection and treatment of pathologically involved regional lymph node involvement led to a regional recurrence rate of 2% compared to 19% if delaying inguinal lymphadenectomy until clinically positive. A 5-year survival rate of greater than 75% was reported for patients undergoing early inguinal lymphadenectomy compared to 6% for those undergoing delayed lymphadenectomy once clinical metastases developed [68]. Once a recurrence in the ILN is diagnosed, the prognosis is grim with a median overall survival of 6 months [69]. The 5-year survival rate is significantly and markedly impacted by LN status with a rate of 93% for patients with negative lymph nodes, 34%–62% for patients with positive ILN nodes, and the lowest survival rates for patients with pelvic lymph node (PLN) involvement [70]. PLN metastases is an ominous finding, with a 5-yr survival rate of 0% to 66% for all cases and 17%-54% for microscopic invasion only, with the mean 5-year survival being approximately 10% [71]. In patients with ILN metastases, 20%-30% will have PLN metastases. This is further characterized by ILN count, as if 2-3 ILN are involved, there is a 23% probability of PLN involvement and if 3 or more are involved, the probability increases to 56% [72]. Most patients who are left untreated will die within 2 years of diagnosis and the cause of death is often secondary to the local effects of tumor growth in addition to their metastatic disease.

Conclusion

Penile cancer is a rare malignancy that remains a significant source of morbidity in the developing world. A wide range of risk factors have been identified, some of which are modifiable. Penile cancer incidence rates as well as outcomes appear to correlate with health awareness and having access to prompt care. HPV vaccination adopted by countries have been successful at reducing rates of female HPV related cancers. The effectiveness for penile cancer has not yet been elucidated, and global rates of this disease remain stable. While neonatal circumcision remains controversial in some countries, education and public health initiatives should be considered to develop healthcare infrastructure and promote smoking cessation, better hygiene, and ubiquitous HPV vaccination.

Key Points

1. Penile cancer remains a significant source of morbidity in the developing world.
2. In the United States and world-wide, penile cancer incidence rates are related to areas of increased economic disparity.
3. On multivariable analysis, a study using the NCDB showed a higher risk of advanced stage disease in uninsured, African-American, Hispanic, less educated and non-metropolitan males.

4. Circumcision has been shown to decrease the incidence of penile cancer through decreased rates of HPV transmission and phimosis.
5. Penile cancer spreads from the primary tumor in a sequential fashion along lymphatic channels.
6. Early identification and treatment significantly improve survival outcomes.
7. Education and public health initiatives in developing countries should be aimed at improving healthcare infrastructure and identifying locally relevant risk factors with the subsequent development of mitigation programs.

REFERENCES

[1] Siegal RL, Miller KD, Jemal A. Cancer Statistics, 2018. *CA Cancer J Clin.* 2018:68(1):7-30. doi:10.3322/caac.21442.

[2] Pow-Sang MR, Ferreira U, Pow-Sang JM, et al. Epidemiology and natural history of penile cancer. *Urology.* 2010:76:S2–6. doi: 10.1016/j.urology.2010.03.003.

[3] Heller DS, Lesions and Neoplasms of the Penis: A Review. *J Low Genit Tract Dis.* 2016;20:107-11. doi: 10.1097/LGT.0000000000000159.

[4] Misra S, Chaturvedi A, Misra NC. Penile Carcinoma: A challenge for the developing world. *Lancet Oncol.* 2004:5:240-7. doi: 10.1016/S1470-2045(04) 01427-5.

[5] Shavit O, Roura E, Barchana M, et al. Burden of human papillomavirus infection and related diseases in Israel. *Vaccine.* 2013;31 Suppl 8:I32-41. doi: 10.1016/j. vaccine.2013.05.108.

[6] Barnholtz-Sloan JS, Maldonado JL, Pow-Sang J, Guiliano AR. Incidence trends in primary malignant penile cancer. *Urol Oncol: Semin Orig Invest.* 2007:25(5):361-367. doi: 10.1016/j.urolonc.2006.08.029.

[7] Hernandez BY, Barnholtz-Sloan J, German RR, et al. Burden of invasive squamous cell carcinoma of the penis in the United States, 1998-2003. *Cancer Suppl.* 2008;113(10):2883-2891. doi: 10.1002/cncr.23743.

[8] Torbrand C, Wigertz A, Drevin L, et al. Socioeconomic factors and penile cancer risk and mortality; a population-based study. *BJU Int.* 2017:199:254-260. doi: 10.1111/bju.13534. Epub 2016 Jul 4.

[9] Couto TC, Arruda RM, Couto MC, et al. Epidemiological study of penile cancer in Pernambuco: experience of two reference centers. *Int Braz J Urol.* 2014:40:738-44. doi: 10.1590/S1677-5538.IBJU.2014.06.04.

[10] Favorito LA, Nardi AC, Ronalsa M, et al. Epidemiologic study on penile cancer in Brazil. *Int Braz J Urol.* 2008:34:587-91; discussion 591-3.

[11] Christodoulidou M, et al. Epidemiology of penile cancer. *Curr Probl Cancer.* 2015:39:126-136. doi: 10.1016/j.currproblcancer. 2015.03.010. Epub 2015 Apr 1.

[12] Wabinga HR, Parkin DM, Wabwire-Mangin F, Nambooze S. Trends in cancer incidence in Kyadondo County, Uganda, 1960-1997. *Br J Cancer*. 2000:82 (9): 1585-1592. doi: 10.1054/bjoc.1999.1071.

[13] Wolbarst A. Circumcision and penile cancer. *The Lancet*. 1932:219(5655):150-153. doi:10.1016/S0140-6736(01)24346-3.

[14] Dean AL Jr. Epithelioma of the Penis 1 1. Read before annual meeting of American Urological Association, Atlantic City, New Jersey, May 22, 1934. *The Journal of Urology.* 1935;33(3):252-276. doi:10.1016/S0022-5347(17)72263-X.

[15] Leiter E, Lefkovitis AM. Circumcision and penile carcinoma. *N Y State J Med.* 1975;75(9):1520-1522.

[16] Maden C, Sherman KJ, Beckmann AM, et al. History of Circumcision, Medical Conditions, and Sexual Activity and Risk of Penile Cancer. *JNCI Journal of the National Cancer Institute*. 1993;85(1):19-24. doi:10.1093/jnci/85.1.19.

[17] Schoen EJ, Oehrli M, Colby CCJ, Machin G. The Highly Protective Effect of Newborn Circumcision against Invasive Penile Cancer. *Pediatrics.* 2000;105(3): e36-e36. doi:10.1542/peds.105.3.e36.

[18] Kochen M, McCurdy S. Circumcision and the risk of cancer of the penis. A life-table analysis. *Am J Dis Child*. 1980;134(5):484-486.

[19] Gray RH, Kigozi G, Serwadda D, et al. Male circumcision for HIV prevention in men in Rakai, Uganda: a randomised trial. *Lancet.* 2007;369(9562):657-666. doi:10.1016/S0140-6736(07)60313-4.

[20] Bailey RC, Moses S, Parker CB, et al. Male circumcision for HIV prevention in young men in Kisumu, Kenya: a randomised controlled trial. *Lancet.* 2007;369(9562):643-656. doi:10.1016/S0140-6736(07)60312-2.

[21] Auvert B, Taljaard D, Lagarde E, Sobngwi-Tambekou J, Sitta R, Puren A. Randomized, controlled intervention trial of male circumcision for reduction of HIV infection risk: the ANRS 1265 Trial. Deeks S, ed. *PLoS Med*. 2005;2(11): e298. doi:10.1371/journal.pmed.0020298.

[22] Tobian AAR, Serwadda D, Quinn TC, et al. Male circumcision for the prevention of HSV-2 and HPV infections and syphilis. *N Engl J Med.* 2009;360(13):1298-1309. doi:10.1056/NEJMoa0802556.

[23] Auvert B, Sobngwi-Tambekou J, Cutler E, et al. Effect of male circumcision on the prevalence of high-risk human papillomavirus in young men: results of a randomized controlled trial conducted in Orange Farm, South Africa. *J Infect Dis.* 2009;199(1):14-19. doi:10.1086/595566.

[24] Gray RH, Serwadda D, Kong X, et al. Male circumcision decreases acquisition and increases clearance of high-risk human papillomavirus in HIV-negative men: a randomized trial in Rakai, Uganda. *J Infect Dis*. 2010;201(10):1455-1462. doi:10. 1086/652184.

[25] Wawer MJ, Tobian AAR, Kigozi G, et al. Effect of circumcision of HIV-negative men on transmission of human papillomavirus to HIV-negative women: a randomised trial in Rakai, Uganda. *Lancet.* 2011;377(9761):209-218. doi:10.1016/S0140-6736(10)61967-8.

[26] Daling JR, Madeleine MM, Johnson LG, et al. Penile cancer: importance of circumcision, human papillomavirus and smoking in in situ and invasive disease. *Int J Cancer*. 2005;116(4):606-616. doi:10.1002/ijc.21009.

[27] Tsen HF, Morgenstern H, Mack T, Peters RK. Risk factors for penile cancer: results of a population-based case-control study in Los Angeles County (United States). *Cancer Causes Control*. 2001;12(3):267-277.

[28] Maiche AG. Epidemiological aspects of cancer of the penis in Finland. *European Journal of Cancer Prevention*. 1992;1(2):153-158. doi:10.1097/00008469-199202000-00008.

[29] Chaux A, Netto GJ, Rodríguez IM, et al. Epidemiologic profile, sexual history, pathologic features, and human papillomavirus status of 103 patients with penile carcinoma. *World J Urol*. 2013;31(4):861-867. doi:10.1007/s00345-011-0802-0.

[30] Morris BJ, Gray RH, Castellsague X, et al. The Strong Protective Effect of Circumcision against Cancer of the Penis. *Adv Urol.* 2011;2011(5):812368–21. doi:10.1155/2011/812368.

[31] Hellberg D, Valentin J, Eklund T, Nilsson S. Penile cancer: is there an epidemiological role for smoking and sexual behaviour? *Br Med J (Clin Res Ed).* 1987;295(6609):1306-1308. doi:10.1136/bmj.295.6609.1306.

[32] Depasquale I, Park AJ, Bracka A. The treatment of balanitis xerotica obliterans. *BJU Int.* 2002;86(4):459-465. doi:10.1046/j.1464-410X.2000.00772.x.

[33] Philippou P, Shabbir M, Ralph DJ, et al. Genital lichen sclerosus/balanitis xerotica obliterans in men with penile carcinoma: a critical analysis. *BJU Int.* 2013;111(6):970-976. doi:10.1111/j.1464-410X.2012.11773.x.

[34] Barbagli G, Palminteri E, Mirri F, Guazzoni G, Turini D, Lazzeri M. Penile carcinoma in patients with genital lichen sclerosus: a multicenter survey. *The Journal of Urology*. 2006;175(4):1359-1363. doi:10.1016/S0022-5347(05)00735-4.

[35] Barnes KT, Smith BJ, Lynch CF, Gupta A. Obesity and invasive penile cancer. *Eur Urol.* 2013;63(3):588-589. doi:10.1016/j.eururo.2012.11.046.

[36] Barnes KT, McDowell BD, Button A, Smith BJ, Lynch CF, Gupta A. Obesity is associated with increased risk of invasive penile cancer. *BMC Urol.* 2016;16(1):42. doi:10.1186/s12894-016-0161-7.

[37] Djajadiningrat RS, van Werkhoven E, Horenblas S. Penile cancer stage, survival and body mass index. *Urol Int*. 2015;94(2):220-224. doi:10.1159/000367927.

[38] Thuret R, Sun M, Budaus L, et al. A population-based analysis of the effect of marital status on overall and cancer-specific mortality in patients with squamous

cell carcinoma of the penis. *Cancer Causes Control.* 2013;24(1):71-79. doi:10. 1007/s10552-012-0091-y.

[39] Attalla K, Paulucci DJ, Blum K, et al. Demographic and socioeconomic predictors of treatment delays, pathologic stage, and survival among patients with penile cancer: A report from the National Cancer Database. Urol Oncol. 2018;36 (1):14.e17-14.e24. doi:10.1016/j.urolonc.2017.09.014.

[40] Solivan GA, SmithL KJ, James WD. Cutaneous horn of the penis: Its association with squamous cell carcinoma and HPV-16 infection. *Journal of the American Academy of Dermatology*. 1990;23(5):969-972. doi:10.1016/0190-9622(90)70315-9.

[41] Miralles-Guri C, Bruni L, Cubilla AL, Castellsague X, Bosch FX, de Sanjose S. Human papillomavirus prevalence and type distribution in penile carcinoma. *Journal of Clinical Pathology*. 2009;62(10):870-878. doi:10.1136/jcp.2008.063149.

[42] Björck M, Athlin L, Lundskog B. Giant condyloma acuminatum (Buschke-Loewenstein tumour) of the anorectum with malignant transformation. *Eur J Surg.* 1995;161(9):691-694.

[43] Arya M, Kalsi J, Kelly J, Muneer A. Malignant and premalignant lesions of the penis. *BMJ.* 2013;346(mar06 1):f1149-f1149. doi:10.1136/bmj.f1149.

[44] Frisch M, Biggar RJ, Engels EA, Goedert JJ, AIDS-Cancer Match Registry Study Group. Association of cancer with AIDS-related immunosuppression in adults. *JAMA*. 2001;285(13):1736-1745.

[45] Tobian AAR, Kigozi G, Gravitt PE, et al. Human papillomavirus incidence and clearance among HIV-positive and HIV-negative men in sub-Saharan Africa. *AIDS.* 2012;26(12):1555-1565. doi:10.1097/QAD.0b013e328353b83c.

[46] Wentzel SW, Vermeulen LP, Beukes CA, Thiart J, Joubert G, Goedhals J. Human immunodeficiency virus (HIV) infection in men with penile carcinoma is associated with increased prevalence of human papilloma virus infection and younger age at presentation. *S Afr J Surg*. 2018;56(3):47-50.

[47] Harish K, Ravi R. The role of tobacco in penile carcinoma. *Br J Urol.* 1995;75(3):375-377. doi:10.1111/j.1464-410X.1995.tb07352.x.

[48] Tam DW. Bowen's Disease and Squamous Cell Carcinoma. *Arch Dermatol.* 1979;115(2):203. doi:10.1001/archderm.1979.04010020049015.

[49] Stern RS, Members of the Photochemotherapy Follow-up Study*. Genital Tumors among Men with Psoriasis Exposed to Psoralens and Ultraviolet A Radiation (PUVA) and Ultraviolet B Radiation. *N Engl J Med.* 1990;322(16):1093-1097. doi:10.1056/NEJM199004193221601.

[50] Stern RS, Bagheri S, Nichols K, PUVA Follow Up Study. The persistent risk of genital tumors among men treated with psoralen plus ultraviolet A (PUVA) for psoriasis. *Journal of the American Academy of Dermatology*. 2002;47(1):33-39.

[51] Archier E, Devaux S, Castela E, et al. Carcinogenic risks of psoralen UV-A therapy and narrowband UV-B therapy in chronic plaque psoriasis: a systematic literature review. *J Eur Acad Dermatol Venereol.* 2012;26 Suppl 3:22-31. doi:10.1111/j.1468-3083.2012.04520.x.

[52] Satterwhite CL. *Incidence, Prevalence, and Cost of Sexuall Transmitted Infection in the United States.* https://www.cdc.gov/std/stats/sti-estimates-fact-sheet-feb-2013.pdf. Published 2013. Accessed October 31, 2018.

[53] Gillison ML, Chaturvedi AK, Lowy DR. HPV prophylactic vaccines and the potential prevention of noncervical cancers in both men and women. *Cancer.* 2008;113(10 Suppl):3036-3046. doi:10.1002/cncr.23764.

[54] Kurdgelashvili G, Dores GM, Srour SA, Chaturvedi AK, Huycke MM, Devesa SS. Incidence of potentially human papillomavirus-related neoplasms in the United States, 1978 to 2007. *Cancer.* 2013;119(12):2291-2299. doi:10.1002/cncr.27989.

[55] Backes DM, Kurman RJ, Pimenta JM, Smith JS. Systematic review of human papillomavirus prevalence in invasive penile cancer. *Cancer Causes Control.* 2009;20(4):449-457. doi:10.1007/s10552-008-9276-9.

[56] Saraiya M, Unger ER, Thompson TD, et al. US assessment of HPV types in cancers: implications for current and 9-valent HPV vaccines. *J Natl Cancer Inst.* 2015;107(6):djv086. doi:10.1093/jnci/djv086.

[57] Zavaski ME, Hanske J, Löppenberg B, et al. Contemporary perceptions of human papillomavirus and penile cancer: Perspectives from a national survey. *Can Urol Assoc J.* 2018;13(2). doi:10.5489/cuaj.5366.

[58] National Cancer Institute. *Online Summary of Trends in US Cancer Control Measures.* https:// progressreport.cancer.gov/ prevention/ hpv_ immunization. Accessed October 31, 2018.

[59] McCammon, KA, Zuckerman JM, Jordan GH. Surgery of the Penis and urethra. *Campbell-Walsh Urology.* 40:907-945.e4. doi: 10.1002/ijc.21961.

[60] Lont AP, Kroon BK, Horenblas S, et al. Presence of high-risk human papillomavirus DNA in penile carcinoma predicts favorable outcome in survival. *Int J Cancer.* 2006:119:1078-1081. doi: 10.1002/ijc.21961.

[61] Willis RA. *The spread of tumors in the human body*, 3rd ed. London: Butterworth, 1973.

[62] Ayyappan K, Ananthakrishnan N, Sankaran V. Can regional lymph node involvement be predicted in patients with carcinoma of the penis? *Br J Urol.* 1994:73:549-553.

[63] Abi-Aad AS, deKernion JB. Controversies in ilioinguinal lymphadenectomy for cancer of the penis. *Urol Clin North Am.* 1992:19:319-324.

[64] Cabanas RM. Anatomy and biopsy of sentinel lymph nodes. *Urol Clin North Am.* 1992;19:267-276.

[65] Burgers JK, Badalament RA, Drago JR. Penile cancer: clinical presentation, diagnosis, and staging. *Urol Clin North Am*. 1992;19:247-256.

[66] Pettaway CA, Pagliaro LC, Theodore C, et al: Treatment of visceral, unresectable, or bulky/unresectable regional metastases of penile cancer. *Urology*. 2010:76:S58-65. doi: 10.1016/j.urology.2010.03.082.

[67] Gao W, Song LB, Yang J, et al. Risk factors and negative consequences of patient's delay for penile carcinoma. *World J Surg Oncol*. 2016:4:124. doi: 10.1186/s12957-016-0863-z.

[68] Fraley, EE, Zhang, G, Manivel C, et al. The role of ilioinguinal lymphadenectomy and significance of histological differentiation in treatment of carcinoma of the penis. *J Urol*. 1989:142:1478-1482. doi: 10.1016/S0022-5347(17)39130-9.

[69] Heyns CF, Fleschner N, Sangar V, et al. Management of the lymph nodes in penile cancer. *Urology*. 2010:76:43-57. doi: 10.1016/j.urology.2010.03.001.

[70] Horenblas S. Lymphadenectomy for squamous cell carcinoma of the penis. Part 2: the role and technique of lymph node dissection. *BJU Int*. 2001:88:473–483.

[71] Lopes A, Bezerra AL, Serrano SV, Hidalgo GS. Iliac nodal metastases from carcinoma of the penis treated surgically. *BJU Int*. 2000:86:690-693. doi: 10.1046/j.1464-410x.2000.00862.x.

[72] Culkin DJ, Beer TM. Advanced penile carcinoma. *J Urol*. 2003:170:359-365. doi: 10.1097/01.ju.0000062829.43654.5e.

In: Penile Cancer: Challenges and Controversies ISBN: 978-1-53615-950-9
Editors: F. E. Martins and M. L. Djordjevic

Chapter 3

PATHOLOGY, PRECURSOR LESIONS, PROGNOSTIC INDICATORS AND GENETICS

***Antonio L. Cubilla*[1,*] *and Alcides Chaux*[2]**

[1]Emeritus of Pathology, Universidad Nacional de Asunción; Director, Instituto de Patología e Investigación. Asunción, Paraguay

[2]Department of Scientific Research, Norte University, Asunción, Paraguay

ABSTRACT

Most penile neoplasms are squamous cell carcinomas, arising predominantly in the glans. Penile carcinomas are classified in HPV-related and HPV-unrelated groups, with subtypes of each group showing distinctive clinicopathologic and outcome features. HPV-unrelated subtypes include usual, verrucous (and hybrid-verrucous), papillary not otherwise specified (NOS), cuniculatum, pseudohyperplastic, sarcomatoid, pseudoglandular, adenosquamous and mucoepidermoid carcinomas. Usual squamous cell carcinoma is the most frequent subtype of penile cancer, showing typical features of squamous differentiation similar to carcinomas elsewhere. Verrucous and papillary carcinomas are exophytic, usually low-grade tumors with a low rate of nodal metastasis. Hybrid-verrucous and cuniculatum are related to verrucous carcinomas with some distinctive features, such as the presence of a usual component the former and deep infiltration of erectile tissues the latter. Pseudohyperplastic carcinoma is a clinicopathologic entity which resembles squamous hyperplasia, observed in the foreskin of elderly men. Sarcomatoid carcinoma shows features resembling sarcomas, similar to tumors elsewhere. Pseudoglandular carcinoma shows tumor nests with clear central spaces due to necrosis, resembling glandular spaces, hence the denomination. Adenosquamous and mucoepidermoid carcinomas are unusual subtypes, showing mixed components such as true glandular differentiation the former and intracellular mucin production the latter. HPV-related subtypes include basaloid, warty, warty-basaloid,

* Corresponding Author's E-mail: antoniocubillaramos@gmail.com.

medullary, clear cell and lymphoepithelioma-like carcinomas. Warty, warty-basaloid and basaloid carcinomas are part of a spectrum of differentiation from low-grade verrucous tumors with koylocytic changes to high-grade aggressive tumors. Medullary carcinoma is composed of anaplastic large cells with prominent nucleoli and intense peritumoral inflammation. Clear cell carcinoma shows solid tumor nests with prominent cytoplasmic clear cell features, koylocytic changes and frequent central necrosis. Lymphoepithelioma-like carcinoma is similar to tumors observed elsewhere, mainly in the nasopharynx. Except for tumors in the warty/basaloid spectrum, the other HPV-related subtypes are unusual.

Pathologic prognostic factors are features observed in the primary tumor of resected specimens used to estimate the likelihood of tumor recurrence, nodal/systemic dissemination and cancer-related death. Evaluation and determination of their statuses should be done in all cases. The 3 main pathologic prognostic factors are histologic grade, perineural invasion and vascular invasion. Histologic grading should be done consistently, using validated and reproducible criteria. A 3-tier grading scale should be preferred, ranging from well-differentiated tumors cells, almost undistinguishable from normal basal/parabasal cells (grade 1) to tumor cells with high-grade features such as nuclear pleomorphism, clumped chromatin, prominent nucleoli, and conspicuous/atypical mitoses (grade 3). Any proportion of grade-3 tumor cells is sufficient to categorize the tumor as grade 3. Presence or absence of vascular invasion, either lymphatic (more frequent) or venous, should also be recorded in every case, taking care of not confusing true vascular invasion with post-fixation retraction artifacts. Similarly, presence or absence of perineural invasion should be determined for each case, paying attention not to confuse true perineural invasion with mere nerve entrapment. Other pathologic prognostic factors include tumor thickness, level of anatomic infiltration, anatomic site of the primary tumor, pattern of growth, and histologic subtype. Pathologic factors can be combined to create risk-scoring systems such as the Penile Prognostic Index, which combines anatomic level of tumor infiltration, histologic grade and perineural invasion.

PART I: PATHOLOGY AND PRECURSOR LESIONS

Squamous Cell Carcinomas

General Features

Over 90% of penile neoplasms are squamous cell carcinomas. Non-epithelial tumors are malignant melanomas, malignant lymphomas and benign or malignant soft tissue tumors. This chapter is restricted to the pathology of squamous cell carcinoma. Squamous cell carcinomas originate predominantly in the mucosal epithelium of glans (about 70%), but preputial and coronal sulcus primary mucosal tumors also occurs (20 and 5%, respectively). Tumors arising in the skin of the shaft or the outer skin of the foreskin are vanishingly rare [1].

According to the 2016 WHO model and the AFIP update, penile squamous cell carcinomas are sub classified in 2 groups, HPV-related and HPV-unrelated (Table 1) [1, 2]. Multiple distinct morphological types with especial clinical, pathological and behavioral features are encountered in each group. Since the seminal studies of Kurman, for vulvar cancer, and Gregoire, for penile cancer, it is known that tumors harboring HPV depict a basaloid or condylomatous morphology and that those negative for the virus does not [3, 4]. This morphological evidence leads to the belief in a bimodal pathway of penile carcinogenesis [5]. Another motive for the separation is the current purported better prognosis of patients with HPV-related tumors [6].

There are 7 types of HPV-related tumors in the modified WHO classification system [2]. These tumors are morphologically distinctive and with some experience most can be recognized by routine H&E stain. Occasionally, p16 immunohistochemistry may be useful. The gold standard for HPV detection is PCR. However, this technique is expensive and not available in most pathology laboratories, whereas p16 can detect HPV in about 85% of the cases. It is used as a surrogate for high risk HPV identification despite the false positive and negative diagnosis [7].

Table 1. Classification of squamous cell carcinoma [1, 2]

HPV-UNRELATED
Usual
Verrucous
Hybrid verrucous
Papillar
Cuniculatum
Pseudohyperplastic
Sarcomatoid
Pseudoglandular
Adenosquamous
Mucoepidermoid
Mixed (combination of HPV-unrelated neoplasms, except verrucous + usual)
Unclassified
HPV-RELATED
Basaloid
Papillary-basaloid
Warty
Warty-basaloid
Medullary
Clear cell
Lymphoepithelioma-like
Mixed (at least one component of HPV-related + other)
Unclassified

HPV-Unrelated Subtypes of Squamous Cell Carcinomas

Usual Squamous Cell Carcinoma

Conventional keratinizing squamous cell carcinoma of various histological grades (Figure 1).

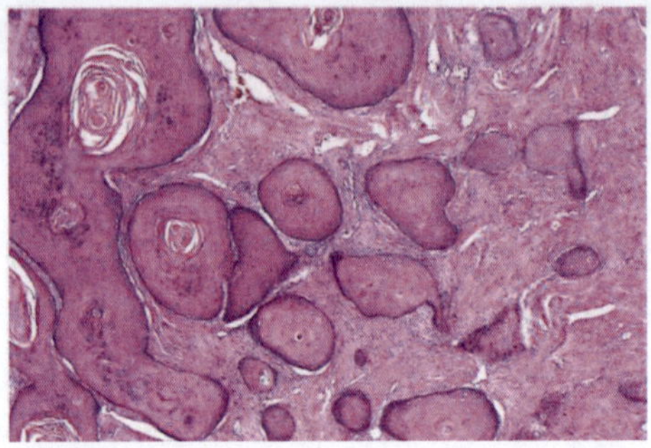

Figure 1. Squamous cell carcinoma, usual.

Clinical Features

Average age is 60 years with a range from the 20s to 90s [8, 9]. Older mean age was reported in Sweden [10] and younger, in Northeastern Brazil [11]. Uncommon in young adults and exceedingly rare in children [12]. A self-appreciated gross abnormality, erhythema, ulcer or mass is the usual presenting symptom. Bleeding and dysuria are infrequent. Rarely, the disease may be recognized after the identification of metastasis to inguinal nodes [13] with the tumor very small concealed under a long phimotic foreskin. HIV positive patients, at higher risk for penile cancer, may present with a penile tumor usually of HPV-related type [14, 15]. Hypercalcemia occurs occasionally, usually in widespread disease [16–18]. In severe phimosis, a mass may be palpated but not visualized. As a result, a primary foreskin carcinoma, usually treatable by circumcision, may be confused with a glans lesion, leading to an unnecessary penectomy. Infiltration of preputial epidermis may be a presenting sign and it is an adverse prognostic factor, except in carcinoma cuniculatum where skin fistulization from deep tumor sinuses are typical and do not affect patient's outcome. Involvement of the skin of the shaft often correlates with infiltration of the corpora cavernosa.

Pathological Features

Macroscopically, tumors are exophytic, exo-endophytic or ulcerative, irregular white-gray nodules or masses measuring from few millimeters to large neoplasms. Larger sizes, from 4 to 5 cm are found in high risk areas, while in low incidence regions the average is 2.0 cm [9, 19]. Cut surface reveals a white tumor compromising lamina propria, dartos, corpus spongiosum or corpora cavernosa.

Microscopically, there are keratinizing squamous tumors and their diagnosis is straightforward. Well-differentiated carcinomas are composed of large irregular or polyhedral squamous sheets or nests next to each other with some intervening reactive fibrous and inflammatory cell stroma. Central keratinization with pearl formation is frequent. The nests must show extreme differentiation to qualify as grade 1. In moderately differentiated squamous cell carcinoma, tumor nests are more irregular in outline and smaller. There is more pleomorphism, nuclear atypia and mitotic figures.

Poorly differentiated carcinomas consist of even smaller nests, cords, trabeculae or isolated anaplastic cells. Keratinization is rare, focal or poorly developed and desmoplastic reaction may be prominent. Nuclear atypia and abundant mitotic figures are the rule. Some tumors are heterogeneous, with more than one histological grade. Many tumors are associated with a stromal reaction and a chronic inflammatory lymphocyte and plasma cell infiltrate [20]. Associated squamous hyperplasia and differentiated PeIN are often present in squamous epithelium adjacent to invasive carcinoma [21]. Lichen sclerosus is present in association with 40% of squamous cell carcinomas of the usual type [22].

Biologic behavior is mainly related to histological grade, depth of infiltration and perineural invasion. Local and regional recurrences, usually due to insufficient surgery, are not uncommon and appear in about 28% of the cases [9]. Recent studies indicate lower recurrent rates around 5% even in conservation surgery procedures as the resurfacing dissection [23]. Inguinal lymph node metastases develop in 28-39% of patients with usual squamous cell carcinoma. Tumors with nodal involvement tend to be larger, thicker, of higher grade and deeply invasive when compared with non-metastasizing squamous cell carcinoma. The mortality rate of usual squamous cell carcinoma ranges from 20% to 38%. The 10-year survival rate for patients with usual squamous cell carcinoma is 78% [8, 9].

Verrucous Carcinoma

Extremely well-differentiated, exophytic tumor with hyperkeratosis, papillomatosis, acanthosis and broadly-based interface between tumor and stroma (Figure 2) [1, 24–26].

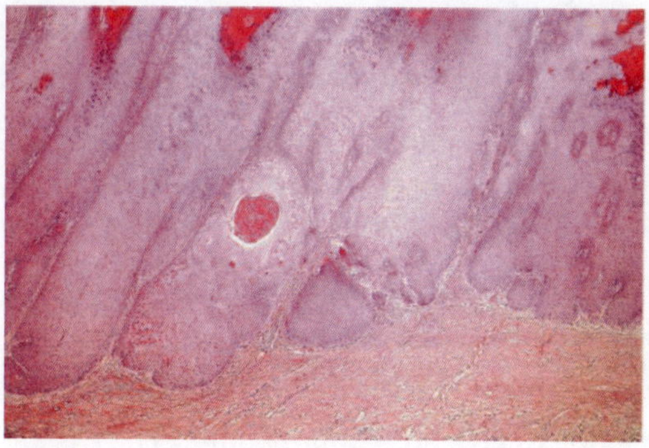

Figure 2. Verrucous carcinoma.

Clinical Features

True verrucous carcinoma (VC) is rare, after exclusion of its morphological simulators, giant condylomas, papillary carcinomas NOS, warty (condylomatus carcinomas) and more typically, the mixed verrucous-squamous hybrid carcinomas [8, 9].

Patients' age is 60 years. Tumor size average is around 3 cm, but larger lesions may be encountered. Most commonly affects the glans, but foreskin cases have been reported.

Pathological Features

Verrucous carcinomas are exophytic verruciform white gray neoplasms. Most tumors are unicentric but multicentric cases are also found. Most of them are superficial or involve up to the corpus spongiosum or preputial dartos. Compromise of corpus cavernosum or lamina propria alone is less frequent. The hallmark is the sharp delineation between a broadly-based tumor and the stroma, which can best be appreciated at the longitudinal cut surface. Tumors are restricted to the epithelium or most commonly penetrate lamina propria or even corpus spongiosum, maintaining its broad base and expansive character. The discussion about the invasiveness of this later presentation is technical or semantic, considering that tumors with these characteristics do not metastasize irrespective of how deep the invasion is. More important is to identify foci of destructive irregular invasion, usually of higher histological grade, findings which will move the classification to the verrucous hybrid category, with potential for nodal metastasis and cancer specific lethality (see below).

Microscopically papillomatosis, hyperkeratosis, and acanthosis are typical. Papillae are not of the condylomatous type; they do not have a central fibrovascular core. Keratohyaline granules, parakeratosis, and vacuolated cells lacking nuclear wrinkling and binucleation, distinct from the koilocytotic cells of warty carcinoma, are noted at the surface. There is extreme differentiation, with prominent intercellular bridges and no or minimal atypia. The base of the tumor is broad in all cases, with pushing, regular expansive borders. Associated lesions are squamous hyperplasia (flat or verrucous), differentiated PeIN and lichen sclerosus [22]. An association with lichen planus hypertrophicus has been reported [24]. Immunohistochemical stains are not useful for the diagnosis. p16, Ki67 and HPV are usually negative [27–30].

In pure verrucous carcinomas, no inguinal metastasis occurs. Recurrences are rare. There is no mortality in properly diagnosed cases.

Hybrid Verrucous Carcinoma

Areas of verrucous carcinoma as described above should be observed, mixed with higher grade usual squamous cell carcinoma (Figure 3). It is more common than pure verrucous carcinomas. It was first recognized and named by Dr. Alberto Ayala, in Houston [25]. A recent series compared clinical, pathological and outcome features of classical (29 cases) and hybrid verrucous carcinomas (30 cases) [31]. The distinction is important because patients' outcome is different in both tumors [32, 33].

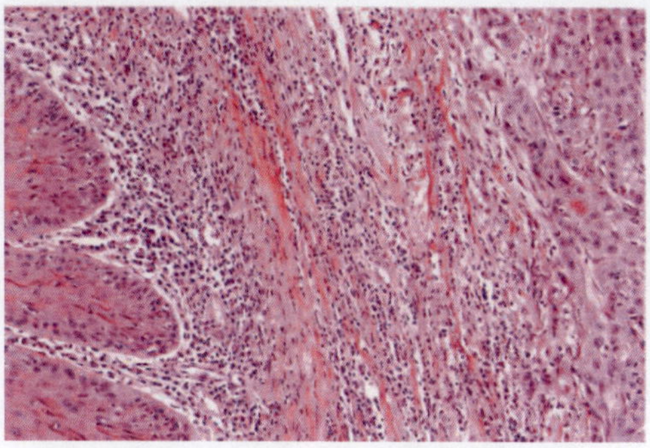

Figure 3. Hybrid verrucous carcinoma.

Clinical Features

Patients' age is 59 years old, similar to classical verrucous carcinomas. The glans is most commonly affected. Presenting symptom is that of a self-appreciated mass in the distal penis.

Pathological Features

An exophytic large white gray mass. The cut surface shows a white neoplasm with a variable irregular to well-defined tumor front. Microscopically hybrid carcinomas, in addition to the presence of classic verrucous carcinoma, show an irregular, destructive invasive front, similar to that of the usual squamous cell carcinoma. The non-verrucous squamous component varies in histological grade, from low to high grade. The invasive pattern is irregular nesting, trabecular or sarcomatoid. Hybrid verrucous carcinomas are usually negative for HPV and p16.

A comparison of classic and hybrid VCs disclosed that the latter are tumors with higher grade, thicker, invade deeper into penile anatomical levels and although rarely, had a potential for nodal metastasis, tumor dissemination and patients' death. Inguinal metastases, usually negative in classic VC were present in 2 of 16 patients with hybrid carcinomas in a report [30]. In the same study none of the classic VC patients died from disease whereas 1 patient with hybrid VC died from metastatic disease and another 2 patients were alive but with metastatic disease at time of last follow up.

Papillary Carcinoma

Exophytic low grade verruciform squamous neoplasm with hyperkeratosis, papillomatosis and a jagged interface between tumor and stroma. No koilocytosis present (Figure 4) [34].

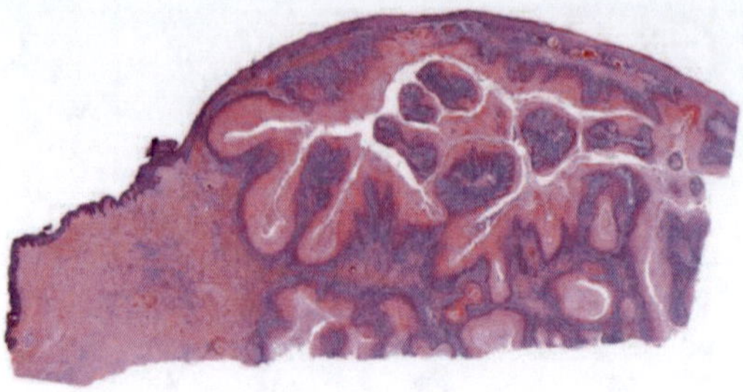

Figure 4. Papillary carcinoma NOS.

Clinical Features

They represent 5-15% of all penile carcinomas [8, 9]. Average age is 63 years. It may occur at all sites, most commonly in the glans and foreskin.

Pathological Findings

They are large, firm, white-gray, granular tumors with a characteristic verruciform pattern of growth. Tumor size is about 5 cm. The cut surface shows a white neoplasm with a serrated surface and a poorly delineated interface between tumor and stroma. More than half of tumors invade up to corpus spongiosum or dartos.

Microscopically it is a well- to moderately-differentiated papillary squamous lesion, with acanthosis and hyperkeratosis. The papillae are highly variable or complex, short or elongated, spiky or blunt, with or without a central fibrovascular core reaching the top. The base of the lesion is jagged, with irregular nests of infiltrating squamous cell carcinoma spreading into subjacent tissue. Most papillary carcinomas are reported as negative for HPV and p16 [4, 35]. The stain may be useful in the differential diagnosis of papillary from the rare low grade warty carcinoma.

Prognosis is good. Recurrence rate is about 12% and the rate for inguinal lymph node metastases is low, ranging from 0% to 12%. The mortality rate ranges from 0% to 6% [8, 9].

Carcinoma Cuniculatum

Complex, deeply penetrating albeit low grade squamous cell carcinomas with some verrucous features with a burrowing growth pattern simulating rabbit nests (Figure 5 A and B) [36, 37].

Clinical Features

Rare tumors, affecting glans and foreskin of older patients (mean age of 77 years). There are several years of evolution. Multiple anatomical compartments are usually affected. Glans and coronal sulcus are usually involved.

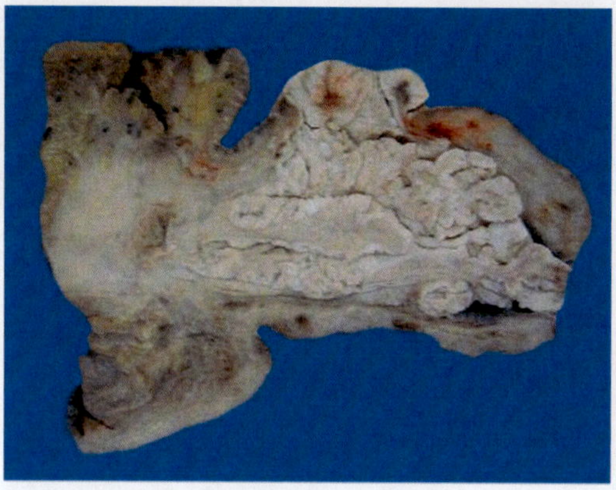

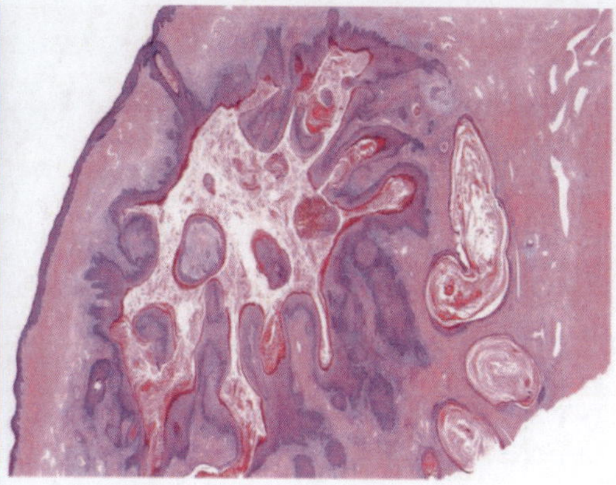

Figure 5. Carcinoma cuniculatum A and B.

Pathological Features

Tumors are white gray exo-endophytic with a verruciform pattern of growth, affecting the glans and extending to coronal sulcus and foreskin. Tumors are among the largest penile carcinomas, with an average size of 6 cm. The cut surface reveals a cerebriform aspect formed by deep invaginations with narrow and elongated neoplastic sinus tracts connecting the surface of the tumor with deep anatomical structures, resembling the architecture of a rabbit's burrow (cuniculus, in Latin). Extension to deep corpus spongiosum and corpus cavernosum is a common finding. Preputial or shaft skin tumor fistulae are present. The boundaries of tumor and stroma, even in deep compromised anatomical levels such as the corpora cavernosa, are sharply delineated.

Microscopically, there is hyperkeratosis, papillomatosis and acanthosis with a low grade verrucoid labyrinthine burrowing pattern with surface fistula formation. The tumor stromal interface is sharply delineated with bulbous expansive borders. The cells are extremely well differentiated and no koilocytes are identified. The sinus and cyst-like lumina contain hyperkeratotic material. Foci of squamous cell carcinoma with destructive invasive pattern are found in some cases with a loss of the verrucous-like features. HPV-DNA using PCR was negative in 2 evaluated cases [35].

The not infrequent focal invasive areas in carcinoma cuniculatum establish a potential for nodal metastases. However, despite the deep penetration, none of the reported cases demonstrated inguinal involvement or systemic dissemination [36, 38].

Pseudohyperplastic Carcinoma

Extremely low grade variant of squamous cell carcinoma simulating pseudoepitheliomatous hyperplasia mostly affecting the foreskin of older patients and associated with lichen sclerosus (Figure 6) [39].

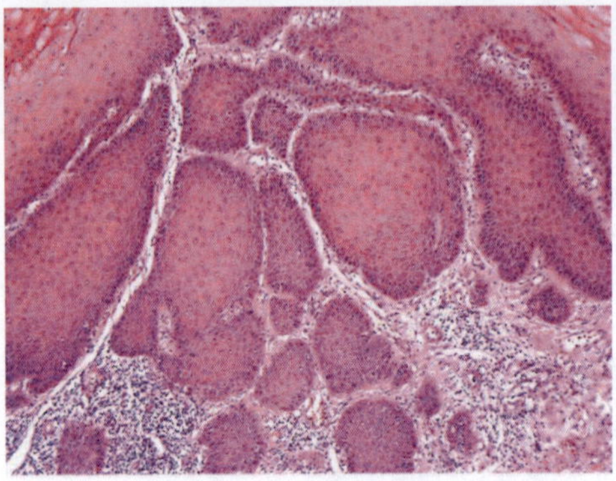

Figure 6. Pseudohyperplastic carcinoma.

Clinical Features

Average age of 69 years is 10 years older than patients with usual squamous cell carcinomas. Tumors are multicentric and mainly affect the foreskin. Verrucous carcinoma is a not an uncommon association. Glans, coronal sulcus and frenulum are affected with lesser frequency. Because of the extreme differentiation and the resemblance of the tumor to pseudoepitheliomatous hyperplasia, a cancer diagnosis may be difficult in small biopsies. The multicentric nature of this process makes the decision of the site of biopsy complicated. The best diagnostic approach is to remove the entire foreskin. In case of a biopsy procedure, the depth must reach at least superficial corpus spongiosum or preputial dartos.

Pathological Features

Macroscopically, tumors are flat or slightly elevated, white and granular, with an average size of 2 cm. Microscopically there is a superficial and orderly downward proliferation of these nests simulating pseudoepitheliomatous hyperplasia. The nests are composed of extremely well differentiated squamous cells with minimal atypia surrounded by a reactive stroma. Tumors usually invade superficial levels, up to dartos in the foreskin and up to lamina propria in the glans but deeper invasion may be present. Separated or continuous foci of squamous hyperplasia, differentiated PeIN, and usual and verrucous squamous cell carcinomas are found in multicentric tumors. Common associated lesions are lichen sclerosus and squamous hyperplasia. Immunohistochemistry for p16 and HPV are usually negative.

The prognosis is excellent with no inguinal nodal metastases. Recurrence in the glans after a circumcision may occur.

Sarcomatoid Carcinoma

Aggressive variant of squamous cell carcinoma composed of spindle, pleomorphic, or polymorphic tumor cells (Figure 7) mixed with areas showing squamous cell features [40]. At least 30% spindle cells are required for the diagnosis. Sarcomatoid carcinomas arises de novo, after recurrence of a usual squamous cell carcinoma, or secondary to sarcomatoid transformation after radiation therapy of a primary penile carcinoma.

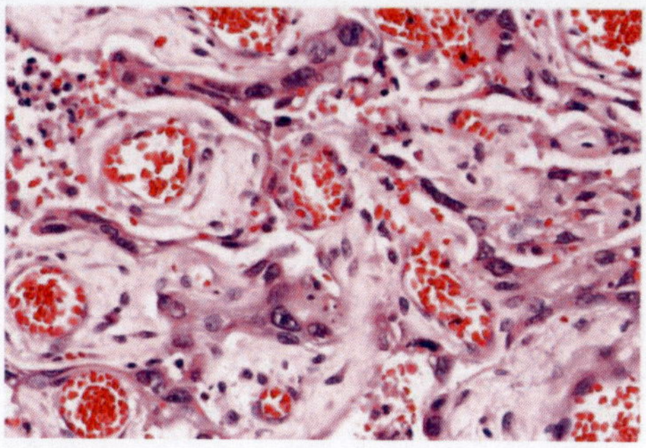

Figure 7. Sarcomatoid carcinoma.

Clinical Features

They are unusual tumors representing about 1-4% of all penile carcinomas [8, 9, 41]. Average patient age is 59 years. Most tumors, due to their large size, affect multiple epithelial compartments, but the glans is the preferred site. Foreskin primary can occur rarely. A previous history of radiation therapy has been linked to the development of sarcomatoid carcinomas [42].

Pathological Features

Macroscopically, they are large (3 to 5 cm), irregular, white-gray or reddish hemorrhagic polypoid masses. The cut surface characteristically shows a dark reddish, sometimes highly necrotic and hemorrhagic neoplasm with deep invasion into corpus spongiosum and corpora cavernosa. Not infrequently, there are satellite nodules of tumor disseminated into deep corpora cavernosa or skin of the penis.

Microscopically there is a variegated appearance in the same case or in other cases. The spindle cell component predominates, with interlacing bundles of atypical spindle cells, resembling fibrosarcoma or leiomyosarcoma. Other patters observed are those of fibrous histiocytoma, myxosarcoma, liposarcoma, hemangiopericytoma, angiosarcoma, rhabdomyosarcoma [43–46]. Foci of osteosarcomatous and chondrosarcomatous differentiation are described. Giant cell features may be prominent. Vascular and perineural invasion, as well as direct urethral extension, are common findings. Necrosis is prominent, and mitoses are numerous. Associated differentiated PeIN and PeIN with warty/basaloid features is commonly found in epithelial areas uninvolved by the carcinoma. Lichen sclerosus is found in a minority of the cases. The pattern of tumor in the nodal metastases is predominantly sarcomatoid.

The best immunohistochemical markers for sarcomatoid carcinomas are vimentin, p53, 34βE12 and p63; EMA, AE1/AE3 and Cam 5.2, which are at least focally positive. Muscle-specific actin, smooth muscle actin, desmin and S-100 are negative (Tables 6.3

and 6.4). Presence of HPV is unusual in sarcomatoid carcinomas [40, 47]. In a study of 5 cases using in situ hybridization, all cases were negative for low and high risk serotypes [40]. In a recent study using PCR 1 of 6 cases was positive for HPV serotypes 6 and 16 [35].

Sarcomatoid carcinoma is the most aggressive primary penile carcinoma. Patients may present initially with simultaneous nodal and systemic metastases. There may be skip systemic dissemination (primary penis tumor with metastasis to multiple organs with sparing inguinal lymph nodes). Inguinal nodal metastasis is seen in 75-89% of the patients and the mortality rate is 40-75%. Local and systemic recurrences are common (67% of the cases) and most of the patients die within a year [48].

Pseudoglandular (Adenoid) Carcinoma

Unusual tumor characterized by acantholysis and formation of pseudoglandular or adenoid spaces (Figure 8). Synonyms are acantholytic and adenoid squamous cell carcinoma [49].

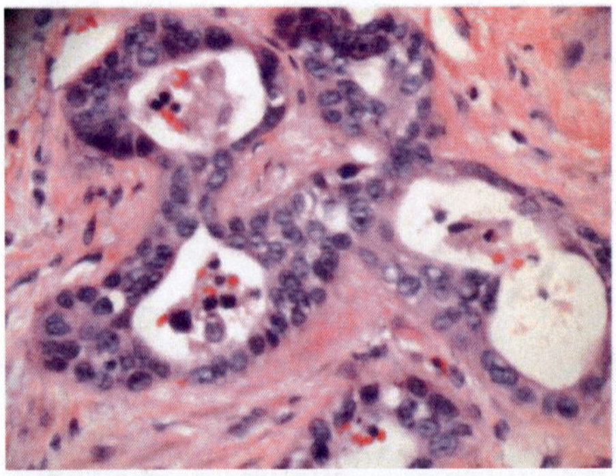

Figure 8. Pseudoglandular carcinoma.

Clinical Features

Aggressive tumors which, compared with the usual type, are of higher grade, invade deeper anatomical structures and are associated with a higher incidence of regional metastases and mortality. Clinical and macroscopic features are those of the usual squamous cell carcinoma. Average age is 54 years. Tumors, due to their size, compromise glans, coronal sulcus and foreskin.

Pathological Features

Macroscopically, tumors are large (4-5 cm), irregular white gray ulcerative or exophytic masses and deeply invading into erectile corpora spongiosa and cavernosa. Microscopically pseudoglandular features comprise 30% to 85% of tumor volume, with a multicystic or honeycomb appearance at low magnification. There are pseudoglands, luminal space lined by atypical flat, cubical or cylindrical cells. The spaces are partially filled with an amorphous eosinophilic material containing keratin, acantholytic cells and necrotic debris. Most tumors demonstrate the histology of poorly differentiated squamous cell carcinoma. Vascular and perineural invasion are frequent. More than half of cases show an associated differentiated PeIN. P16 and HPV are usually negative. Pseudoglandular carcinomas disclose more adverse pathological factors comparing with usual squamous cell carcinomas.

Adenosquamous Carcinoma

There is a biphasic population of squamous and true glandular elements (Figure 9), which are mucinous and CEA positive [50–53]. The glandular component may be related to embryologically misplaced mucous cells occasionally encountered in the perimeatal squamous epithelium of the glans, to goblet cells in the squamous epithelium of the foreskin, or to aberrant differentiation of neoplastic squamous epithelium.

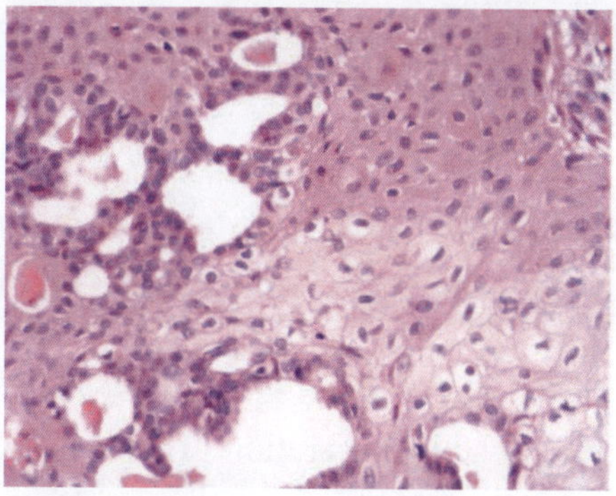

Figure 9. Adenosquamous carcinoma.

Clinical Features

Patients mean age is 55 years. Tumors are large (about 7 cm) and involve the glans, with extension to coronal sulcus and foreskin.

Pathological Features

Macroscopically, it is a granular white-gray, firm neoplasm. The cut surface reveals an irregular tumor replacing most of glans. Microscopically, the squamous cells usually predominate over the glands. Both components are usually discrete, but admixtures are also noted. The glands are lined by cubical or cylindrical epithelium and have intraluminal and intracellular mucin. To establish their surface site of origin, there are foci of penile intraepithelial neoplasia (PeIN) in mucosa adjacent to the invasive carcinoma. Immunohistochemistry for CEA is positive in the glandular component; 34βE12 has also been reported positive in both components [50].

There is limited experience with clinical behavior of these rare neoplasms. Local recurrence is observed in up to 25% of the patients [9]. Inguinal nodal metastatic rate ranges from 43% to 50%. However, mortality rate is low, ranging from 0% to 14%% [9, 48].

Mucoepidermoid Carcinoma

Intracellular mucin secreting squamous cell carcinoma without evidence of gland formation (Figure 10). Unusual tumors with 6 cases reported [54–56].

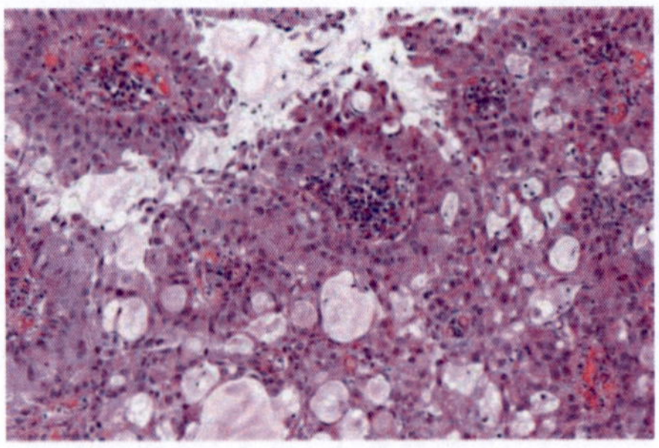

Figure 10. Mucoepidermoid carcinoma [56].

Clinical Features

They occur in the 7th decade usually in the distal penis or glans.

Pathological Features

Macroscopically, they are irregular white gray masses affecting glans and extending into sulcus or foreskin with epithelial ulceration. The cut surface shows an infiltrating tumor affecting corpus spongiosum. Microscopically there is a moderately differentiated keratinizing infiltrating squamous cell carcinoma with the usual features, except that in areas groups of mucin-secreting cells are present. Extracellular mucinous lakes may be present. There is no glandular differentiation. In a reported case, areas of warty (condylomatous) pattern were also noted. In adjacent epithelia, foci of PeIN with features of stratified mucin producing intraepithelial lesion (SMILE), can be observed. In one case we found cytokeratin 7 positive, cytokeratin 5, p63 and p16 negatives. HPV was negative. Three patients of the reported 6 had inguinal nodal metastasis. In our reported case the patient is free of disease after 3 years of radical surgical treatment with nodal metastasis.

HPV-Related Subtypes of Squamous Cell Carcinomas

Basaloid Carcinoma

Basaloid carcinoma is an HPV-related tumor composed of small or intermediate size basophilic cells (Figure 11 A-C) [57].

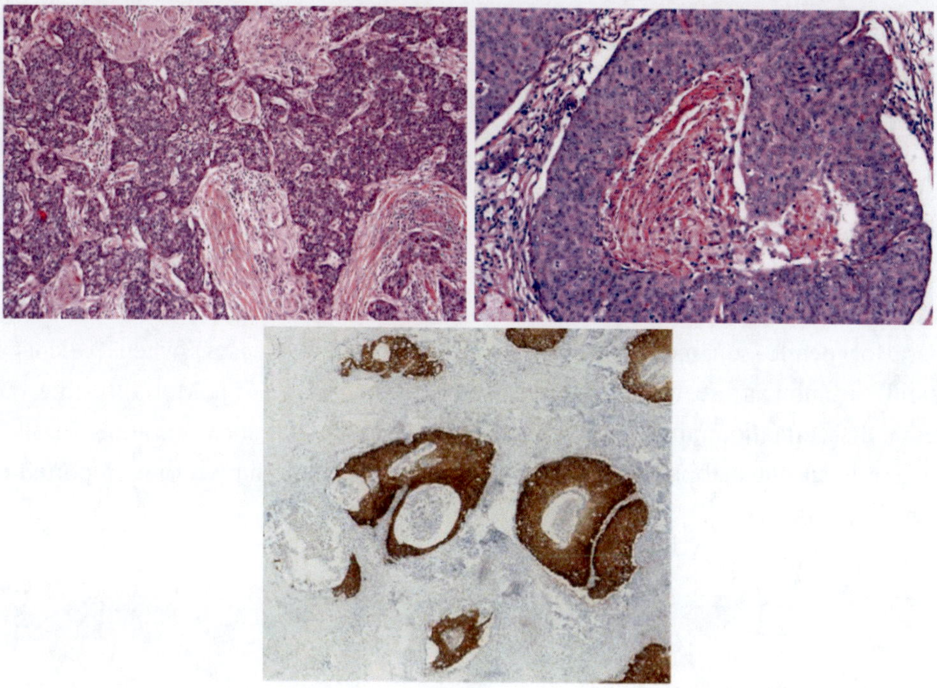

Fig 11. Basaloid carcinoma A, B and C. P16.

Clinical Features

It accounts for 10-14% of penile squamous cell carcinomas. Average age is 52-54 years, younger than patients with usual squamous cell carcinoma. Clinical presentation is that of a large ulcerated non-exophytic mass. The glans is the most frequent affected anatomical. Primary preputial location rarely occurs. One half to two thirds of patients have enlarged, positive inguinal lymph nodes at the time of diagnosis.

Pathological Features

Macroscopically, there is an ulcerated, irregular, mass with an average diameter of 3-4.5 cm [8, 9, 57]. Basaloid carcinomas have distinctive tan, solid appearance with a rounded or slightly lobulated contour at cut surface. Minute necrotic foci can be grossly appreciated.

Microscopically there is a downward proliferation of packed solid nests of cells separated by scant intervening stroma. Or there is a nesting pattern each nest surrounded by a clear space composed of uniform, small, poorly differentiated cells with a high nuclear to cytoplasmic ratio and scant cytoplasm. Mitoses are numerous. Nucleoli are inconspicuous. There is limited or no squamous maturation. Abrupt central keratinization may also be present. Centrally, the nest typically contains necrotic cells or keratin debris in a comedocarcinoma-like pattern. Basaloid carcinomas are usually deeply invasive, extending into erectile penile tissues. Invasion of corpus cavernosum is evident in 79-83% of the cases. Superficial basaloid squamous cell carcinomas invading only lamina propria are rare. Vascular and perineural invasion are frequent findings (69% and 50% of the cases, respectively). PeIN of basaloid or warty histology is prevalent in tissues adjacent to invasive basaloid carcinomas. Basaloid carcinomas are positive for p16 and HPV. CK 34βE12 (high molecular weight cytokeratin) is positive. HPV-16 is the most commonly found serotype, representing 82% of all HPV genotypes identified in this variant [57].

Basaloid carcinoma is considered an aggressive neoplasm with a high incidence of nodal metastasis present in 50-100% of the patients. Local recurrence is among the highest for penile squamous cell carcinoma (36% of the cases) when patients with basaloid carcinomas are treated with partial penectomy [9, 45]. Mortality rate due to systemic dissemination ranges from 21% to 67%. The 10-year survival rate is 76% [1].

There is an unusual papillary variant of basaloid carcinoma with few reported cases (Figure 12 A and B) [1].

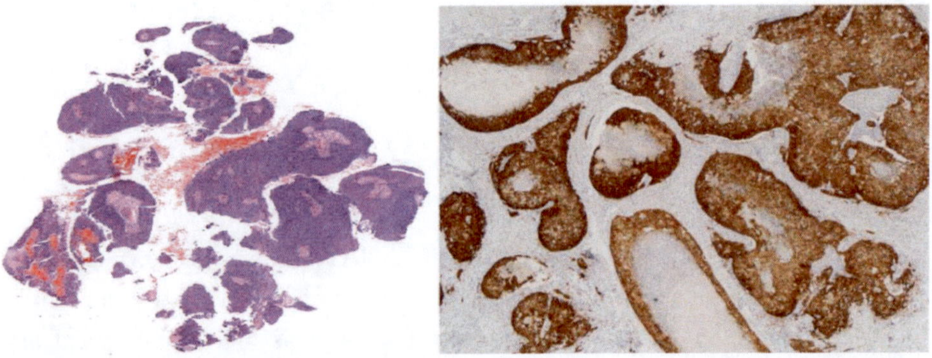

(a) (b)

Figure 12. Papillary basaloid carcinoma A and B. P16.

Warty Carcinoma

Exophytic cauliflower-like verruciform, moderately differentiated neoplasm composed of condylomatous papillae (Figure 13 A-D) [58, 59].

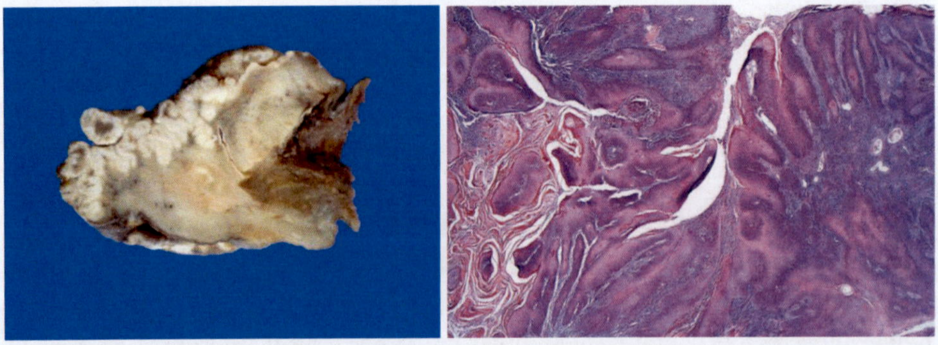

Figure 13. (Continued).

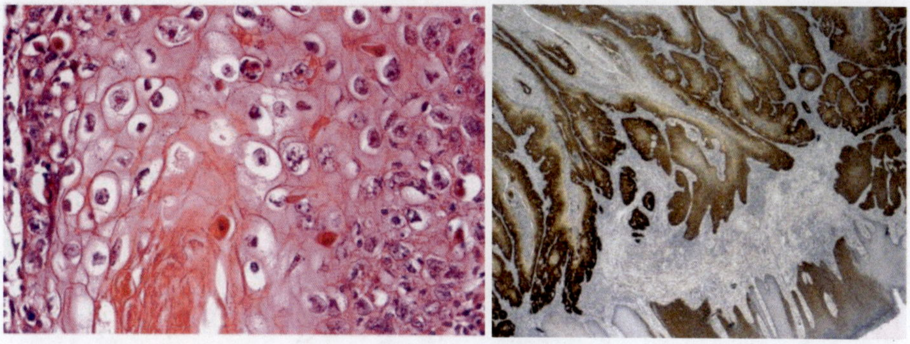

Figure 13. Warty (condylomatous) carcinoma A, B, C and D. P16.

Clinical Features

It represents 6-10% of all penile squamous cell carcinomas [8, 58]. Warty carcinomas are slow-growing lesions and a history of genital warts is common. The median age is 48-55 years, about 10 years younger than the usual squamous cell carcinoma. They involve multiple anatomical compartments Tumors may exclusively involve either glans or foreskin.

Warty carcinomas can be recognized at macroscopic examination. It shows a characteristic cauliflower or cobblestone-like, firm, white-gray granular mass. There are similarities with common or giant condylomas. The nodularity varies from uniformly small and symmetrical to flatter mosaic-like to coarser, less uniform, granular and nodular, asymmetrical. The cut surface shows a papillary neoplasm with condylomatous papillae which at cut surface appear as a nodule with a dark core surrounded by a tan white tumor tissue. There is usually gross involvement of lamina propria and corpus spongiosum and occasionally corpora cavernosa.

Microscopically the condylomatous papillae are long and undulating with a central fibrovascular core and a jagged tumor front. The most conspicuous microscopic finding is the presence of nuclear pleomorphism of koilocytotic type, which is not present in other verruciform penile carcinomas. The nuclei are increased in size, wrinkled, and hyperchromatic, with frequent binucleation or multinucleation. Perinuclear clear halos and individual cell necrosis are common. Clear cell features may predominate. Invasion to erectile tissues is common. Tumors limited to lamina propria are infrequent. Vascular and perineural invasion are uncommon. Warty carcinomas are positive for p16 and HPV in more than half of the cases. Local recurrence after penectomy occurs in 10% of warty carcinomas and inguinal lymph node metastasis in about 17%-18%. Systemic dissemination is rare and mortality rate is low (0-9%) [8, 9, 58, 59].

Warty-Basaloid Carcinoma

An HPV-related tumor with mixed warty and basaloid features (Figure 14 A-C) [60].

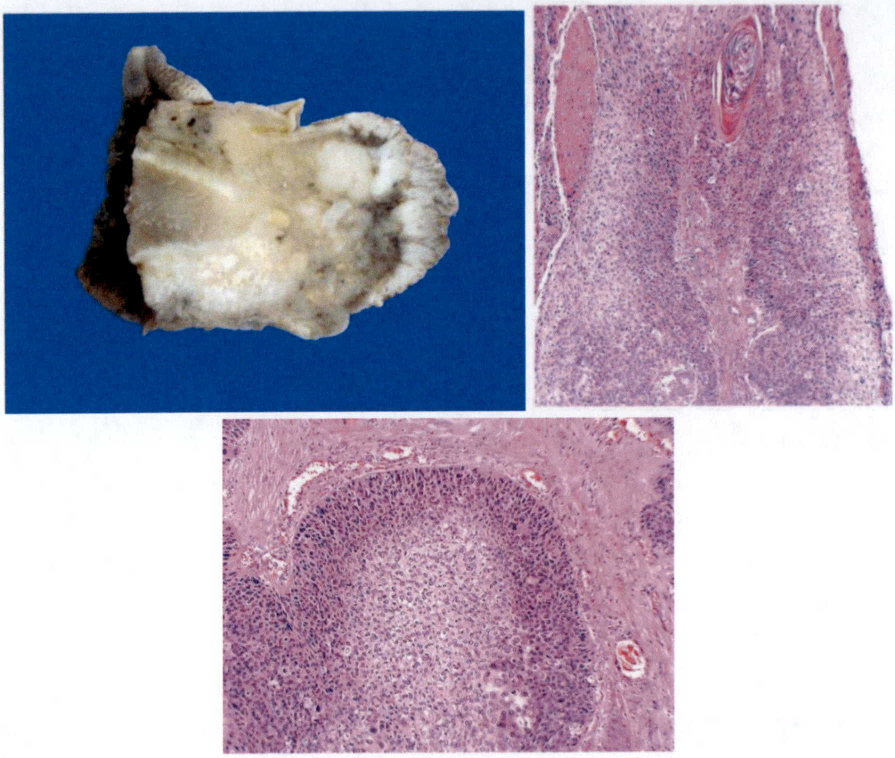

Figure 14. Warty-basaloid carcinoma A, B and C.

Clinical Features

Clinical presentation is that of a large penile mass in most cases. The median age is of 62 years. About two-thirds of tumors affect multiple anatomical compartments, glans, coronal sulcus and foreskin.

Pathological Features

Macroscopically, tumors are exoendophytic, white-gray large (5 cm) irregular masses affecting multiple compartments. The cut surface is tan-to-white solid or mixed papillomatous on the surface and solid in deeper invasive areas. In most cases, deeply penetrating tumor is noted in corpus spongiosum, dartos or corpora cavernosa.

Microscopically, tumors are biphasic with variable proportions of warty and basaloid components. There are various patterns: the most common, observed in two-thirds of the cases, shows a condylomatous aspect on the surface and basaloid features in deep areas. In 15% of the cases there is a non-papillomatous invasive nesting pattern with central warty clear cells and peripheral basaloid cells. Rarely tumors are papillary, and each papilla has a biphasic warty and basaloid cell. Vascular invasion is noted in one-half and perineural invasion in one-quarter of the cases. HPV is detected in most cases either by PCR or by p16 immunohistochemistry.

Prognosis is intermediate between pure warty and basaloid carcinomas. In one study inguinal nodal metastases were present in 52% of patients who received groin dissection and 33% died from disseminated carcinoma. The estimated survival rates at 5- and 10-years are 69% and 61%, respectively.

Medullary Carcinoma

A poorly differentiated solid carcinoma composed of anaplastic large cells with prominent nucleoli and characteristically rich in inflammatory cells (Figure 15 A and B) [61].

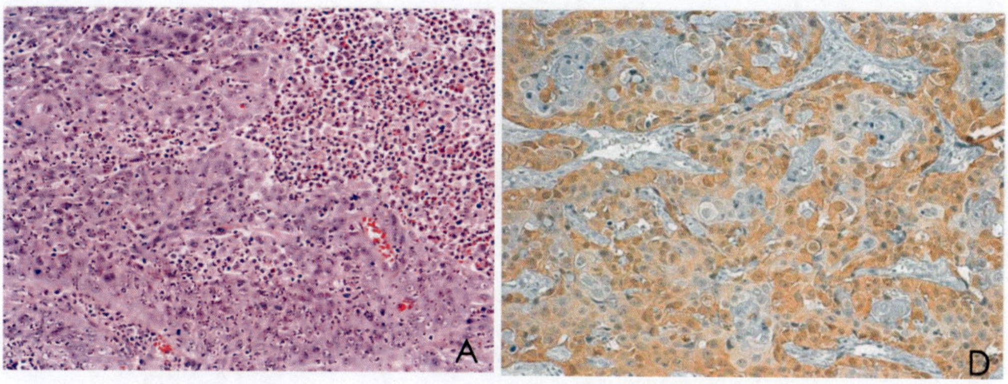

Figure 15. Medullary carcinoma A and B. P16.

Clinical Features

There is scanty information about the clinical features. Patient's median age is 71 years with a range of 42 to 92 years old. Most primary tumors are located in the glans, but foreskin and sulcus are also rarely affected.

Pathological Features

Tumors are macroscopically large, irregular white gray masses destroying most of the glans and secondarily extending to coronal sulcus and inner foreskin surface, which is frequently ulcerated.

Microscopically tumors grow in large sheets, solid nests, or are trabecular. In some cases, cells are less cohesive and small groups are surrounded by inflammatory cells. Individual cell or tumor geographic necrosis is common. Cytologically, there are anaplastic features without squamous maturation. Focal keratinization is rarely observed. Nuclei are large polymorphic with prominent eosinophilic nucleoli. Mitoses exceed 10 per 10 high power fields. Associated lesions are changes of PeIN, differentiated or warty/basaloid types. Lichen sclerosus is observed in some cases. A noteworthy pathological feature is the presence of dense inflammatory cell infiltrate within the tumor or stroma. HPV was detected by DNA PCR in all the reported cases. HPV 16 was the most common genotype found but others genotypes - 33, 58 and 66 - were also identified

[61]. Using the mRNA technology, HPV was detected in 75% of the cases. Immunohistochemistry for p16 is usually positive.

Clinical and follow up information of patients with medullary carcinomas is not available. However, adverse pathological prognostic features present in these tumors, such as high histological grade and deep invasion of corpora cavernosa, would indicate a probable aggressive clinical behavior.

Clear Cell Carcinoma

Aggressive tumors growing in confluent sheets or nests composed of clear cells originating in the mucosal squamous epithelium of the penis (Figure 16 A-C) [62]. Histologically similar HPV positive cases of clear cell carcinoma in the foreskin thought by their authors to originate from adnexal glands of penile skin were reported in Austria [63].

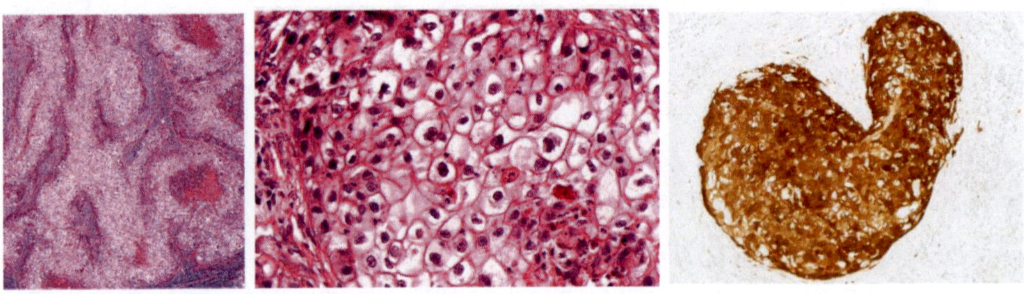

Figure 16. Clear cell carcinoma A, B and C. P16.

Clinical Features

Patients' mean age is 78 years with a range of 52 to 95 years. They present as a large tumor mass in the distal part of the penis or as distant systemic metastasis. Tumors involve preferentially the glans with extension to coronal sulcus or foreskin.

Pathological Features

Macroscopically, tumors are large white gray granular firm irregular masses with ulceration of glans epithelial surface. The cut surface shows a replacement of the normal anatomical architecture of the glans, with massive tumor occupation of erectile tissues, up to corpora cavernosa. They measure 6 cm in largest dimensions.

Microscopically there is a solid nesting growth with central comedo-necrosis composed of clear cells. At high power, nuclei are hyperchromatic, rounded, ovoid or wrinkled some with duplication. There are prominent cytoplasmic clear cell features. They are also confluent nests with central and geographical-like necrosis. Warty and warty-basaloid PeIN are found in adjacent glans epithelium. Adverse microscopic pathological prognostic factors are noted: high histological grade, tumor thickness averaging 40 mm, deep invasion of corpora cavernosa and vascular and perineural invasion. Immunohistochemical staining shows p16 and GATA 3 positivity. HPV16 was detected by PCR in one of the reported 3 cases.

Inguinal node metastases are frequent. Of the 3 reported cases two patients died from disseminated disease 9 and 12 months after penectomy. The third patient was alive with metastatic disease 15 months until the moment of last follow up.

Lymphoepithelioma-Like Carcinoma

Poorly differentiated squamous cell carcinoma with poorly cohesive cells immersed and obscured by inflammatory cells, resembling "lymphoepithelial-like carcinoma" of the nasopharynx. Only 2 cases have been reported (Figure 17 A and B) [64].

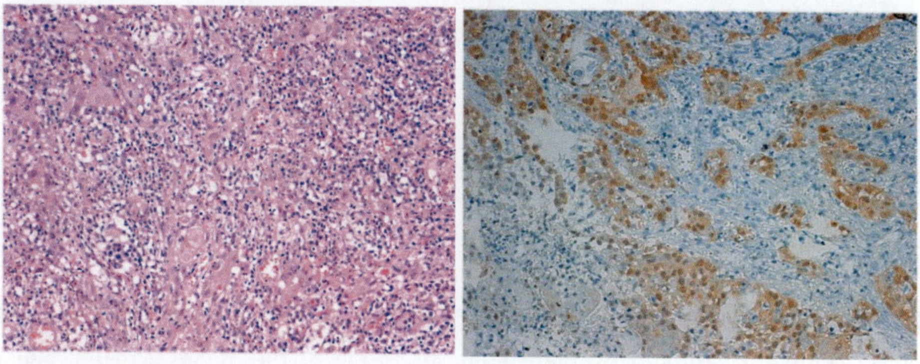

Figure 17. Lymphoepithelioma like carcinoma A and B. P16.

Clinical Features

Uncircumcised 50-70-year-old males with tumors in the glans extending into coronal sulcus and foreskin.

Pathological Features

Macroscopically, they are well to poorly circumscribed, white gray tumor masses mainly affecting the glans. A syncytial microscopic growth pattern is present, with irregular sheets, nests, trabecules, cords or individual cells within a dense lymphoplasmocytic and eosinophilic matrix, which obscures tumor cell boundaries. There is no keratinization, and cells are poorly cohesive, some presenting individually isolated from other epithelial cells and surrounded and obscured by inflammatory cell infiltrate. Immunostain P63 is useful for the identification of the epithelial cells. p16 is usually positive in these tumors indicating their HPV relation.

Adverse prognostic pathological factors are present: invasion of erectile tissues, vascular and perineural invasion, and high histological grade. Metastasis was present in one of the 2 reported cases. Both patients underwent surgical treatment with penectomies and died from causes other than penile cancer.

Mixed Carcinomas

The denomination of mixed carcinoma, other than verrucous hybrid and warty-basaloid carcinomas, is restricted to penile squamous cell carcinomas in which two or more clearly recognized histological variants coexist. One of the subtypes should represent at least 20% of the tumor mass for the tumor to be placed in this category. There are mixed tumors in the HPV-unrelated and HPV-related groups [65].

Unclassified Carcinoma

Rarely, there are penile epithelial squamous neoplasms which are difficult to classify in any of the above described categories. In such cases, the report should include at least histologic grade, vascular/perineural invasion, and infiltration of anatomic levels.

Precursor Lesions

Current nomenclature for penile precancerous lesions is Penile Intraepithelial Neoplasia (PeIN). Histologically there is an alteration of the mucosal penile squamous epithelium characterized by dysplastic changes with an intact basement membrane. There are various subtypes accepted by the 2016 WHO/ AFIP classification systems (Table 2) [1, 2].

Table 2. WHO/AFIP histological classification of Penile Intraepithelial Neoplasia [1, 2]

HPV-unrelated
-Differentiated
HPV-related
-Warty -Basaloid -Warty-basaloid
Other

General Features

PeIN subtypes are precursors of invasive carcinomas and they can be presented as a solitary (unicentric) or multiple (multicentric) lesions or in association with invasive carcinomas. In countries with low incidence of penile cancer most patients present with solitary lesions whereas in countries with a high incidence of penile cancer they are most commonly diagnosed in association with invasive cancer [66, 67]. This apparent paradox is explained by the higher clinical stages in the latter regions, due to cultural factors resulting patients neglect and late diagnosis, and the identification and early treatment of precancerous lesions in more developed regions preventing or down staging invasive cancers. Differentiated PeIN is associated with low grade keratinizing variants of invasive carcinomas whereas basaloid/warty PeIN are frequent in specimens with invasive basaloid or warty carcinoma [21]. Basaloid and warty basaloid PeINs are usually associated with HPV16 whereas in warty PeIN HPV genotypes are more heterogeneous [68]. Differentiated PeIN is commonly associated with lichen sclerosus [21, 22] but the pathogenesis of this relation is not well understood [69].

Clinical and Pathological Features

Warty/basaloid PeIN occur in patients about 10 years younger than differentiated PeIN (fourth to fifth and fifth to seven decades respectively) [70]. HPV-related PeIN preferentially affects the glans and differentiated PeIN prefers the foreskin. Differentiated PeIN present as a solitary white plaque usually in the foreskin whereas basaloid PeIN is characterized by an erythematous nodular or diffuse lesion, uni or multifocal.

Table 3. HPV genotypes in PeIN subtypes [68]

PeIN	HPV genotypes
Basaloid	16, 18, 35, 44(2), 52, 56, 58
Warty-basaloid	16, 18, 30, 33, 35, 52, 56, 44/51/59
Warty	16, 18, 30, 33, 39, 56, 66, 73, 11, 84, 87

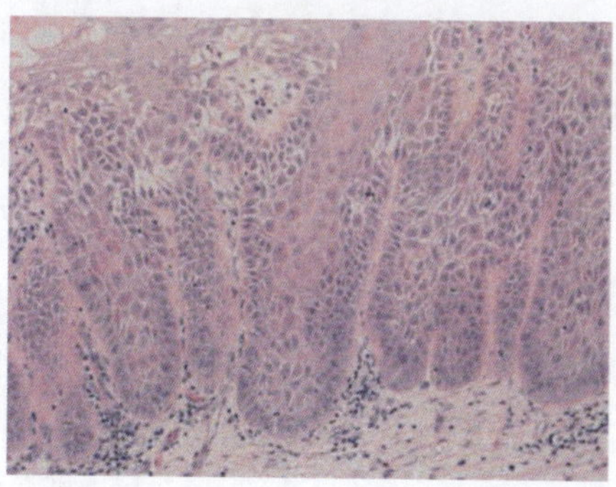

Figure 18. Differentiated PeIN.

Histologically, HPV-unrelated differentiated PeIN is characterized by a thickened epithelium, maturing eosinophilic cytoplasm, dyskeratosis and basal cell atypias (Figure 18). Warty PeIN has a low papillary appearance, cell maturation and pleomorphic koilocytosis. Warty-basaloid PeIN show basaloid and warty features. HPV-related basaloid PeIN show smaller anaplastic cells involving the full epithelial thickness (Figures 19-21). Other types of PeIN are rarely present. K1 67 and p53 separates PeIN from squamous hyperplasia. p16 is negative in differentiated PeIN and positive in warty/basaloid PeIN [71, 72]. HPV 16 is the most common genotype detected in PeIN, but there is some variation according to subtypes of PeIN. HPV 16 is the preferential genotype present in basaloid PeIN but warty PeIN depict a heterogeneous array of HPV genotypes. There are other rare intraepithelial lesions like pagetoid, spindle, clear cells, pleomorphic, which need more studies. (Table 3) [68].

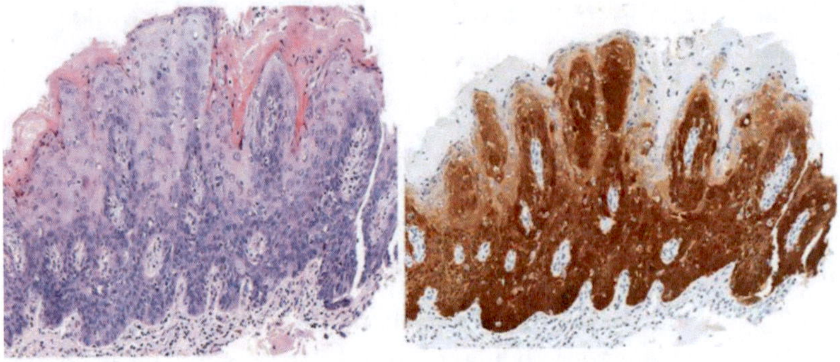

Figure 19. Warty PeIN.

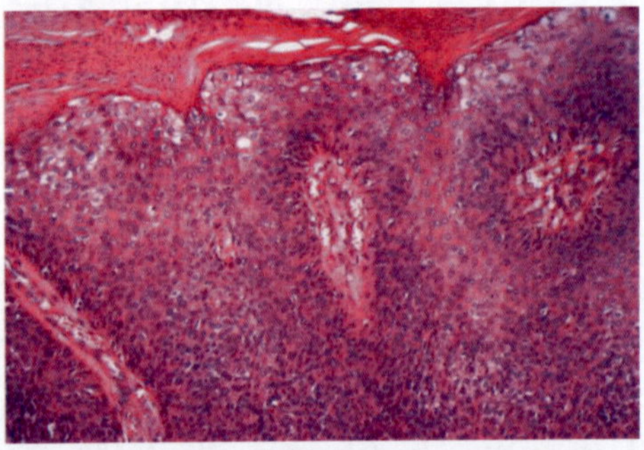

Figure 20. Warty-basaloid PeIN.

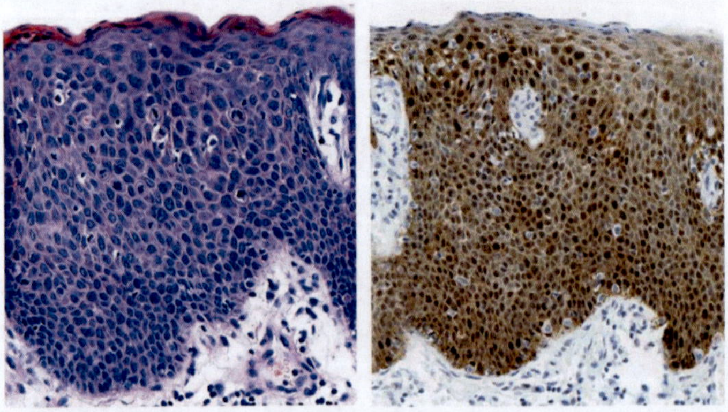

Figure 21. Basaloid PeIN.

Follow-Up Studies

There is scant information regarding biological behavior of PeIN. There is more information on conversion of HPV infection in general population into clinical lesions, such as condylomas or PeIN [73, 74].

PART II: PROGNOSTIC FACTORS

Certain pathologic features observed in primary tumors have been proposed as prognostic factors, i.e., variables that can be used to predict the likelihood of an outcome, such as tumor recurrence, nodal metastasis or cancer-related death. These variables can be used in isolation or, more sensibly, as part of prognostic indexes [75, 76]. The proper evaluation of these pathologic features usually requires the assessment of surgical specimens, as biopsies are mostly inadequate for such matters [77].

In spite of several studies evaluating the use of molecular biomarkers as predictors of outcome in penile cancer, [78] no clear and consistent biomarker has been found to have clinically significance and reproducible value as a prognostic factor. Until further and more robust evidence emerges, molecular profiling should be considered of limited clinical usefulness.

It has to be noted that, besides pathologic features of the primary tumor, events such as insufficient resection margins of the surgical specimen can also impact prognosis and predict outcome [79]. In this regard, it is desirable to obtain negative resection margins to avoid local tumor recurrence, which would increase the risk of nodal metastasis and systemic dissemination [48]. The use of standardized guidelines for handling specimens and reporting features is encouraged.

In this section, we first introduce the pathologic features that have been shown more robustness in predicting outcome, and then we describe in detail one of the risks scores than have been proposed, the Penile Prognostic Index. Even though other risk scores have been proposed, [75] enough evidence points about their limited clinical usefulness [80].

Pathologic Features

Histologic Grade

Histologic grade is one of the more consistent prognostic factors. High-grade tumors metastasize and disseminate more frequently than low-grade tumors, regardless of other pathologic features. To preserve its prognostic power, histologic grading should be done consistently, using a validated morphologic system. At one end of the differentiation spectrum, grade 1 tumors are those composed by neoplastic cells almost undistinguishable from normal squamous cells, except for a minimal basal or parasabal atypia. At the other end of the spectrum, grade 3 tumors are those composed by any proportion of anaplastic cells (nuclear pleomorphism, coarse chromatin, prominent nucleolus, irregular and thickened nuclear membrane, abundant and atypical mitoses). Then, grade 2 tumors include the remaining cases not fitting criteria for grades 1 or 3, with neoplastic cells showing evident but not extreme nuclear atypia and ample eosinophilic cytoplasm with a clear tendency towards squamous maturation. It should be emphasized that any proportion of anaplastic cells carries implicit a risk for nodal metastasis. Tumors with more than one histologic grade (i.e., heterogeneous tumors) should be graded according to the highest grade found, regardless of its proportion.

Perineural Invasion

Perineural invasion is defined as the presence of tumor cells in the perineural space. Presence of perineural invasion is an important predictor of nodal metastasis and cancer-related mortality. Its presence or absence should always be noted in the pathologic examination of surgical specimens. Caution should be paid for a proper differential diagnosis of perineural invasion versus nerve entrapment.

Vascular Invasion

Vascular invasion, either lymphatic or venous, is associated with an increased risk for nodal metastasis. Lymphatic vascular invasion is more frequently observed, although venous invasion and invasion of vascular erectile tissues can also be seen in some cases. The presence or absence of vascular invasion should always be noted. As with perineural invasion, caution should be paid for a proper differential diagnosis of true vascular invasion and retraction artifacts (endothelial markers can be used in such cases but are seldom required).

Other Prognostic Features

Some other features of the primary tumor are also associated with outcome, although to a lesser degree when compared to histologic grade, perineural invasion and vascular invasion. These features include tumor thickness, anatomic level of infiltration, anatomic location, pattern of growth and histologic subtype.

Tumor thickness should be measured from the non-necrotic non-keratinized tumor surface to its deepest point of infiltration. Tumor thickness is moderately associated with nodal metastasis. Tumors invading up to 5 mm show a low risk for metastasis while those invading more than 10 mm are more likely to have nodal involvement. In tumors invading from 5 to 10 mm other pathological features, especially perineural invasion and histological grade, should be used for predicting the likelihood of nodal involvement.

Tumors invading only lamina propria or superficial corpus spongiosum are at lower risk for nodal metastasis than those invading deep corpus spongiosum or corpora cavernosa. Tumors exclusively located at the foreskin have a better prognosis than those arising in the glans, especially because they tend to be of lower grade and invade superficial anatomical layers. Verruciform tumors are associated with good prognosis while tumors with vertical pattern of growth are more likely to present nodal metastasis, systemic dissemination and cancer-related death.

Finally, penile carcinomas can be stratified in 3 risk groups for nodal metastasis: low risk (verrucous, papillary, low-grade warty, pseudohyperplastic and low-grade mixed carcinomas, as well as carcinoma cuniculatum), intermediate risk (low-grade usual, high-grade warty and high-grade mixed carcinomas) and high risk (high-grade usual, sarcomatoid, pseudoglandular, adenosquamous and basaloid carcinomas).

The Penile Prognostic Index

The Penile Prognostic Index aims at predicting the likelihood of nodal metastasis based on pathologic features of the surgical specimen [81]. It can be used for therapeutic planning to define which patients are likely to benefit from an inguinal dissection. The Penile Prognostic Index combines 3 prognostic factors (histologic grade, anatomic level of infiltration, and perineural invasion) to classify a patient into a risk group category. This score is built adding up 3 values assigned to each one of the variables involved.

1. Histologic grade: 1 point to well differentiated (grade 1), 2 point to moderately well differentiated (grade 2) and 3 points to poorly differentiated (grade 3) tumors.
2. Anatomic level:
   a. Glans tumors: 1 point for invasion up to lamina propria, 2 points for invasion of corpus spongiosum and 3 points for invasion of corpora cavernosa, including its tunica albuginea.
   b. Foreskin tumors: 1 point for invasion up to lamina propria, 2 point for invasion of preputial dartos and 3 point for invasion of preputial skin, either dermis or epidermis.
3. Perineural invasion: 0 points if perineural invasion is absent and 1 point if perineural invasion is present.

A value from 2 to 7 is then obtained. For patients in the low-risk category (scores 2 to 3) the probability of nodal metastasis is very low. If there is no clinical evidence of nodal involvement (e.g., palpable inguinal nodes, imaging studies), a surveillance program should suffice. Inguinal dissection is likely to be unnecessary. For patients in the high-risk group (scores 5 to 7) the probability of nodal metastasis is high. These patients should receive prophylactic inguinal lymphadenectomy, regardless of the clinical status of the inguinal nodes. Patients in the intermediate category (score 4) are problematic to handle and other clinicopathological features (clinical status of inguinal nodes, imaging studies, histological subtype, vascular invasion) should be evaluated.

Conclusion

Most penile neoplasms are squamous cell carcinomas, arising predominantly in the glans. Penile carcinomas are classified in HPV-related and HPV-unrelated groups, with subtypes of each group showing distinctive clinicopathologic and outcome features. HPV-unrelated subtypes include usual, verrucous (and hybrid-verrucous), papillary, cuniculatum, pseudohyperplastic, sarcomatoid, pseudoglandular, adenosquamous and mucoepidermoid carcinomas. HPV-related subtypes include basaloid, warty, warty-basaloid, medullary, clear cell and lymphoepithelioma-like carcinomas. Pathologic prognostic factors are features observed in the primary tumor of resected specimens used to estimate the likelihood of tumor recurrence, nodal/systemic dissemination and cancer-related death. Evaluation and determination of their statuses should be done in all cases. The 3 main pathologic prognostic factors are histologic grade, perineural invasion and vascular invasion. Histologic grading should be done consistently, using validated and reproducible criteria. Presence or absence of vascular or perineural invasion should also be recorded in every case. Other pathologic prognostic factors include tumor thickness, level of anatomic infiltration, anatomic site of the primary tumor, pattern of growth, and histologic subtype. Pathologic factors can be combined to create risk-scoring systems such as the Penile Prognostic Index.

Key Points

- Most penile tumors correspond to squamous cell carcinomas arising in the distal penis.
- Penile carcinomas are grouped in HPV-related and HPV-unrelated subtypes, depending on their association with HPV infection, with each subtype showing distinctive clinicopathologic and outcome features.
- HPV-unrelated subtypes include usual (the most frequent), verrucous, hybrid-verrucous, papillary, pseudohyperplastic, sarcomatoid, pseudoglandular, adenosquamous, and mucoepidermoid carcinomas.
- HPV-related subtypes include basaloid, warty, warty-basaloid, medullary, clear cell, and lymphoepithelioma-like carcinomas.

- Penile Intraepithelial Neoplasia (PeIN) is the precursor lesion of penile carcinomas. Depending on their morphology, PeIN is classified as differentiated (HPV-unrelated) and warty/basaloid (HPV-related).
- Pathologic prognostc factors are features of the primary tumor evaluated in resected specimens that can be used to estimate the likelihood of tumor recurrence, nodal metastasis, and systemic dissemination.
- The 3 main prognostic factors are histologic grade, vascular (lymphatic or venous) invasion, and perineural invasion. Other prognostic factors include tumor thickness, anatomic level of infiltration, anatomic location, pattern of growth, and histologic subtype.
- Prognostic factors can be combined into risk-scoring systems such as the Penile Prognostic Index, which combines histologic grade, anatomic level of infiltration, and perineural invasion. The risk categories can be used for therapeutic planning (e.g., timing for inguinal nodal dissection) and follow-up strategies.

References

[1] Epstein JI, Cubilla AL, Magi-Galluzzi C. Tumors of the Penis. In: *Tumors of the Prostate Gland, Seminal Vesicles, Penis, and Scrotum*. 5th ed.; 2019.

[2] Cubilla, AL, Dillner J, Amin, MB, et al. Tumours of the Penis. In: Moch, H, Humphrey, PA, Ulbright TM, et al., eds. *World Health Organization Classification of Tumours of the Urinary System and Male Genital Organs*. Fourth. Lyon: IARC; 2016:259–286.

[3] Kurman RJ, Toki T, Schiffman MH. Basaloid and warty carcinomas of the vulva. Distinctive types of squamous cell carcinoma frequently associated with human papillomaviruses. *Am. J. Surg. Pathol.* 1993;17:133–145.

[4] Gregoire L, Cubilla AL, Reuter VE, et al. Preferential association of human papillomavirus with high-grade histologic variants of penile-invasive squamous cell carcinoma. *J. Natl. Cancer Inst.* 1995;87:1705–1709.

[5] Rubin MA, Kleter B, Zhou M, et al. Detection and typing of human papillomavirus DNA in penile carcinoma: evidence for multiple independent pathways of penile carcinogenesis. *Am. J. Pathol.* 2001;159:1211–1218. doi:10.1016/S0002-9440(10)62506-0.

[6] Djajadiningrat RS, Jordanova ES, Kroon BK, et al. Human papillomavirus prevalence in invasive penile cancer and association with clinical outcome. *J. Urol.* 2015;193:526–531. doi:10.1016/j.juro.2014.08.087.

[7] Cañete-Portillo S, Sanchez D, Alemany L, et al. The Relative Value of P16 for HPV Detection in Penile Carcinomas. A Study of 219 of the Most Common HPV-Related Neoplasms. *Mod Pathol (in press)* 2019.

[8] Cubilla AL, Reuter V, Velazquez E, et al. Histologic classification of penile carcinoma and its relation to outcome in 61 patients with primary resection. *Int. J. Surg. Pathol.* 2001;9:111–120. doi:10.1177/106689690100900204.

[9] Guimarães GC, Cunha IW, Soares FA, et al. Penile squamous cell carcinoma clinicopathological features, nodal metastasis and outcome in 333 cases. *J. Urol.* 2009;182:528–534; discussion 534. doi:10.1016/j.juro.2009.04.028.

[10] Persson B, Sjödin J-G, Holmberg L, et al. The National Penile Cancer Register in Sweden 2000-2003. *Scand. J. Urol. Nephrol.* 2007;41:278–282. doi:10.1080/00365590601183709.

[11] Favorito LA, Nardi AC, Ronalsa M, et al. Epidemiologic study on penile cancer in Brazil. *Int Braz J Urol* 2008;34:587–591; discussion 591-593.

[12] Hemal AK, Kumar R, Wadhwa SN. Carcinoma penis in a young boy. A case report. *Indian J Cancer* 1996;33:108–110.

[13] Pizzocaro G, Piva L, Bandieramonte G, et al. Up-to-date management of carcinoma of the penis. *Eur. Urol.* 1997;32:5–15.

[14] Kreuter A, Brockmeyer NH, Weissenborn SJ, et al. Penile intraepithelial neoplasia is frequent in HIV-positive men with anal dysplasia. *J. Invest. Dermatol.* 2008; 128:2316–2324. doi:10.1038/jid.2008.72.

[15] Théodore C, Androulakis N, Spatz A, et al. An explosive course of squamous cell penile cancer in an AIDS patient. *Ann. Oncol.* 2002;13:475–479.

[16] Chaux A, Reuter V, Lezcano C, et al. Autopsy findings in 14 patients with penile squamous cell carcinoma. *Int. J. Surg. Pathol.* 2011;19:164–169. doi:10.1177/1066896909333781.

[17] Ayyathurai R, Webb DB, Rowland S, et al. Humoral hypercalcemia of penile carcinoma. *Urology* 2007;69:184.e9–10. doi:10.1016/j.urology.2006.10.012.

[18] Videtic GM, Ago CT, Winquist EW. Hypercalcemia and carcinoma of the penis. *Med. Pediatr. Oncol.* 1997;29:576–577.

[19] Lam KY, Chan KW. Molecular pathology and clinicopathologic features of penile tumors: with special reference to analyses of p21 and p53 expression and unusual histologic features. *Arch. Pathol. Lab. Med.* 1999;123:895–904. doi:10.1043/0003-9985(1999)123<0895:MPACFO>2.0.CO;2.

[20] Chaux A, Torres J, Pfannl R, et al. Histologic grade in penile squamous cell carcinoma: visual estimation versus digital measurement of proportions of grades, adverse prognosis with any proportion of grade 3 and correlation of a Gleason-like system with nodal metastasis. *Am. J. Surg. Pathol.* 2009;33:1042–1048. doi:10.1097/PAS.0b013e31819aa4c9.

[21] Cubilla AL, Velazquez EF, Young RH. Epithelial lesions associated with invasive penile squamous cell carcinoma: a pathologic study of 288 cases. *Int. J. Surg. Pathol.* 2004;12:351–364. doi:10.1177/106689690401200408.

[22] Velazquez EF, Cubilla AL. Lichen sclerosus in 68 patients with squamous cell carcinoma of the penis: frequent atypias and correlation with special carcinoma variants suggests a precancerous role. *Am. J. Surg. Pathol.* 2003;27:1448–1453.

[23] Corbishley CM, Tinwell B, Kaul A, et al. Glans resurfacing for precancerous and superficially invasive carcinomas of the glans penis: Pathological specimen handling and reporting. *Semin Diagn Pathol* 2015;32:232–237. doi:10.1053/j.semdp.2014.12.016.

[24] Alvarez Alvarez C, Meijide Rico F, Rodríguez González L, et al. [Verrucous carcinoma of the penis arising from a lichen planus. A true preneoplastic lesion?]. *Actas Urol Esp* 2006;30:90–92.

[25] Johnson DE, Lo RK, Srigley J, et al. Verrucous carcinoma of the penis. *J. Urol.* 1985;133:216–218.

[26] Seixas AL, Ornellas AA, Marota A, et al. Verrucous carcinoma of the penis: retrospective analysis of 32 cases. *J. Urol.* 1994;152:1476–1478; discussion 1478-1479.

[27] Masih AS, Stoler MH, Farrow GM, et al. Penile verrucous carcinoma: a clinicopathologic, human papillomavirus typing and flow cytometric analysis. *Mod. Pathol.* 1992;5:48–55.

[28] Stankiewicz E, Kudahetti SC, Prowse DM, et al. HPV infection and immunochemical detection of cell-cycle markers in verrucous carcinoma of the penis. *Mod. Pathol.* 2009;22:1160–1168. doi:10.1038/modpathol.2009.77.

[29] Dai B, Ye DW, Kong YY, et al. Predicting regional lymph node metastasis in Chinese patients with penile squamous cell carcinoma: the role of histopathological classification, tumor stage and depth of invasion. *J. Urol.* 2006;176:1431–1435; discussion 1435. doi:10.1016/j.juro.2006.06.024.

[30] Cubilla AL, Lloveras B, Alejo M, et al. The basaloid cell is the best tissue marker for human papillomavirus in invasive penile squamous cell carcinoma: a study of 202 cases from Paraguay. *Am. J. Surg. Pathol.* 2010;34:104–114. doi:10.1097/PAS.0b013e3181c76a49.

[31] Sanchez DF, Soares FA, Alvarado-Cabrero I, et al. Comparison of Pathologic and Outcome Features of Classical vs. Mixed (Hybrid) Verrucous Carcinoma (VC) of Penis. A Study of 59 Cases. *Mod. Pathol.* 2017:255A.

[32] Kato N, Onozuka T, Yasukawa K, et al. Penile hybrid verrucous-squamous carcinoma associated with a superficial inguinal lymph node metastasis. *Am J Dermatopathol* 2000;22:339–343.

[33] Clemente Ramos LM, García González R, Burgos Revilla FJ, et al. Hybrid tumor of the penis: is this denomination correct? *Arch. Esp. Urol.* 1998;51:821–823.

[34] Chaux A, Soares F, Rodríguez I, et al. Papillary squamous cell carcinoma, not otherwise specified (NOS) of the penis: clinicopathologic features, differential diagnosis, and outcome of 35 cases. *Am. J. Surg. Pathol.* 2010;34:223–230. doi:10.1097/PAS.0b013e3181c7666e.

[35] Cubilla AL, Velazquez EF, Young RH. Distinctive association of HPV with special types of penile squamous cell carcinoma and giant condyloma. A study of 211 cases. *Mod Pathol* 2009;22:164A.

[36] Barreto JE, Velazquez EF, Ayala E, et al. Carcinoma cuniculatum: a distinctive variant of penile squamous cell carcinoma: report of 7 cases. *Am. J. Surg. Pathol.* 2007;31:71–75. doi:10.1097/01.pas.0000213401.72569.22.

[37] Lau P, Li Chang HH, Gomez JA, et al. A rare case of carcinoma cuniculatum of the penis in a 55-year-old. *Can Urol Assoc J* 2010;4:E129-132.

[38] Vinson MA, Okorji O, Gagucas R. Extensive Presentation of Penile Carcinoma Cuniculatum a Variant of Squamous Cell Carcinoma with Low Malignant Potential. *Urol Case Rep* 2016;8:18–20. doi:10.1016/j.eucr.2016.05.004.

[39] Cubilla AL, Velazquez EF, Young RH. Pseudohyperplastic squamous cell carcinoma of the penis associated with lichen sclerosus. An extremely well-differentiated, nonverruciform neoplasm that preferentially affects the foreskin and is frequently misdiagnosed: a report of 10 cases of a distinctive clinicopathologic entity. *Am. J. Surg. Pathol.* 2004;28:895–900.

[40] Velazquez EF, Melamed J, Barreto JE, et al. Sarcomatoid carcinoma of the penis: a clinicopathologic study of 15 cases. *Am. J. Surg. Pathol.* 2005;29:1152–1158.

[41] Lont AP, Gallee MPW, Snijders P, et al. Sarcomatoid squamous cell carcinoma of the penis: a clinical and pathological study of 5 cases. *J. Urol.* 2004;172:932–935. doi:10.1097/01.ju.0000136363.90911.e5.

[42] Fukunaga M, Yokoi K, Miyazawa Y, et al. Penile verrucous carcinoma with anaplastic transformation following radiotherapy. A case report with human papillomavirus typing and flow cytometric DNA studies. *Am. J. Surg. Pathol.* 1994;18:501–505.

[43] Urdiales Viedma M, Fernández Rodríguez A, Romero Díaz JA, et al. Squamous carcinoma of the penis with a rhabdoid phenotype. *Arch. Esp. Urol.* 2003;56:425–427.

[44] Morinaga S, Nakamura S, Moro K, et al. Carcinosarcoma (carcinoma with sarcomatous metaplasia) of the penis. *J Urol Pathol* 3:369–376.

[45] Antonini null, Zucconelli null, Forgiarini null, et al. Carcinosarcoma of penis. Case report and review of the literature. *Adv Clin Path* 1997;1:281–285.

[46] Qi X-P, Lin G-B, Zhu Y-L, et al. Pseudoangiosarcomatous squamous cell carcinoma of the penis: a case report with clinicopathological and human papilloma virus analyses. *Zhonghua Nan Ke Xue* 2009;15:134–139.

[47] Poblet E, Pascual A, Godínez JM, et al. Human papillomavirus-associated penile sarcomatoid carcinoma. *J. Cutan. Pathol.* 2008;35:559–565. doi:10.1111/j.1600-0560.2007.00867.x.

[48] Chaux A, Reuter V, Lezcano C, et al. Comparison of morphologic features and outcome of resected recurrent and nonrecurrent squamous cell carcinoma of the penis: a study of 81 cases. *Am. J. Surg. Pathol.* 2009;33:1299–1306. doi:10.1097/PAS.0b013e3181a418ae.

[49] Cunha IW, Guimaraes GC, Soares F, et al. Pseudoglandular (adenoid, acantholytic) penile squamous cell carcinoma: a clinicopathologic and outcome study of 7 patients. *Am. J. Surg. Pathol.* 2009;33:551–555. doi:10.1097/PAS.0b013e31818a01d8.

[50] Romero FR, de Castro MG, Garcia CRC, et al. Adenosquamous carcinoma of the penis. *Clinics (Sao Paulo)* 2006;61:363–364.

[51] Cubilla AL, Ayala MT, Barreto JE, et al. Surface adenosquamous carcinoma of the penis. A report of three cases. *Am. J. Surg. Pathol.* 1996;20:156–160.

[52] Jamieson NV, Bullock KN, Barker TH. Adenosquamous carcinoma of the penis associated with balanitis xerotica obliterans. *Br J Urol* 1986;58:730–731.

[53] Masera A, Ovcak Z, Volavsek M, et al. Adenosquamous carcinoma of the penis. *J. Urol.* 1997;157:2261.

[54] Layfield LJ, Liu K. Mucoepidermoid carcinoma arising in the glans penis. *Arch. Pathol. Lab. Med.* 2000;124:148–151. doi:10.1043/0003-9985(2000)124<0148:MCAITG>2.0.CO;2.

[55] Costa MR, Sugita DM, Vilela MHT, et al. Mucoepidermoid carcinoma of the penis: Case report and literature review. *Can Urol Assoc J* 2015;9:E27-29. doi:10.5489/cuaj.2126.

[56] Yorita K, Kuroda N, Naroda T, et al. Penile warty mucoepidermoid carcinoma with features of stratified mucin-producing intra-epithelial lesion and invasive stratified mucin-producing carcinoma. *Histopathology* 2018;72:867–873. doi:10.1111/his.13438.

[57] Cubilla AL, Reuter VE, Gregoire L, et al. Basaloid squamous cell carcinoma: a distinctive human papilloma virus-related penile neoplasm: a report of 20 cases. *Am. J. Surg. Pathol.* 1998;22:755–761.

[58] Cubilla AL, Velazques EF, Reuter VE, et al. Warty (condylomatous) squamous cell carcinoma of the penis: a report of 11 cases and proposed classification of "verruciform" penile tumors. *Am. J. Surg. Pathol.* 2000;24:505–512.

[59] Bezerra AL, Lopes A, Landman G, et al. Clinicopathologic features and human papillomavirus dna prevalence of warty and squamous cell carcinoma of the penis. *Am. J. Surg. Pathol.* 2001;25:673–678.

[60] Chaux A, Tamboli P, Ayala A, et al. Warty-basaloid carcinoma: clinicopathological features of a distinctive penile neoplasm. Report of 45 cases. *Mod. Pathol.* 2010;23:896–904. doi:10.1038/modpathol.2010.69.

[61] Cañete-Portillo S, Clavero O, Sanchez DF, et al. Medullary Carcinoma of the Penis: A Distinctive HPV-related Neoplasm: A Report of 12 Cases. *Am. J. Surg. Pathol.* 2017;41:535–540. doi:10.1097/PAS.0000000000000779.

[62] Sanchez DF, Rodriguez IM, Piris A, et al. Clear Cell Carcinoma of the Penis: An HPV-related Variant of Squamous Cell Carcinoma: A Report of 3 Cases. *Am. J. Surg. Pathol.* 2016;40:917–922. doi:10.1097/PAS.0000000000000607.

[63] Liegl B, Regauer S. Penile clear cell carcinoma: a report of 5 cases of a distinct entity. *Am. J. Surg. Pathol.* 2004;28:1513–1517.

[64] Mentrikoski MJ, Frierson HF, Stelow EB, et al. Lymphoepithelioma-like carcinoma of the penis: association with human papilloma virus infection. *Histopathology* 2014;64:312–315. doi:10.1111/his.12248.

[65] Cañete-Portillo S, Alemany L, Sanchez D, et al. Detection of HPV and P16 in Mixed Squamous Cell Carcinoma of the Penis. A Study of 101 cases. *Mod Pathol (in press)* 2019.

[66] Oertell J, Caballero C, Iglesias M, et al. Differentiated precursor lesions and low-grade variants of squamous cell carcinomas are frequent findings in foreskins of patients from a region of high penile cancer incidence. *Histopathology* 2011;58:925–933. doi:10.1111/j.1365-2559.2011.03816.x.

[67] Soskin A, Vieillefond A, Carlotti A, et al. Warty/basaloid penile intraepithelial neoplasia is more prevalent than differentiated penile intraepithelial neoplasia in nonendemic regions for penile cancer when compared with endemic areas: a comparative study between pathologic series from Paris and Paraguay. *Hum. Pathol.* 2012;43:190–196. doi:10.1016/j.humpath.2011.04.014.

[68] Fernández-Nestosa MJ, Guimerà N, Sanchez DF, et al. Human Papillomavirus (HPV) Genotypes in Condylomas, Intraepithelial Neoplasia, and Invasive Carcinoma of the Penis Using Laser Capture Microdissection (LCM)-PCR: A Study of 191 Lesions in 43 Patients. *Am. J. Surg. Pathol.* 2017;41:820–832. doi:10. 1097/xPAS.0000000000000821.

[69] Pietrzak P, Hadway P, Corbishley CM, et al. Is the association between balanitis xerotica obliterans and penile carcinoma underestimated? *BJU Int.* 2006;98:74–76. doi:10.1111/j.1464-410X.2006.06213.x.

[70] Alemany L, Cubilla A, Halec G, et al. Role of Human Papillomavirus in Penile Carcinomas Worldwide. *Eur. Urol.* 2016;69:953–961. doi:10.1016/j.eururo.2015. 12.007.

[71] Chaux A, Pfannl R, Lloveras B, et al. Distinctive association of p16INK4a overexpression with penile intraepithelial neoplasia depicting warty and/or basaloid

features: a study of 141 cases evaluating a new nomenclature. *Am. J. Surg. Pathol.* 2010;34:385–392. doi:10.1097/PAS.0b013e3181cdad23.

[72] Chaux A, Pfannl R, Rodríguez IM, et al. Distinctive immunohistochemical profile of penile intraepithelial lesions: a study of 74 cases. *Am. J. Surg. Pathol.* 2011;35:553–562. doi:10.1097/PAS.0b013e3182113402.

[73] Sudenga SL, Ingles DJ, Pierce Campbell CM, et al. Genital Human Papillomavirus Infection Progression to External Genital Lesions: The HIM Study. *Eur. Urol.* 2016;69:166–173. doi:10.1016/j.eururo.2015.05.032.

[74] Fernández-Nestosa MJ, Cubilla AL. Infectious disease: The natural history of HPV infection in men. *Nat Rev Urol* 2015;12:478–480. doi:10.1038/nrurol.2015.200.

[75] Chaux A, Cubilla AL. Stratification systems as prognostic tools for defining risk of lymph node metastasis in penile squamous cell carcinomas. *Semin. Diagn. Pathol.* 2012;29:83–9.

[76] Sanchez DF, Soares F, Alvarado-Cabrero I, et al. Pathological factors, behavior, and histological prognostic risk groups in subtypes of penile squamous cell carcinomas (SCC). *Semin Diagn Pathol* 2015;32:222–231. doi:10.1053/j.semdp.2014.12.017.

[77] Velazquez EF, Barreto JE, Rodriguez I, et al. Limitations in the interpretation of biopsies in patients with penile squamous cell carcinoma. *Int. J. Surg. Pathol.* 2004;12:139–146. doi:10.1177/106689690401200207.

[78] Vuichoud C, Klap J, Loughlin KR. The Emerging Role and Promise of Biomarkers in Penile Cancer. *Urol. Clin. North Am.* 2016;43:135–143. doi:10.1016/j.ucl.2015.08.012.

[79] Velazquez EF, Soskin A, Bock A, et al. Positive resection margins in partial penectomies: sites of involvement and proposal of local routes of spread of penile squamous cell carcinoma. *Am. J. Surg. Pathol.* 2004;28:384–9.

[80] Chaux A. Risk group systems for penile cancer management: A study of 203 patients with invasive squamous cell carcinoma. *Urology* 2015;86:790–6. doi:10.1016/j.urology.2015.03.050.

[81] Chaux A, Caballero C, Soares F, et al. The prognostic index: a useful pathologic guide for prediction of nodal metastases and survival in penile squamous cell carcinoma. *Am. J. Surg. Pathol.* 2009;33:1049–1057. doi:10.1097/PAS.0b013e31819d17eb.

In: Penile Cancer: Challenges and Controversies
Editors: F. E. Martins and M. L. Djordjevic
ISBN: 978-1-53615-950-9

Chapter 4

CLINICAL EVALUATION, IMAGING AND STAGING

Natália Martins*[1], *MD*, *Liliya Tryfonyuk*[2], *MD* and *Francisco E. Martins*[3]*, *MD

[1]Unidade Local de Saúde do Norte Alentejano, Portalegre, Portugal
[2]Rivne Regional Clinical Hospital, Rivne, Ukraine
[3]Department of Urology, University of Lisbon, School of Medicine, CHLN/Hospital Santa Maria, Lisbon, Portugal

ABSTRACT

Penile cancer is an uncommon malignancy in the USA and Europe. It has a devastating effect on the patient and may be a challenge to diagnose and treat accurately. Early detection plays a crucial role in disease control and proper diagnostic modalities must be employed to accurately identify the cancer, characterize its progression and define its prognosis. Penile cancer is generally an aggressive malignancy characterized by early locoregional lymph node (LN) involvement and later metastatic spread. Appropriate management and treatment outcomes of penile cancer depend critically upon a correct diagnosis, grading and staging of the primary lesion and locoregional lymph node involvement. Unfortunately, there is still a significant delay between initial symptoms and seeking medical advice, sometimes this interval exceeding one year. A high index of suspicion for penile cancer is important in men with penile lesions, particularly if risk factors are present. The use of proper diagnostic imaging modalities, especially the use of imaging modalities in combination with biopsy, is of paramount importance to correctly identify the disease and predict its progression. Over the past few decades, the diagnostic and staging modalities of penile cancer have improved patient risk stratification, thus enabling identification of those patients at higher risk for disease progression with impact on treatment outcomes. Nonetheless, the relatively low incidence of penile cancer, the small patient samples in the published literature, and the almost nonexistent prospective,

* Corresponding Author's E-mail: faemartins@gmail.com.

randomized clinical trials have maintained numerous unresolved controversies about optimal methods for accurate diagnosis and staging of penile cancer.

Keywords: penile cancer, diagnosis, imaging, staging, magnetic resonance, computed tomography, ultrasound, PET computed tomography

INTRODUCTION

Penile cancer (PC) is rare in developed countries, occurring in approximately 1 in 100,000 men in the Western industrialized world and accounts for less than 0,6% of all male cancers [1, 2]. However, higher incidence rates are observed in developing countries where it may represent as much as 10% of male malignancies in parts of Asia, Africa and South America with significant geographic variation, which is mainly explained by circumcision, sexual practices and socioeconomic patterns [3, 4, 5]. Penile cancer occurs most commonly in the sixth to eighth decades of life [5]. In 2010, approximately 1,250 new cases of PC were diagnosed in the United States with 310 deaths, with an incidence rate of 0.3-0.5 per 100,000 [6]. In Sweden, a slightly higher incidence of 0.6-2.1 was registered [7]. Squamous cell carcinoma represents more than 95% of all cases of PC [2].

Over the past few decades, the staging of penile cancer has improved patient risk stratification, enabling identification of patients at high risk of progression in localized disease with positive impact on management, therapeutic outcomes, quality of life and prognosis. However, patients with extensive metastatic disease still have dismal prognoses.

Imaging and other clinical staging modalities have improved dramatically and play a major role in the initial assessment, treatment planning and follow-up of patients with penile cancer. Although clinical evaluation of the primary lesion may be quite straightforward, posing problems in the differential diagnosis of penile squamous cell carcinoma with basal cell carcinoma, Kaposi sarcoma, malignant melanoma, extramammary Paget's disease, urethral carcinoma and metastasis, locoregional lymph node staging pose important and difficult issues. Several techniques have been used to deal with these difficulties, such as ultrasound with fine needle aspiration cytology (US-FNAC), dynamic sentinel node biopsy and axial imaging including computed tomography (CT), magnetic resonance imaging (MRI), and positron emission tomography (PET) imaging with fluorodeoxyglucose (FDG) combined with CT (PET/CT with FDG).

In this chapter, we provide a comprehensive description of the clinical evaluation, diagnostic work-up, and locoregional and metastatic staging of penile cancer.

Clinical Diagnosis

Accurate clinical, histological and staging of both the primary neoplasm and regional lymph nodes are of paramount importance for choosing the most appropriate treatment.

Primary Tumor

Clinically, penile cancer usually presents as a palpable induration, or a visible, exophytic, nodular, or flat and ulcerative, or fungating lesion that alerts the patient to its presence (Figure 1). Penile cancer involves primarily the glans penis (34.5% - 48%) of patients followed by the prepuce (4.5% - 21%), penile shaft (<2% - 5.3%), overlapping on the glans and prepuce (4.5% - 9.0%) and unspecified (42.5%) [8-10]. This distribution may be related to constant exposure of the glans, coronal sulcus and inner prepuce to toxic substances, such as smegma and human papilloma virus (HPV) infection within the preputial sac, being the shaft of the penis relatively spared. Very uncommonly, a nodular, ulcerative or suppurative lesion in the groin may result from lymphatic metastatic involvement from a primary tumor concealed within a long-standing phimotic foreskin.

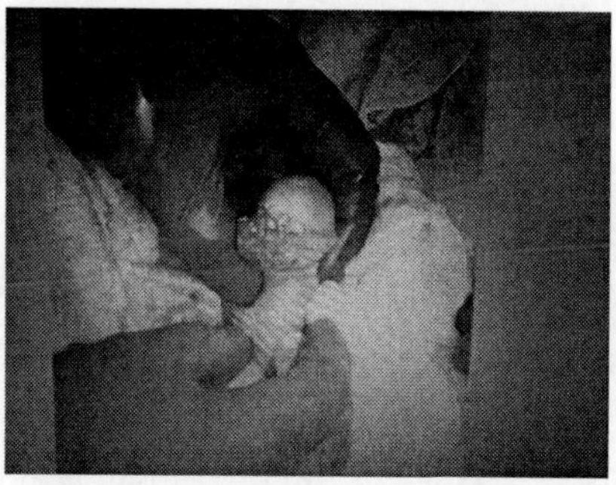

Figure 1. Penile carcinoma exhibiting exophytic growth involving the glans and coronal sulcus.

Penile cancer is not commonly associated with significant symptoms in an early stage of evolution. Pain is infrequent and is not proportional to the severity or extent of the local destructive process and very rarely is an inaugural complaint. If chronic suppuration is present, constitutional symptoms, such as malaise, fever, weight loss, anorexia and fatigue may occur. Occasionally, bleeding from the primary penile lesion, the groin nodes, or both may occur. However, because these symptoms are associated with advanced, metastatic stages of the disease, they are rarely seen initially.

The initial diagnostic workup of penile cancer should start with physical examination of the primary penile lesion by visual inspection and palpation as well as accurate assessment of the groins for presence of lymph nodes. Physical examination of the primary penile lesion should address number and dimensions of the tumor, sites involved (prepuce, glans, shaft, or in combination), morphology (flat, exophytic, ulcerating, fungating), relationship with adjacent structures (corpus spongiosum, corpora cavernosa, urethra), and boundaries or edges of the tumor, including fixation to surrounding tissues.

Penile cancer patients seem to delay seeking medical attention for correct diagnosis. Unfortunately, this delay is occasionally caused by medical erroneous diagnosis, such as balanitis, cutaneous infections, warts, etc. In some reports, in 15% to 50% of the patients the diagnosis was delayed for more than one year (Figure 2) [11-15]. Explanations and factors inconsistently reported as being associated with patients' delay are age, marital status, education, embarrassment, fear, ignorance and personal neglect [15-17].

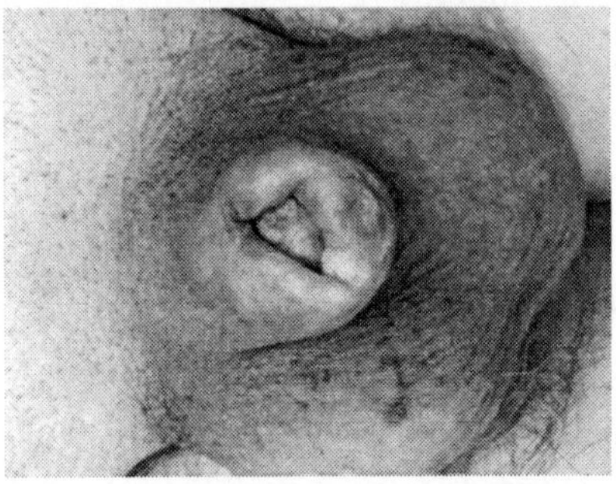

Figure 2. Phimotic prepuce resulting from lichen sclerosus. A hard, ulcerative lesion is visible on the glans and noted by the patient for more than 6 months.

Regional Lymph Nodes

Clinical evaluation of the regional lymph nodes is also very important as involvement of the inguinal nodes, including number and site of positive nodes and extracapsular involvement provide relevant indications of biologic aggressiveness and prognostic factors of survival (Figure 3). Careful bilateral palpation of the inguinal areas for enlarged adenopathies is critical. Palpation of the groins should be the initial workup of regional involvement by penile cancer.

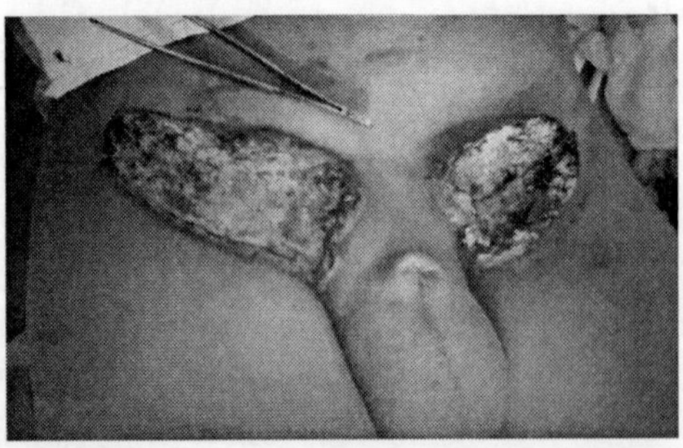

Figure 3. Patient with ulcerating bilateral inguinal metastases following penile amputation and radiotherapy.

Differential Diagnosis

Penile malignant lesions should be differentiated from other benign, premalignant or malignant lesions. These include balanitis, lichen sclerosus, abscess, lymphedema, Bowenoid papulosis, Bowen's disease, erythroplasia of Queyrat, the latter three being recognized manifestations of penile intra-epithelial neoplasia (carcinoma *in situ*) and are histologically indistinguishable. Other malignant tumors are basal cell carcinoma, malignant melanoma, Kaposi sarcoma, extramammary Paget's disease, urethral carcinoma, and metastatic deposits [18-20] (Table 1). The WHO classified squamous cell carcinoma of the penis for subtypes as basaloid carcinoma, warty (condylomatous) carcinoma, verrucous carcinoma, nonspecified papillary carcinoma, sarcomatous carcinoma, adenosquamous carcinoma, and mixed carcinomas [19] (Table 2). These subtypes vary with respect to metastatic potential.

Table 1. Differential diagnosis of penile cancer

Benign Conditions	
	Condylomata acuminate
	Buschke-Löwenstein tumor
	Sexually transmitted diseases
	Benign pigmented warts
	Seborrheic keratosis
	Melanocytic nevi
	Angiokeratoma
	Lichen planus
	Psoriasis
	Balanitis
	Eczema
	Contact dermatitis
Precancerous skin lesions or carcinoma in situ lesions	
	HPV -related
	Giant condyloma
	Bowen's disease
	Erythroplasia of Queyrat
	Bowenoid papulosis
	Chronic inflammation related
	Verrucous cutaneous hyperplasia
	Cutaneous horn
	Lichen sclerosus
	Leukoplakia
	Peudoepitheliomatous, Keratotic and Micaceous Balanitis (PKMB)
Malignant Conditions	
	Malignant melanoma
	Paget's disease
	Basal cell carcinoma
	Kaposi sarcoma

Table 2. Penile SCC subtypes according to WHO

Squamous cell carcinoma
Basaloid carcinoma
Warty (condylomatous) carcinoma
Verrucous carcinoma
Papillary carcinoma, NOS (not otherwise specified)
Sarcomatous carcinoma
Mixed carcinomas
Adenosquamous carcinoma

Biopsy

Squamous cell carcinoma (SCC) accounts for more than 95% of the cases of penile cancer. All suspicious penile lesions that do not respond to a short trial of antibiotic therapy should undergo histologic confirmation. This can be achieved by one of the following methods: incisional biopsy, tissue core biopsy, fine needle aspiration cytology (FNAC), brush biopsy, or excisional biopsy [21, 22].

Erythroplasia of Queyrat has the highest risk of developing SCC and Bowenoid papulosis is known to have the lowest risk. Balanitis xerotica obliterans, a misnomer that should be replaced by lichen sclerosus et atrophicus (LSA) is a common lesion that has been associated with SCC but has no proven direct causal link.

Incisional biopsy is preferable, taking a wedge of tissue that includes tumor and adjacent normal-looking tissue. Small or superficial penile biopsies may be difficult to evaluate in terms of histologic type, grade, depth of invasion, and other pathologic parameters related to prognosis [23]. Velasquez et al. reported that the histologic type and grade could be misinterpreted in 30%, the depth of invasion in 91%, and vascular invasion could be missed in 88% of cases [23]. However, it has been suggested that treatment decision and prognosis should preferably be based on histopathologic parameters of a resected specimen [24]. The pathology report should include all details relevant for choice of treatment, risk of metastatic spread, and prognosis assessment, such as anatomic location, dimensions, histologic type or subtype, grade, growth pattern, direction and depth of invasion, resection margins, lymphovascular invasion and perineural invasion [21]. The details of histopathologic diagnosis have been described in other chapters of this book and, therefore, to avoid redundancy they will not be discussed here.

Molecular Biology

Several molecular biology markers have been identified for better correlation with prognosis. However, currently these markers have not found clinical utility on a routine basis [20]. SCC antigen is neither sensitive enough as a marker of tumor burden nor has shown prognostic significance for survival in penile cancer patients treated with surgery [25].

IMAGING

Imaging and other diagnostic and staging techniques have improved significantly the risk stratification of penile cancer (Table 3). Patients with advanced and metastatic disease still have dismal prognoses. However, advances in imaging and staging have enabled identification of a cohort of patients with localized penile cancer at high risk of progression. These techniques include ultrasonography, axial imaging with computed tomography (CT), MRI and PET with CT (PET/CT) using the radiotracer fluorodeoxyglucose (FDG). Surgical lymph node assessment techniques, such as (dynamic) sentinel node sampling biopsy (SNB) and modified inguinal node dissection have also contributed significantly for better staging of the disease. The latter (surgical) modalities will be discussed in the following section (staging).

PET/CT-FDG imaging is based on cellular uptake of the radiotracer fluorodeoxyglucose, which is elevated in cancerous cells as well as other tissues with a high glycolytic rate [26].

The depth or extent of tumor infiltration cannot be accurately determined by physical examination in most cases. Therefore, MRI plays a critical role in this setting as it may help identify invasion into the corpora cavernosa or corpus spongiosum, urethra and prostate [27]. CT is usually not indicated for newly diagnosed penile tumors without clinically positive inguinal lymph nodes [28].

Table 3. Imaging techniques for clinical diagnosis and staging of penile cancer

Ultrasonography (US)
Computed tomography (CT)
Magnetic resonance imaging (MRI)
Positron emission tomography/computed tomography (PET and PET/CT)
18F-Fluorodeoxyglucose PET/CT (FDG-PET/CT)
Single-photon emission computed tomography-CT (SPECT-CT)

Ultrasonography

Ultrasonography of the primary tumor has been recommended by the EAU Guidelines for local assessment of the primary penile tumor suspected to infiltrate the corpora cavernosa [29]. However, ultrasonography often underestimated tumor thickness and could not delineate accurately invasion into subepithelial connective tissue of the glans penis from corpus spongiosum involvement (i.e., glanular stage T1 vs glanular stage T2). Nonetheless, some studies have shown the potential of ultrasonography in clearly visualizing the extent of primary tumor, in identifying the tunica albuginea separating from the corpus cavernosum and in revealing high sensitivity for detecting corpus cavernosum invasion [30, 31].

MRI

This imaging modality has been recommended if ultrasonography findings remain inconclusive [29]. Lont et al. studied the accuracy of physical examination and compared it with ultrasonography and MRI imaging in assessing the extent of the primary tumor in squamous cell carcinoma of the penis. The positive predictive value was 100%, 67% and 75%, respectively for physical examination, ultrasonography and MRI, respectively [32]. They concluded that physical examination is a reliable method for estimating penile tumor size and predicts corpus cavernosum infiltration with a high positive predictive value, leaving imaging modalities for those tumors for which the infiltration of the corpora could not be determined properly by physical palpation alone. Because of its finer soft-tissue contrast resolution, MRI has also showed to be superior to CT scan in the evaluation of primary penile tumor. Depth of invasion, involvement of the tunica albuginea, the corpora cavernosa, and the penile urethra is more accurately determined on T2-weighted and contrast-enhanced T1-weighted MRI (Figure 4) [29, 33].

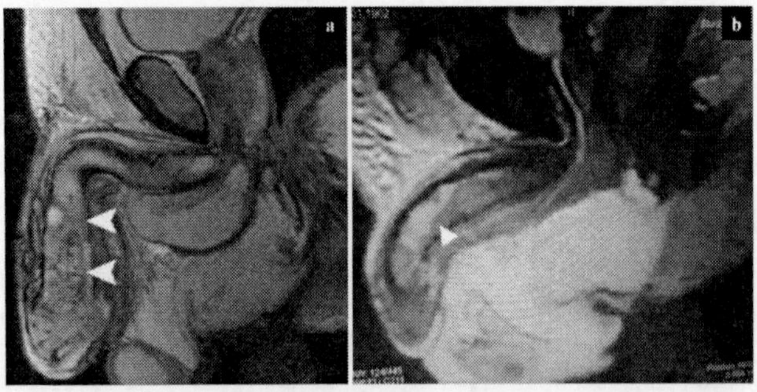

Figure 4. Verrucous carcinoma of the penis. Sagittal T2-weighted MR image demonstrates a mass with heterogeneous signal intensity (arrowheads) involving the glans penis and the corpora cavernosa. (Reprinted with permission from RadioGraphics 2005; 25: 1629-1638).

Local staging of penile cancer based on MRI with artificial erection, obtained by intracavernosal injection of 10 ug Prostaglandin E1 (PGE1) showed higher definition of penile cancer tissue compared to corpora cavernosa on both T1- and T2-weighted images with enhancement on gadolinium-contrasted images [34]. The study concluded that the penile MRI combined with pharmacologically induced erection was reliable and highly accurate and performed better than clinical examination alone for local staging of penile cancer [27, 29, 35]. In summary, for small-volume glans tumors, imaging studies add little relevant information to physical examination. For lesions suspicious for cavernosal invasion, MRI with gadolinium enhancement, and eventually augmented with pharmacologically induced erection, may add very useful information, especially when organ-sparing surgery is contemplated.

PET and PET/CT

Positron emission tomography imaging with fluorodeoxyglucose combined with computed tomography (FDG-PET/CT) provides important functional imaging in combination with useful anatomic information, which improves diagnostic accuracy and confidence. A high FDG-uptake by most primary penile lesions and lymph node metastases suggest that FDG-PET/CT is a very suitable tool for penile cancer staging [36]. In this study, Scher et al. reported that primary penile tumor exhibited a pattern of FDG uptake characteristic for malignancy, with both sensitivity and specificity of 75%. However, it may be argued that primary penile cancer is readily and accurately diagnosed by physical examination and confirmed by biopsy and histopathology, and any additional assessment should be directed at tumor staging. Tumor staging of penile malignancy requires clear distinction of tumor from surrounding anatomical structures and tissue layers, and this is better and more accurately assessed by ultrasound scan and MRI, but not by PET or PET/CT. FDG-PET/CT appears to be most useful for detecting pelvic and distant metastases in clinically node-positive patients.

Sentinel Lymph Node Biopsy

The original lymphatic drainage of the penis was described by Ramon Cabanas in 1977 after performing one hundred lymphangiograms in men with both benign and malignant penile pathologies [37]. In his lymphangiogram studies, the sentinel lymph node (SLN) was mapped to inguinal region in the antero-medial border of the epigastric-saphenous junction. However, it was shown later that the use of Cabanas' anatomic landmarks alone could yield false-negative results due to altered lymphatic drainage [38].

In penile cancer, the SLN can be located by injecting a blue dye and a radioactive tracer in and around the primary tumor [39]. Preoperative localization of the SLN by scintigraphy helps intraoperative dissection and tracking. Additionally, dynamic lymphoscintigraphic imaging may improve the static modality by showing the route of drainage to the lymph nodes in a so-called dynamic sentinel lymph node biopsy (DSLNB) procedure [40]. The recent introduction of a hybrid tracer, which is both radioactive (99mTechnetium-nanocolloid) and fluorescent (indocyanine green), has allowed intraoperative visual navigation to sentinel nodes [41]. The detection rate of the hybrid tracer appears to be higher than the one achieved with the blue dye alone.

The contemporary SLN procedure is a reliable staging modality with minimal morbidity and reasonably good sensitivity (7% false-negative rate and 93% sensitivity) [42].

Dynamic sentinel lymph node biopsy is indicated in penile cancer patients with intermediate to high risk of having occult, clinically negative (non-palpable) metastases to the inguinal lymph nodes [33]. This detection procedure should be performed bilaterally to prevent the morbidity of bilateral inguinal lymphadenectomy. In case the DSLNB is positive, a complete lymphadenectomy should be carried out.

Further combinations of lymphoscintigraphy with CT technology to perform single-photon emission computed tomography (SPECT-CT) were developed. Studies using this combination technology revealed high sensitivity and specificity of 86% each [43].

STAGING

Historically, several staging systems have been used to assess local, regional and distant involvement by carcinoma of the penis. The chronologic evolution of the penile carcinoma staging began in 1966 with the introduction of the Jackson system followed by the introduction of the TNM classification in 1968 and revisions in 1978, 1987, and 2002 [44-46]. Penile cancer should be staged clinically and pathologically and preferably according to the American Joint Committee on Cancer/Union for International Cancer Control (AJCC/UICC) seventh edition TNM classification (Figure 5) (Table 4) [47].

Due to the strong predictive value of lymph node (LN) involvement in terms of overall survival, an accurate evaluation of regional lymph node is critical. The presence and extent of this LN involvement are known to be the most important predictors of survival in patients with squamous penile cell carcinoma [48].

Lymphatic drainage of the penile prepuce and skin is directed to superficial inguinal nodes, while lymphatics from the glans penis go to the deep inguinal and external iliac nodes. The corpora cavernosa, penile urethra, and corpus spongiosum drain to the internal iliac lymph nodes [49]. Metastatic spread, therefore, follows a predictable and stepwise pattern of progression from the primary lesion to the inguinal lymph nodes and then on to the pelvic nodes and ultimately systemic, distant sites [50].

Table 4. American Joint Committee on Cancer TNM Classification for penile cancer

Primary tumor (T)	
Tis	Carcinoma in situ
Ta	Non-invasive localized verrucous carcinoma
T1	Tumor invades subepithelial connective tissue
T1a	Without lymphovascular invasion and well differentiated
T1b	With lymphovascular invasion or poorly differentiated
T2	Tumor invades corpus spongiosum with or without invasion of the urethra
T3	Tumor invades corpus cavernosum without or with invasion of the urethra
T4	Tumor invades other adjacent structures
Regional lymph nodes (N) (clinical)	
N0	No palpable or visibly enlarged inguinal lymph nodes
N1	Palpable mobile unilateral lymph node
N2	Palpable mobile multiple or bilateral inguinal lymph nodes
N3	Fixed inguinal nodal mass or pelvic lymphadenopathy, unilateral or bilateral
Regional lymph nodes (pN) (pathological)	
pN0	No regional lymph node metastasis
pN1	Metastasis in up to two regional lymph nodes
pN2	Metastases in three or more unilateral lymph nodes or bilateral inguinal lymph nodes
pN3	Metastasis in pelvic lymph nodes, unilateral or bilateral, or extranodal extension of any regional lymph node metastasis
Distant metastasis (M)	
M0	No distant metastasis
M1	Distant metastasis

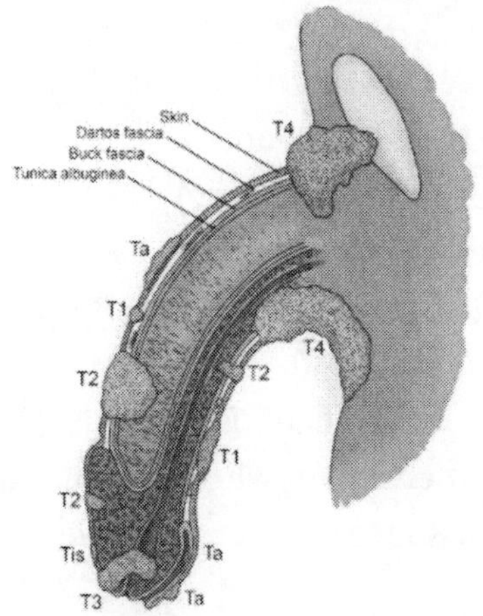

Figure 5. TNM staging of penile cancer.

Although the role of imaging in the staging of penile cancer has been vaguely defined due to its low prevalence, many institutions, nonetheless, have included it as an integral part of the initial evaluation of the disease.

Accurate staging of the disease at first inspection/diagnosis provides important information for choice of treatment and assessment of critical predictors of survival which has improved patient risk stratification over the past few decades. Some of these staging techniques are invasive and include ultrasound-guided fine needle aspiration biopsy, dynamic sentinel node biopsy, and various forms of lymph node dissections which have improved lymph node staging.

Predictors of Lymph Node Involvement

Lymphovascular infiltration at the primary tumor site is one of the strongest predictors of occult lymph node metastatic spread [51, 52]. Other predictive factors include perineural invasion, grade of differentiation superoxide dismutase-2 expression, tumor depth and clear cell differentiation [53-55]. Nomograms have been developed to predict lymph node invasion but due to their complexity and lack of external validation they did not gain much popularity for routine use [56, 57]. Unfortunately, prediction lacks enough accuracy for reliable clinical lymph nodal staging. Intermediate and high-risk cancers (pT1 grade ≥ 2) need further clinical and pathological evaluation. Metastatic invasion of pelvic lymph nodes is best predicted by pathologic characteristics of the inguinal lymphadenectomy specimen [58].

Primary Penile Tumor

Clinical staging of the primary lesion has traditionally relied on physical examination. Visual inspection and palpation have usually been considered sufficient to clinically stage the primary tumor [33]. Physical examination alone can assess infiltration of the tumor into the corpora cavernosa. Ultrasonography can also give further information about infiltration of the corpora cavernosa. However, ultrasonography of the penis has limited yield given it poor soft-tissue resolution [59]. CT scan has also limited utility given its poor soft-tissue resolution [32]. In doubt as to the presence of corpora cavernosa invasion and to better assess whether penile-sparing surgery is appropriate, MRI has far superior soft-tissue resolution, particularly if combined with artificial erection with PGE1 [27, 35].

Although almost all primary penile tumors are FDG-avid, FDG-PET/CT is not very useful for staging of the primary penile lesion due to its limited spatial resolution which makes it unsuitable for the evaluation of ingrowth into the surrounding structures. Also,

FDG is excreted via urine, which potentially interferes with imaging accuracy of the primary lesion. Thus, physical examination and, in selected cases, MRI show excellent accuracy for staging primary penile tumors [32, 33].

Regional Lymph Nodes

Accurate lymph node staging is of utmost importance to determine the best treatment and prognosis. Involvement of inguinal nodes, the number and site of positive nodes and extracapsular nodal invasion are the strongest prognostic factors of survival. Cure rates in patients without lymph node metastases exceed 80%, whereas they decrease progressively with higher stages of lymphatic involvement (Figure 6 A and B) [33, 60].

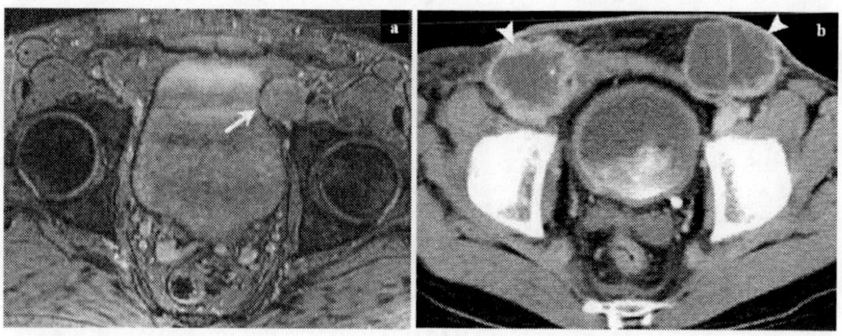

Figure 6. A) Metastatic left groin lymphadenopathy from penile carcinoma.T2*-weighted MR image obtained before the administration of ultrasmall superparamagnetic iron oxide particles shows an enlarged lymph node in the left groin (arrow); B) Lymph node metastases from penile carcinoma. Contrast-enhanced CT scan shows bilateral metastatic lymph node involvement (arrowheads) in the form of inguinal and right common iliac lymphadenopathy. (Reprinted with permission from RadioGraphics 2005; 25: 1629-1638).

Careful inspection and palpation of both groins to detect enlarged inguinal lymph nodes is a critical part of the initial physical examination of any penile cancer patient. Unfortunately, at the time of presentation, approximately 20% of patients have locally advanced disease with clinically palpable inguinal nodes [61].

Non-Palpable Inguinal Lymph Nodes

The likelihood of the presence of micrometastatic disease averages 25% in the absence of groin abnormalities (cN0) [33]. Nonetheless, current imaging techniques cannot reliably detect micro-metastases. Inguinal ultrasound can detect pathologic nodes with some enlargement. Ultrasonographic nodal features have been reported to have relatively high specificity [62]. In cN0 disease patients, dynamic sentinel node biopsy (DSNB) is indicated in intermediate (T1G2) or high-risk (T1G3 or worse) disease. Early detection of lymph node metastases by DSNB and subsequent resection in clinically node negative T2-3 penile tumor improves survival compared to surveillance (63). DSNB is a less morbid approach compared with prophylactic ILND and was shown in a meta-analysis to be a method with high detection rate of sentinel nodes [64]. If DSNB is unavailable, US-guided FNAC of visualized nodes can be used [25].

CT or MRI scans cannot reliably detect micrometastases [29]. FDG-PET/CT imaging also cannot detect small-volume (<10 mm) lymph node metastases [65].

Diagnostic lymphadenectomy, involving radical lymph node dissection, has been suggested as the most reliable staging tool in penile cancer [66]. Contemporary superficial and modified groin dissection in combination with intraoperative frozen section histopathology has been considered "standard" approach to LN staging in penile carcinoma [67]. However, inguinal lymphadenectomy entails high morbidity, such as severe lymphedema of the lower limb, wound suppurative infection and abscess, seroma formation, skin flap necrosis after cutaneous reconstruction of the groin and mortality rate greater than 1% [20, 49, 68]. It is important to note that the prognosis of penile cancer is strictly linked to lymph node invasion and, in this way, radical lymphadenectomy can be curative [66]. Unfortunately, subjecting all penile cancer patients to bilateral inguinal lymph node dissection would be deemed "overkill" for most patients (29)! This is a true dilemma for oncologic urologists as they are faced with the difficult task of selecting the most appropriate candidates for bilateral groin dissections, specifically patients at intermediate risk of developing lymph node metastases, i.e., those patients whose primary tumor is classified as T1G2. Currently, with the advent of new imaging modalities, such as CT and MRI that are useful to delineate the morphological significance of the lymph nodes, FDG-PET/CT, DSLNB, SPECT-CT, intraoperative lymphatic mapping (IOLM), and MRI enhanced with lymphotrophic nanoparticles may help differentiate lymph nodes functionally [29].

Palpable Inguinal Lymph Nodes

Ultrasound combined with FNAC (US-guided FNAC) has been indicated in patients with palpable inguinal nodes (93% sensitivity; 91% specificity; 20%-30% false-negative rate), but its value is unclear and unreliable in cN0 disease (39% sensitivity; 100% specificity) [69, 70]. Thus, in clinically suspicious cases of lymphadenopathy, the EAU guidelines recommend US-guided FNAC to confirm the etiology of the clinically palpable lymph nodes [33]. If a positive node is detected, radical inguinal lymph node dissection (ILND) with excision of the overlying skin and needle biopsy is highly recommended to prevent malignant cell seeding into healthy tissue [71].

Pelvic Lymph Nodes

Literature is scarce on pelvic lymph nodes. In one study involving 18 patients with clinical inguinal nodal metastases, FDG-PET/CT provided high diagnostic accuracy with sensitivity of 91%, specificity of 100% and negative and positive predictive values of 94% and 100%, respectively. Its correct prediction was 96% [72].

The 5-year survival rate for patients with pelvic lymph node invasion was 0% in one study [73]. Other studies reported a median 5-year survival of approximately 10% [74, 75, 76]. Patients with microscopic pelvic lymphatic involvement might benefit from early pelvic lymphadenectomy [77].

Historically, the prognostic factors for pelvic lymph node invasion were the number of positive inguinal nodes, involvement of Cloquect's node, the lymph node ratio (nº of positive lymph nodes/total lymph nodes removed), extranodal extension, p53 expression, >3 enlarged inguinal nodes on preoperative CT imaging, and lymph node size ≥3.5 cm [22]. However, in a single-institution study, Hegarty reported that pelvic lymphadenectomy was positive in only 17% of patients, emphasizing the need for better indicators of prognosis to improve patient selection [78].

Distant Metastases

Hematogenous spread is rare and, therefore, distant metastases of penile cancer are uncommon at presentation (less than 3%-5%). In most of these patients, regional lymph node involvement is also present [79]. Thus, routine diagnostic imaging to assess distant metastatic involvement of penile cancer is neither cost-effective nor recommended. Staging of distant metastases is only indicated and reserved for selected high-risk patients, especially those with inguinal and/or pelvic nodal invasion, or in patients with clinical manifestations of metastatic disease such as pain, cachexia, hepatomegaly, lung metastases and pleural effusion. The most common metastatic sites in patients who succumb to disseminated penile cancer are (in order of frequency): lymph nodes (including inguinal, pelvic and retroperitoneal), liver, lungs, heart, kidneys, adrenal glands, bone, skin, thyroid, brain, pancreas, spleen, and pleura [22, 80, 81]. Malignant hypercalcemia has also been reported [82].

Table 5. Staging, incidence and outcomes in penile cancer

Stage[a]	2012 incidence in US	2012 incidence in US	~5-year survival (%)
0 (Tis or Ta, N0M0)	NA	NA	100
1 (T1aN0M0)	NA	NA	90
2 (T1b–T3N0M0)	NA	NA	50
3 (T1–T3N1–N2M0)	NA	NA	30
4 (any T4, any N3 or M1)	NA	NA	5
All stages	1570 (1)	310	NA

[a]Adapted from American Joint Committee on Cancer (AJCC) Staging Manual, seventh edition (2012) published by Springer, New York, Inc.

In selected cases where imaging of distant penile cancer metastases is necessary, several modalities can be employed today, such as CT, PET/CT, FDG-PET/CT, and MRI. Unfortunately, most information has been obtained from case reports and small series [83]. However, results suggest that PET/CT, for example, is a useful tool for accurate M staging [72]. The whole-body imaging aspect provided by PET/CT scanning can be critical in clinical decision making. If distant metastases are detected in patients scheduled for locoregional treatment protocol, systemic or palliative regimens should be indicated instead [84].

Hematogenous metastases usually occur late in the disease course and are closely associated with poor prognosis. Because distant metastases imply a dismal prognosis, M staging is critical to avoid potentially invasive, harmful and certainly futile therapeutic interventions. Attempts were made to correlate staging, incidence and outcomes in penile cancer (Table 5) [1, 5].

Patterns of Recurrence after Surgery

The rate of recurrence after surgical treatment was compared between patients undergoing penile-sparing therapeutic modalities and partial or total amputation in a retrospective study including 700 patients [85]. Patients were divided into two groups: those surgically staged as pN0 or pN+ and clinically node-negative (cN0) patients and regional (inguinal) recurrences were compared. The latter (cN0) group had opted for a watchful waiting approach. Of these 700 patients, 205 (29.3%) developed a recurrence, local in 18.6%, regional in 9.3% and distant in 1.4%. Most of the recurrences (86%) occurred within 2 years. Local recurrences were more common (27.7%) after penile-sparing therapy compared with amputation (5.3%), although survival did not seem to be compromised due to the efficacy of surgical salvage. The regional recurrence rate was 2.3% in patients with pN0, 19.1% with pN+ and 9.1% undergoing a watchful waiting approach. The 5-year disease-specific survival rate was 92% after a local recurrence and 32.7% after regional recurrence, while all patients with a distant recurrence died within 22 months.

Conclusion

Penile cancer is a rare but aggressive malignancy. The initial clinical evaluation should be a thorough history and physical examination followed by a biopsy of the primary lesion to confirm a pathologic diagnosis. Accurate clinical staging, involving detection of loco-regional disease, requires a combined approach including physical examination, imaging studies and eventually surgical intervention. This is crucial for selecting the best treatment of penile cancer and in the proper sequence. Due to its location, traditional surgical intervention for penile cancer is associated with devastating consequences on anatomical, functional and psychosocial domains of patients' quality of life. Rigorous assessment of the extent of primary tumor as well as involvement of loco-regional lymph nodes and distant metastatic spread are the most decisive prognostic indicators and crucial for treatment planning. With the advent of modern imaging modalities, such as MRI as a more sensitive staging tool for T-staging of the primary tumor and other modalities for the more complex N-staging of loco-regional disease, such as FNAC, DSLNB, FDG-PET/CT, SPECT-CT, intraoperative lymphatic mapping (IOLM), and MRI enhanced with lymphotrophic nanoparticles have been proven useful. For detection of microscopic nodal metastases, the dynamic sentinel node biopsy is recommended as it provides accurate pathological staging, avoiding the morbidity of inguinal lymph node dissection. Furthermore, DSLNB can be preceded by ultrasonography-guided FNAC to avoid undetected macrometastases. FNAC can also be used to confirm metastatic disease in suspicious groins. Nonetheless, no noninvasive or minimally invasive or currently highly sophisticated tool will be 100% accurate in the exact locoregional staging of penile cancer. Additional efforts should be carried out to further decrease false-negative rates.

For M-staging, conventional imaging should be recommended according to currently existing guidelines. Although FDG-PET/CT has been associated with high sensitivity, its role in clinical practice needs further study.

Follow-up and surveillance protocols have relied mostly on physical examination and ultrasound-guided FNAC. However, PET/CT may have a role in localizing suspected recurrence foci but has not been adopted for routine use yet.

Although several imaging and surgical modalities have been developed, the identification of suspicious regional and distant metastatic disease calls for physician's clinical astuteness based on the primary tumor pathology and stage, which will ultimately guide management decisions.

KEY POINTS

- Initial clinical evaluation of penile cancer mandates for a thorough history and physical examination to determine the morphological and physical characteristics of the primary lesion and inguinal region involvement
- Due to the strong predictive value of lymph node involvement in terms of overall survival, an accurate evaluation of regional lymph node status is critical. The presence and extent of this involvement are the most important predictors of survival in patients with SCC of the penis.

- MRI with artificial erection induced by intracavernosal injection of PGE1 is useful for the evaluation of the primary tumor
- Examination of both the penile primary lesion and bilateral inguinal regions is critical to staging and subsequent treatment planning
- Adequate histologic characterization through biopsy, and preferably with a resected specimen, is mandatory to determine accurate histopathologic grading and staging
- Squamous cell carcinoma (SCC) with its histologic variant accounts for >95% of malignant penile tumors
- Penile cancer should be staged according to the TNM system of the American Joint Committee on Cancer/Union for International Cancer Control (AJCC/UICC)
- Ultrasound-guided FNAC is indicated for both palpable and non-palpable inguinal nodes. Inguinal lymphadenectomy is indicated in node-positive disease. If negative, DSLNB should be recommended.
- In clinically negative inguinal lymph node disease, imaging with CT or MRI cannot reliably detect micrometastases. FDG-PET/CT imaging also cannot detect small-volume (<10 mm) lymph node metastases. PET/CT and FDG-PET/CT imaging may be particularly useful in detecting pelvic lymph node metastases and occult distant metastases, improving patient selection for systemic chemotherapy and/or extensive surgical resection. However, in routine clinical practice, these imaging studies should only be requested if CT of the pelvis is negative
- Although several imaging and surgical modalities have been developed, the identification of suspicious regional and distant metastatic disease calls for physician's clinical astuteness based on the primary tumor pathology and stage, which will ultimately guide management decisions.

References

[1] Siegel R, Naishadham D, Jemal A. Cancer statistics. *CA Cancer J Clin* 2012; 62: 10-29.

[2] Chaux A, Netto GJ, Rodriguez IM et al. Epimediologic profile, sexual history, pathologic features, and human papillomaviruss status of 103 patients with penile carcinoma. *World J Urol* 2013; 13: 861-867.

[3] Narayana AS, Olney LE, Loening SA, Weimar GW, Culp DA. Carcinoma of the penis: analysis of 219 cases. *Cancer* 1982; 49: 2185-2191.

[4] Ornellas AA, Seixa AL, Marota A, et al. Surgical treatment of invasive quamous cell carcinoma of the penis: retrospective analysis of 350 cases. *J Urol* 1994; 151: 1244-1249.

[5] Barnholtz-Sloan JS, Maldonado JL, Pow-Sang J, et al. Incidence, survival and mortality of primary malignant penile cancer. *Urol Oncol* 2007; 25: 361-367.

[6] National Cancer Institute, *Penile Cancer*, http://www.cancer.gov/cancertopic/type/penile.

[7] Kirrander P, Sherif A, Friedrich B, et al. Swedish National Penile Cancer Register: incidence, tumour characteristics, management and survival. *BJU Int* 2016; 117: 287-292.

[8] Sufrin G, Huben R. Benign and malignant lesions of the penis. In: Gillenwater JY editor(s). *Adult and Pediatric Urology*. 2nd Edition. St. Louis: Mosby Year Book, 1991.

[9] Mosconi AM, Roila F, Gatta G, et al. Cancer of the penis. *Crit Rev Oncol Hematol* 2005; 53:165-77. 10.1016/j.critrevonc.2004.09.006.

[10] Hernandez HY, Barnholtz-Sloan J, German RR et al. Burden of invasive squamous cell carcinoma of the penis in the United States, 1998-2003. *Cancer* 2008; 113: 2883-2891.

[11] Hardner, G. J., et al.: Carcinoma of the penis: analysis of therapy in 100 consecutive cases, *ibid*. 108: 428 (1972). 22.

[12] Gursel, E. O., Georgountzos, C., Uson, A. C., Melicow, M. M., & Veenema, R. J. Penile cancer Clinicopathologic study of 64 cases. *Urology* 1973: 1(6), 569–578. doi:10.1016/0090-4295(73)90517-7.

[13] Skeppner E, Windahl T, Andersson SO, Fugl-Meyer KS. Treatment-seeking, aspects of sexual activity and life satisfaction in men with laser-treated penile carcinoma. *Eur Urol* 2008; 54:631–9.

[14] Skeppner E, Andersson SO, Johanssons JE, Windhal T. Initial symptoms and delay in patients with penile carcinoma *Scandinavian Journal of Urology and Nephrology,* 2012; 46: 319–325.

[15] Smith LK, Pope C, Botha JL. Patients' help-seeking experiences and delay in cancer presentation: a qualitative synthesis. *Lancet* 2005; 366:825–31.

[16] Ristvedt SL, Trinkaus KM. Psychological factors related to delay in consultation for cancer symptoms. *Psychooncology* 2005; 14:339–50.

[17] Pettaway CA, Lance RS, Davis JW. Tumors of the penis. In: Wein A, Kavoussi LR, Novick AC, Partin AW, Peters CA (Eds). *Campbell-Walsh Urology*. Tenth International Edition. Philadelphia: Elsevier Saunders Inc.2012, pp: 901-933.

[18] Sarkar FH, Mile BJ, Plieth DH, Crisman JD. Detection of human papillomavirus in squamous cell neoplasm of the penis. *J Urol* 1992; 147: 389-392.

[19] Eble JN, Sauter G, Epstein JI, Sesterhenn I, World Health Organization Classification of Tumours. Pathology and genetics of tumours of the urinary system and male genital organ. 2004. Lyon: IARC Press.

[20] Van Poppel H, Watkin NA, Oanto A, Moonen L, Horwich A, Kataja V, on behalf of ESMO Guidelines Working Group. Penile cancer: ESMO clinical practice guidelines for diagnosis, treatment and follow-up. *Annals of Oncology* 2013; 24(Suppl 6): vi115-vi124.

[21] Mikuz G, Winstanley AM, Schulman CC, et al. Handling and pathology reporting of circumcision and penectomy specimens. *Eur Urol* 2004; 46: 434-439.

[22] Heyns CF, Mendoza-Valdés A, Pompeo ACL. Diagnosis and staging of penile cancer. *Urology* 2010; 76 (Suppl 2A): S16-S23.

[23] Velasquez EF, Barreto JE, Rodriguez I, et al. Limitations in the interpretation of biopsies in patients with penile squamous cell carcinoma. *Int J Surg Pathol* 2009; 12: 139-146.

[24] Cubilla AL. The role of pathologic prognostic factors in squamous cell carcinoma of the penis. *World J Urol* 2009; 27: 169-177.

[25] Pizzocaro G, Algaba F, Horenblas S et al. EAU Penile cancer guidelines 2009. *Eur Urol* 2010; 57: 1002-1012.

[26] Fletcher JW, Djulbegovic B, Soares HP, et al. Recommendations on the use of 18F-FDG PET in oncology. *J Nucl Med* 2008; 49: 480-508.

[27] Petralia G, Villa G, Scardino E, et al. Local staging of penile cancer using magnetic resonance imaging with pharmacologically induced penile erection. *Radiol Med* (Torino) 2008; 113: 517-528.

[28] Clark P, Spiess P, Agarwal N, et al. Penile cancer Version 1.2014. *National Comprehensive Cancer Network Websit*e. www.nccn.org/professionals/physician_gls/pdf/penile.pdf. Assessed April 27, 2014.

[29] Mueller-Lisse UG, Scher B, Scherr MK, Seitz M. Functional imaging in penile cancer: PET/computed tomography, MRI and sentinel lymph node biopsy. *Curr Opin Urol* 2008; 18: 105-110.

[30] Yamashita T, Ogawa A. Ultraound in penile cancer. *Urol Radiol.* 1989;11(3):174-177.

[31] Dorak AC, Ozkan GA, Tamac NI, Saray A. Ultrasonography in the recognition of penile cancer. *J Clin Ultrasound* 1992; 20: 624-626.

[32] Lont AP, Besnard AP, Gallee MP, van Tinteren H, Horenblas S. A comparison of physical examination and imaging in determining the extent of primary penile carcinoma. *BJU Int.* 2003 Apr;91(6):493-5.

[33] Hakenberg OW, Comperat EM, Minhas S et al. EAU Guidelines on penile cancer: 2014 update. *Eur Urol* 2015; 67: 142-150.

[34] Scardino E. Villa G, Bonomo G, et al. Magnetic resonance imaging combined with artificial erection for local staging of penile cancer. *Urology* 2004; 63: 1158-1162.

[35] Kayes O, Minhas S, Allen C, et al. The role of magnetic resonance imaging in the local staging of penile cancer. *Eur Urol* 2007; 51: 1313-1319.

[36] Scher B, Seitz M, Reiser M, et al. 18F-FDG PET/CT for staging of penile cancer. *J Nucl Med* 2005; 46: 1460-1465.

[37] Cabanas RM. An approach for the treatment of penile carcinoma. *Cancer* 1977; 39: 456-466.

[38] Perinetti E, Crane DB, Catalona WJ. Unreliability of entinel lymph node biopsy for staging penile carcinoma. *J Urol* 1980; 124: 734-735.

[39] Ottenhof SR, Leone AR, Horenblas S, Spiess PE, Vegt E. Advancements in staging and imaging for penile cancer. *Curr Opin Urol* 2017; 27(6): 612-620.

[40] Horenblas S, Jansen L, Meinhardt W, et al. Detection of occult metastasis in squamous cell of the penis using a dynamic sentinel node procedure. *J Urol* 2000; 163: 100-104).

[41] KleinJan GH, van denBerg NS, van Oosterom MN, et al. Toward (hybrid) navigation of a fluorescent camera in an open surgery setting. *J Nucl Med* 2016; 57: 1650-1653.

[42] Leijte JAP, Kroon BK, Valdés Olmos RA, et al. Reliability and safety of current dynamic sentinel node biopsy for penile carcinoma. *Eur Urol* 2007; 52: 170-177.

[43] Lutzen U, Naumann CM, Marx M, et al. A study on the value of computer-assisted assessment for SPECT/CT-scans in sentinel lymph node diagnostics of penile cancer reliability and morbidity of this procedure. *Cancer Imaging* 2016; 16: 29.

[44] Jackson SM. The treatment of carcinoma of the penis. *Br J Surg* 1966; 53: 33-35.

[45] Leijte JA, Gallee M, Antonini N et al. Evaluation of current TNM classification for penile carcinoma. *J Urol* 2008; 180: 933-938.

[46] Leijte JA, Horenblas S. Shortcomings of the current TNM classification for penile carcinoma: time for a change? *World J Urol* 2009; 27: 151-154.

[47] Sobin L, Gospodariwics M, Witterkin C. *TNM Classification of Malignat Tumors. UICC International Union against Cancer*, 7th edition. West Sussex, Uk. Willy-Blackwell 2009; 239-242.

[48] Emerson RE, Ulbright TM, Elbe JN, et al. Predicting cancer progression in patients with penile squamous cell carcinoma: the importance of depth of invasion and vascular invasion. *Mod Pathol* 2001; 14: 963-968.

[49] Singh AK, Saokar A, Hahn PF, Harisinghani MG. Imaging of penile neoplasm. *Radiographics* 2005; 25: 1629-1638.

[50] Dewire D, Lepor H. Anatomic considerations of the penis and its lymphatic drainage. *Urol Clin North Am* 1992; 19: 211-219.

[51] Winters BR, Mosssanen MN, Holt SK, et al. Predictors of nodal upstaging in clinical node negative patients with penile carcinoma: a national cancer database analysis. *Urology* 2016; 96: 29-34.

[52] Bhagat SK, Gopalkrishnan G, Kekre NS, et al. Factors predicting inguinal node metastasis in squamous cell cancer of penis. *World J Urol* 2010; 28: 93-98.

[53] Termini L, Fregnani JH, Boccardo E, et al. SOD2 immunoexpression predicts lymph node metastases in penile cancer. *BMC Clin Pathol* 2015; 15: 3.

[54] Mannweiler S, Sygulla S, Tsybrovskyy O, et al. Clear-cell differentiation and lymphatic invasion, but not the revised TNM classification, predict lymph node metastases in pT1 penile cancer: a clinicopathological study of 76 patients from a low incidence area. *Urol Oncol* 2013; 31: 1378-1385.

[55] Graafland NM, Lam W, Leijte JAP, et al. Prognostic factors for occult inguinal lymph node involvement in penile carcinoma and assessment of the high-risk EAU subgroup: a two-institution analysis of 342 clinically node-negative patients. *Eur Urol* 2010; 58: 742-747.

[56] Ficarra V, Zattoni F, Artibani W et al. Nomogram predictive of pathological inguinal node involvement in patients with squamous cell carcinoma of the penis. *J Urol* 2006; 175: 1700-1704; discussion 1704-1705.

[57] Chaux A, Caballero C, Soares F et al. The prognostic index: a useful pathologic guide for prediction of nodal metastases and survival in penile squamous cell carcinoma. *Am J Surg Pathol* 2009; 33: 1049-1057.

[58] Zhu Y, Zhang HL, Ye DW, et al. Predicting pelvic lymph node metastases in penile cancer patients: a comparison of computed tomography, Cloquet's node, and disease burden of inguinal lymph nodes. *Onkologie* 2008; 31: 37-41.

[59] Bertolotto M, Serafini G, Dogliotti L, et al. Primary and secondary malignancies of the penis: ultrasound features. *Abdom Imaging* 2005; 30: 108-112.

[60] Djajadiningrat RS, Graafland NM, van Werkhoven E. et al. Contemporary management of regional nodes in penile cancer – improvement of survival? *J Urol* 2014; 191: 68-73.

[61] Persson B, Sjödin JG, Holmberg L et al. The National Penile Cancer Register in Sweden 2000-2003. *Scand J Urol Nephrol* 2007; 41: 278-282.

[62] Krishna RP, SSistia SC, Smile R, et al. Sonography: an underutilized diagnostic toll in the assessment of metastatic groin nodes. *J Clin Ultrasound* 2008; 36(4): 517-528.

[63] Lont AP, Horenblas S, Tanis PJ, et al. Management of clinically node negative penile carcinoma: improved survival after the introduction of dynamic sentinel node biopsy. *J Urol* 2003; 170: 783-786.

[64] Sadeghi R, Gholami H, Zakavi SR, et al. Accuracy of sentinel lymph node biopsy for inguinal lymph node staging of penile squamous cell carcinoma: Systematic review and meta-analysis of the literature. *J Urol* 2012; 187: 25-31.

[65] Leijte JA, Graafland NM, Valdé Olmos RA, et al. Evaluation of hybrid 18F-fluorodeoxyglucose positron emission tomography/computed tomography in

staging clinically node-negative patients with penile carcinoma. *BJU Int* 2009; 104:640-644.

[66] Hungerhuber E, Schlenker B, Karl et al. Risk stratification in penile carcinoma: 25-year experience with surgical inguinal lymph node staging. *Urology* 2006; 68: 621-625.

[67] Izawa J, Kedar D, Wong F, Pettaway CA. Sentinel lymph node biopsy in penile cancer: evolution and insights. *Can J Urol* 2005; 12 (Suppl 1): 24-29.

[68] Ravi R. Morbidity following groin dissection for penile carcinoma. *Br J Urol* 1993; 72: 941-945.

[69] Saison I, Lawrentschuk N, Leewansangtong S, et al. Fine-needle aspiration cytology predicts inguinal lymph node metastasis without antibiotic pretreatment in penile carcinoma. BJU Int 2006; 97: 1225-1228 cancer guidelines 2009. *Eur Urol* 2010; 57: 1002-1012.

[70] Kroon BK, Horenblas S. Deurloo EE, et al. Ultrasonography-guided fine-needle aspiration cytology before sentinel node biopsy in patients with penile carcinoma. *BJU Int* 2005; 95: 517-521.

[71] Goldberg BB, Merton DA, Liu JB, et al. Contrast-enhanced sonographic imaging of lymphatic channels and sentinel lymph nodes. *J Ultrasound Med* 2005; 24: 953-965.

[72] Graafland NM, Leijte JA, Valdés Olmos RA et al. Scanning with 18F-FDG-PET/CT for detection of pelvic nodal involvement in inguinal node-positive penile carcinoma. *Eur Urol* 2009; 56: 339-345.

[73] Pandey, Mahajan V, Kannan RR. Prognostic factors in node-positive carcinoma of the penis. *J Surg Oncol* 2006; 93: 133-138.

[74] Lopes A, Hidalgo G, Kowalki LP, et al. Prognostic factors in carcinoma of the penis: multivariate analysis of 145 patients treated with amputation and lymphadenectomy. *J Urol* 1996; 156: 1637-1642.

[75] Srinivas V, Morse MJ, Herr HW, Sogani PC, Whitmore WF Jr. Penile cancer: relation of extent of nodal metastasis to survival. *J Urol* 1987; 137: 880-882.

[76] Ravi R. Morbidity following groin dissection for penile carcinoma. *Br J Urol* 1993; 72: 941-945.

[77] Lopes A, Bezerra AL, Serrano SV, Hidalgo GS. Iliac nodal metastasis from carcinoma of the penis treated surgically. *BJU Int* 2000; 86: 690-693.

[78] Hegarty PK, Kayes O, Freeman A, et al. A prospective study of 100 cases of penile cancer managed according to European Association of Urology guidelines. *BJU Int* 2006; 98: 526-531.

[79] Rippentrop JM, Joslyn SA, Konety BR. Squamous cell carcinoma of the penis: evaluation of data from the Surveillance, Epidemiology, and End Results program. *Cancer* 2004; 101: 1357-2108.

[80] Chaux A, Reuter V, Lezcano C, et al. Autopsy findings in 14 patients with penile squamous cell carcinoma. *Int J Surg Pathol. Epub* 2009 May 1.

[81] Van der Merwe A, Zarrabi A, Bason J, et al. Distant cutaneous metastases secondary to squamous carcinoma of the penis. *Can J Urol* 2009; 16: 4498-4501.

[82] Ho CC, Nazri J, Zulkifli MZ, et al. Metastatic penile cancer presenting as hypercalcemia and pathological fracture of the humerus: a rare event. *Med J Malays* 2006; 61: 503-505.

[83] Ottenhof SR, Vegt E. The role of PET/CT imaging in penile cancer. *Trans Androl Urol 2017*; 6(5): 833-838. Doi:

[84] Zhang S, Li W, Liang F. Clinical value of fluorine-18-2-fluoro-2-deoxy-D-glucose positron emission tomography/computed tomography in penile cancer. *Oncotarget* 2016; 7: 48600-6.

[85] Leijte JA, Kirrander P, Antonini N et al. Recurrence patterns of squamous cell carcinoma of the penis: recommendations for follow-up based on a two-centre analysis of 700 patients. *Eur Urol* 2008; 54: 161–168.

Section B. Surgical Management of Penile Cancer

In: Penile Cancer: Challenges and Controversies
Editors: F. E. Martins and M. L. Djordjevic
ISBN: 978-1-53615-950-9

Chapter 5

MANAGEMENT OF LOCALIZED DISEASE: THE ROLE OF PENILE-PRESERVING SURGERY

Mohamed Kamel[1,*], MD and Nabil Bissada[2], MD
[1]Department of Urology, University of Arkansas for Medical Sciences, Little Rock, Arkansas, US
[2]Department of Urology, Baylor College of Medicine, The Michael E. Debakey, Veterans Affairs Hospital, Houston, Texas, US

ABSTRACT

Traditional treatment of penile cancer with penile amputation leads to significant psychological and functional limitations to the patient. Penis Conserving Surgery (PCS) is an appealing alternative that aims to preserve urinary and sexual functions, avoids the detrimental psychological impact of penile amputation and in the meantime does not compromise oncological control. In this book chapter, we describe the role, advantages, disadvantages and limitations of the various PCS techniques. PCS in the appropriately selected patient; as we describe in this book chapter; provides comparable oncological outcomes to penile amputation. The superior urinary, sexual and psychological outcomes of PCS over penile amputation are described as well.

ABBREVIATIONS

CIS	Carcinoma in situ
CO2	Carbon Dioxide
EAU	European Association of Urology

[*] Corresponding Author's E-mail: mkamel@uams.edu

FS	Frozen Section
IIEF-15	International Index of Erectile Function
MMS	Mohs Micrographic Surgery
NCCN	National Comprehensive Cancer Network
Nd: YAG	Neodymium-doped: Yttrium Aluminium Garnet (Nd:YAG)
Pca	Penile Cancer
PCS	Penis Conserving Surgery
PGR	Partial Glans Resurfacing
STSG	Split Thickness Skin Graft
TGR	Total Glans Resurfacing
WLE	Wide Local Excision.

1. Introduction

Penile amputation has long been the traditional treatment for penile cancer (Pca). The psychological and functional implications of this form of treatment are devastating with reported cases of post-traumatic stress disorder in those patients [1]. Penis conserving surgery (PCS) is an alternative that is attractive to the patient because of its obvious psychological and functional advantages over penile amputation. The most common locations for Pca are the glans and prepuce (47.7%) which makes PCS a feasible option [2]. In addition to the favorable location, most Pca are well to moderately differentiated (65%), localized to the penis at diagnosis (62%) and with superficial spreading as the most common form of tumor spread (42%) [2, 3]. All these pathological features helped to increase the acceptance of PCS. Pca is a disease of the elderly with the highest incidence in the 6th and 7th decades of life [2]. The desire to continue to be able to perform sexual intercourse among elderly males is documented. One study reported that men with Pca were willing to trade a treatment with lower life expectancy for the sake of maintaining potency [4]. Similarly the Massachusetts Male Aging study showed that over 50% of men in that age group can attain an erection sufficient for sexual intercourse [5]. The challenge with PCS, as with any other organ sparing surgery, is to maintain adequate organ function without compromising oncological control. Also, as expected follow-up after PCS will likely be more intense than penile amputation since the recurrence rates are higher. In this chapter we will focus on the indications, contraindications, outcomes and the various techniques of PCS.

2. The Indications of PCS

Since the follow-up for PCS is more intense than those receiving penile amputation, a compliant well-informed patient is an important requisite for PCS. Pathologically, the ideal candidate for PCS will be the patient with low stage disease, Tis/Ta or T1. In some patients with T2 disease and with well to moderately differentiated tumor grade, PCS may be offered [6, 7]. Also, in a few patients with urethral involvement that is confined to the glans and with negative intraoperative frozen section (FS), PCS can be offered [8]. Usually tumors that are amenable to PCS are located on the distal portion of the penis, that is, in the prepuce, glans or distal penile shaft.

3. The Contraindications to PCS

Patients in whom complete tumor excision with visibly and pathologically negative margins as confirmed by intraoperative FS is not feasible should not be offered PCS. Similarly, patients in whom the remaining penile stump is inadequate for a forwarded directed urine stream, and the suggested length to achieve that is a minimum of 3-4 cms penile stump, should not be offered PCS.

4. Intraoperative FS in PCS

Intraoperative FS from both corporal and deep urethral margin are essential in PCS. The advantages of performing the FS is to reduce the risk of local recurrence and in the meantime reduce the length of the safety margin, thereby maximizing penile length. The importance of performing intraoperative FS has been demonstrated in various studies. In one large study of Pca patients treated by PCS, 12% (22/179) had positive margin in the final pathology specimen, none had intraoperative FS. The authors suggest as long as intraoperative FS are negative, the final length of safety margin may not be important [9]. Also, residual microscopic disease was an independent prognostic factor for local recurrence with increased risk of regional recurrence for T1 lesions [10]. Recurrence rate in studies where FS is consistently performed as a part of PCS (excluding partial amputation) is 4-10% compared to 29% in studies where intraoperative FS was not routinely performed [10-12].

5. Current Recommendations for Safety Margins in PCS

Traditional teaching in performing PCS, as partial penectomy, was to excise the tumor and to extend the margin to 2 cms of normal tissue of the penis. However, and like other genitourinary cancers as kidney cancers, such an extent of safety margins has been questioned. This is supported by research that 2 cms safety margin may not be necessary if intraoperative FS is negative. Agrawal et al. examined 64 partial/total penectomy specimens for microscopic tumor extension. The authors found the maximum tumor extension to be 5mm beyond visible growth for well/moderately differentiated tumors and 10 mm for poorly differentiated tumors. No skip lesions were identified [13]. Minhas et al. reported a local recurrence rate of only 4% in a study of 51 patients treated with glansectomy and wide local excision with 0-10 mm safety margin in 48% of patients and less than 2cm margins in 98% of patients [12]. Based on these studies, the European Association of Urology (EAU) recommended that a 5 mm margin is accepted [14]. We recommend as well performing intraoperative FS and if positive repeat excision till a negative FS should be obtained.

6. Follow-Up after PCS

The follow up after PCS includes physical exam of both the penis and the groin. In some patients, physical exam of the groin is challenging in the morbidly obese patient, patients with previous inguinal surgery and those who received previous groin radiation. In these circumstances, a groin ultrasound or computerized tomography scan or magnetic resonance imaging may be helpful. Most recurrences (92%) after PCS occurred in the first 5 years in one study [15]. Consequently, the current recommendations for follow-up after PCS is every 3 months in the first 2 years after surgery, then every 6 months for years 3-5 and then annually till 10 years. It is possible to allow the well-informed patient to discontinue follow-up after 5 years if the patient can do self-exam. In patients who had partial penectomy, the follow-up can be every 6 months for the first 2 years then annually between 3-5 years [14, 16].

7. Local Recurrence after PCS

Djajadiningrat et al. reported the experience of the Netherlands Cancer Institute on local recurrence following PCS. The authors studied 859 patients classified into 2 groups; partial penectomy group and other organ sparing surgery group. They reported an overall 20% recurrence rate (local, and/or regional, and/or distant) in the partial penectomy group compared to 27% in those receiving a more conservative surgical approach [17].

Table 1. Summary of oncological/functional outcomes of selected penile conserving surgery studies

Study	N	Type of PCS	F/U (m)	Recur. (%)	TTR (m)	LRM	CSS (%) 5-years	Complications (%)	Functional outcomes
DjajadinIngrate [17]	859	PP:408 OPCS: 451	65	PP: L:4, L+R:4, L+D:1 R+/-D:20 OPCS: L:27, L+R:5 L+D: 0, R+/-D:9	10	PP§	L:88 R:33 M:13	N/A	N/A
Philippou [9]	179	Cir: 13 WLE:29 GL: 87 PP: 50	42.8	L: 8.9 R:10.6 M:5	L:26.1 R:26.8 M:11.7	PP TP	L:91.7 R:38.4	Infection:0.6 Graft loss:1.8 Corporal tip necrosis:0.6 Short penile Stump:1.2	All patients able to void upright
Veeratterapillay [18]	65	GL (Total): 46 GL (Partial): 1 GR: 3 GL+ distal corporectomy: 15	40	GL: 4 GL+ distal corpore-ctomy:13	15	WLE:2 GL: 1 PP: 1	N/A	Graft loss:1.5 Graft Contra-cture:4.5 Meatal Stenosis: 7.5	5% poor cosmoses 85%: Good erections at 1 year
Feldman [19]	56	WLE: 25 PG: 14 Circ: 11 Biopsy+ Topical TTT: 4 MMS: 2	65.6	¶21.4	51.4	N/A	N/A	No urethral or meatal stenosis	All patients able to void upright Preserved potency
Bissada [11]	30	Tailored excisions	†12-360	L: 10	N/A	WLE:3	N/A	N/A	Preserved potency
Bandiera-monte [38]	224	Laser: CO2+/- Chemotherapy	66	↓L:17.5	-N/A	Laser: 30 PP:8 TP:1 RT:1	N/A	Bleeding<1% Urethral stenosis <1% Preputial adhesions:2.7%	Preserved potency

Table 1. (Continued)

Study	N	Type of PCS	F/U (m)	Recur. (%)	TTR (m)	LRM	CSS (%) 5-years	Complications (%)	Functional outcomes
Shindel [37]	33	MMS	58	L: 32	N/A	MMS:7TP:1	96	Infection: 3%- PE:3% Meatal stenosis: 6%	N/A
Shabbir [25]	25	GR+STSG	39	L:4	^14	Topical-Chemo therapy (n = 1)	N/A	Graft take failure:1.4%	-Preserved potency
Smith [8]	72	GL+STSG	27	L: 4	N/A	-WLE (n = 3)	*17	Graft loss: 2.7 Meatal stenosis: 1.3	-Preserved potency
Parnham [29]	177	GL+STSG	41.4	9.3%	8.7	N/A	Near 90% at 50 m	Graft Loss Partial: 20% Total:3.4% Meatal Stenosis: 2.8%	N/A

Circ: circumcision; WLE: Wide local excision; GL: Glansectomy; CSS: Cancer specific survival; F/U follow-up; GR: Glans resurfacing; L: Local recurrence; LRM: Local recurrence management; M: metastasis/distant recurrence; M: months; N/A: Not available; N: number; OPCS: Other penis conserving surgery; PCS: Penis conserving surgery; PE: Pulmonary embolus; PP: Partial penectomy; R: Regional recurrence; RT: Radiotherapy; STSG: Split Thickness Skin Graft; TP: Total penectomy; TTR: Time to Recurrence.

§PP performed in 70/185 recurrences in OSSS group. PP performed in 33/120 recurrences in PP group.

¶ 25% of recurrences after 5 years of follow up.

† described as range.

^Only one recurrent CIS at 14 months F/U.

↓Local recurrences as single event in 20 patients and multiple in 12 patients.

*3 recurrences at 4, 19 and 28 months.

We will discuss individual recurrence rates following each PCS technique later in this chapter. The oncological outcomes of the pertinent studies on PCS are summarized in Table1.

8. Management of Local Recurrence in PCS

Risk factors for local recurrence following PCS included T stage, N status and the presence of lymphovascular invasion. Local recurrence after PCS is considered if such a recurrence occurred ≥3 months from the PCS. Recurrence after PCS, in which the pathology of the initial tumor removed did not reveal corpora cavernosa invasion, can still be managed by another PCS. In one study for patients with Pca and stage T1/T2 disease who underwent PCS, local control was achieved in 94% of patients after another PCS and with no increased risk of nodal disease or reducing survival [10]. There is agreement in several studies that local recurrence after OSS, promptly treated, does not affect overall patient survival [9, 10, 15, 17-19]. However, it is agreed that local recurrence after PCS, in which the initial tumor invaded the corpora cavernosa, should be managed by partial or total penile amputation [14, 16].

9. Role of PCS as Salvage Option Following Failed Penile Radiation

Preliminary data from the United Kingdom Supra-regional centers treating Pca demonstrated that salvage PCS surgery may be considered in select patients who received radiation therapy as a primary treatment for their Pca and failed. Shabbir et al. reported on 17 patients who had chronic ulceration following radiation therapy for Pca. Recurrent cancer was present in 15/17 patients. Management was with glansectomy+ STSG in 14, WLE + full thickness skin graft in 1, partial and radical penectomy each in 1 patient. 16/17 of their patients are recurrence-free at a mean follow up of 3 years and with no problem regarding graft uptake despite previous radiation [20].

10. Advantages of PCS

There are many advantages for penile sparing surgery. It is better than amputation since the patient may be able to urinate standing and in reasonable percentage of patients able to have sexual intercourse. The psychological benefits over total amputation are obvious. Our review included the outcomes of studies reporting on functional outcomes, that is, both urinary and sexual as well as psychological benefits of performing a PCS.

10.1. Urinary Function

Patients who underwent PCS are usually able to void while standing and less likely to leak urine than those who received penile amputation. In patients in whom spraying of urine continues to be a problem, the use of a small funnel placed on the remaining penile stump may be helpful. In one study, patients who underwent PCS (excluding partial penectomy) were less likely to leak during urination compared to partial/total penectomy (43% vs 83%) [21].

10.2. Sexual Function

Studies using the International Index of Erectile Function (IIEF-15) questionnaire revealed a clear advantage in terms of potency and sexual function in patients receiving PCS than amputation. Such benefits were even more pronounced in the less aggressive PCS when compared to partial penectomy. Gulino et al. studied 42 patients with PCS, not including partial penectomy, with IIEF-15 completed 6 months after surgery. Results showed 73% of patients reported spontaneous rigid erection, and 60% reported spontaneous coital activity and 19/25 (76%) patients reported normal ejaculation after glansectomy with urethral advancement [22]. Sansalone et al. compared pre- and post-operative IIEF-15 surveys in patients who had partial penectomy with urethral advancement to cover the corporal tips (n = 25). Although, a majority reported a reduction in sexual intercourse frequency, 68% reported high confidence in achieving erection, and 68% achieved the same level of orgasm and ejaculation as prior to surgery [23]. Kieffer et al. studied 90 patients with Pca with 54 patients receiving partial or total penectomy and 36 who received PCS. The PCS group reported better orgasmic function, but no difference was observed between the 2 groups in the remaining domains of IIEF-15. The type of "more conservative" OSS (laser/local excison/circumcision/glansectomy) did not affect the outcomes of the IIEF-15; however, the group that had the "more aggressive" PCS, partial penectomy, reported worse orgasmic function after surgery [21].

10.3. Psychological Function

There are few studies and with small number of patients that assessed the psychological impact of Pca surgical treatments. Maddineni et al. conducted a systematic review on 6 studies with a total of 128 patients. Surgical treatment in the form of PCS was offered in 101 patients: partial penectomy (n = 78), glansectomy (n = 8), and laser therapy (n = 5). The results showed an incidence of 53% mental illness, 25% avoidance behavior, and 40% impaired overall well-being. Post-traumatic stress disorder was also reported in 2 of 30 patients in one study [1]. In a more contemporary report, patients who underwent PCS compared favorably to the general population using the standardized Short-Form-36 (SF-36®) assessing the mental health related quality of life issues which was believed to relate to the coping mechanisms developed by cancer survivors [21].

11. Surgical Techniques Utilized in PCS

11.1. Circumcision

Uncircumcised elderly patients presenting with phimosis associated with bleeding or a palpable lump under the foreskin should be suspected for having Pca. It is not uncommon that the diagnosis of Pca is achieved following circumcision. If the tumor is small and in the distal portion of the prepuce, then circumcision is likely to be enough. However, in patients in whom the tumor is larger and more proximal, circumcision with distal corporotomy is warranted. Intraoperative FS is essential. Penile cancers developing in a circumcision scar usually occur after ritual circumcision with extensive scarring. Bissada et al. reported that these cancers tend to be low/intermediate grade and surgical excision appeared to be the only effective treatment. This included local excision, tailored resections and occasionally up to total penectomy or more extensive surgery. Most important is that radiotherapy did not provide cure in that group of patients [24].

11.2. Glandular Resurfacing

In this procedure, the glandular epithelium and subepithelium are excised. If less than 50% of the glandular surface is excised, this is termed partial glandular resurfacing (PGR) and total glandular resurfacing (TGR) if >50% [25]. The procedure gained its roots from the management of lichen sclerosis of the glans penis and is indicted in patients with CIS [25 26]. Reports on the oncological outcome of glandular resurfacing are few and mostly encompassing small number of patients and consequently the results should be interpreted with caution. Ayres et al. reported GR on 36 patients with T1a lesions, citing a recurrence rate of only 6% and positive margin rate of 11%; however median follow up was only 21 months [27]. Shabbir et al. reported on 25 patients with CIS (TGR n = 10/PGR n = 15), the positive surgical margin rate was 48% and re-operation rate was 28%. However, the overall recurrence was only 4%, and there was no effect on survival at 29 months of mean follow up [25]. The procedure is associated with quick recovery, rapid return of glandular sensation, and preservation of preoperative penile function [25, 26, 28]. However, patients should be warned that additional procedures may be needed.

11.2.1. Technique of GR

1. A tourniquet is placed at the base of the penis. This is followed by 2 circular incisions at the perimeatal area and the coronal sulcus and the glans is divided into 4 quadrants (Figure 1).
2. The epithelium and subepithelium are excised with deep spongiosal biopsies taken for FS (Figure 2). Circumcision is also performed in uncircumcised patients, and the shaft skin is approximated 10mm proximally from the coronal sulcus.
3. The defect is covered with Split Thickness Skin Graft (STSG), quilted with 5-0 vicryl for graft stabilization (Figure 3). Bedrest is advised for 48 hours. Non-adhesive dressing and catheter are removed after 5 days [25, 26].

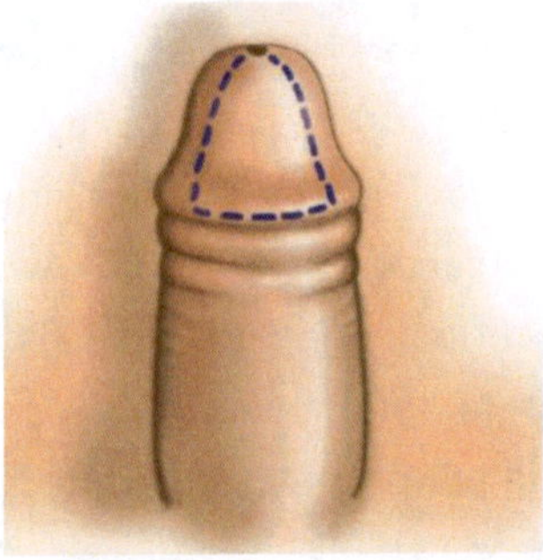

Figure 1. Circular perimeatal and coronal incisions and division of the glans into quadrants.

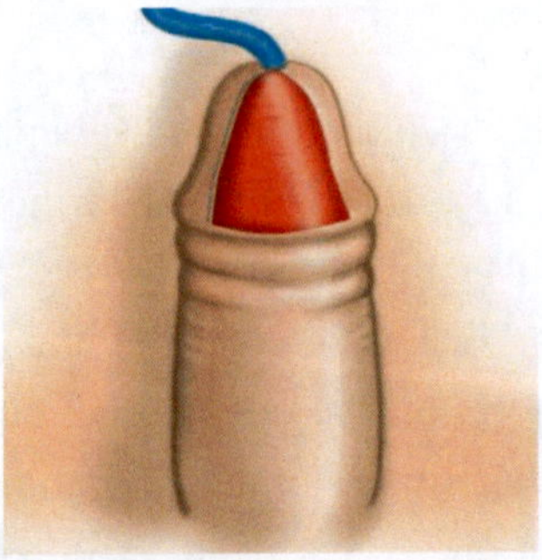

Figure 2. Excision of epithelium and subepithelial tissues of the glans.

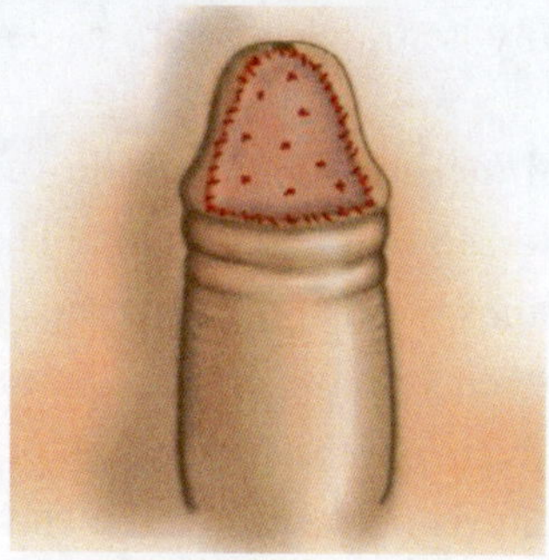

Figure 3. Split Thickness Skin Graft (STSG) is used to cover the defect.

11.3. Glansectomy

Nearly 50% of Pca encountered are located on the glans penis. Large tumors involving the glans penis, and when sometimes additionally involving the glandular urethra, should be managed by glansectomy. The corporal tips may need to be excised if an adequate safety margin is in question. The corporal tips can be covered by advancing the penile skin, or urethral advancement with spatulation, or the use of STSG. In our experience, we recommend the STSG to be 30% larger than the defect to compensate for graft contraction. The STSG is selected from a non-hairy donor site, typically the medial side of the thigh. Also, a good dressing to stabilize the graft allows for adequate take of the graft. Full thickness skin graft has a poor cosmetic outcome and poor graft site intake and consequently not commonly used [11]. Similarly, buccal mucosa is not recommended as it is more accustomed to a humid rather than dry environment [28]. Partial glansectomy or wedge excision is indicated in small glandular tumors. The defect is covered with STSG if primary anastomosis is not possible or, if performed, will cause a tilt to the urethral meatus and a deviated urinary stream.

Parnham et al. reported on 177 patients who underwent glansectomy and STSG in a tertiary referral center in the United Kingdom with a mean follow up of 41 months. The authors reported impressive results with local recurrence rate of 9.3%, mortality rate of 10.7% and reoperation rate for complications as meatal stenosis and graft loss in 9% [29]. In another smaller study, Smith et al. reported on 72 patients who had glansectomy and the local recurrence rate was only 4% at 27 months mean follow up [8]. Regarding the sexual function following glansectomy, Sedigh et al. reported on patients who underwent glansectomy and 59.1% experienced reduction of genital sensation and a 9.1% loss of erogenous sensation. Ejaculatory reflex was preserved in 68.2%. A reduction in erectile function, orgasmic function, and overall satisfaction was reported on IIEF-15 questionnaires [30]. There have been reported cases of female partners experiencing pain during intercourse following glansectomy, likely due to the loss of the cushion effect of the glans [31].

The technique of glansectomy is straightforward as described below:

1. Circumferential coronal incision is made followed by dissection deep to Buck's fascia and control of dorsal venous complex. The dissection continues between urethra and corporal bodies without dividing the urethra (Figure 4).
2. This leaves the glans attached to the urethra, that is divided followed by covering the corporal tips with advancing the penile skin or STSG.
3. If urethral advancement is used to cover the corporal tips, the urethra is mobilized off the corporal bodies (Figure 5) and spatulated to cover the corporal ends (Figure 6). Urethral catheter is removed after 10 days.

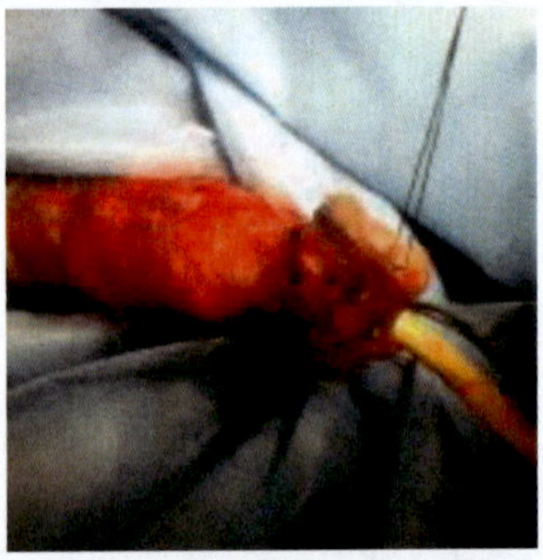

Figure 4. Dissection of glans off the corporal tips.

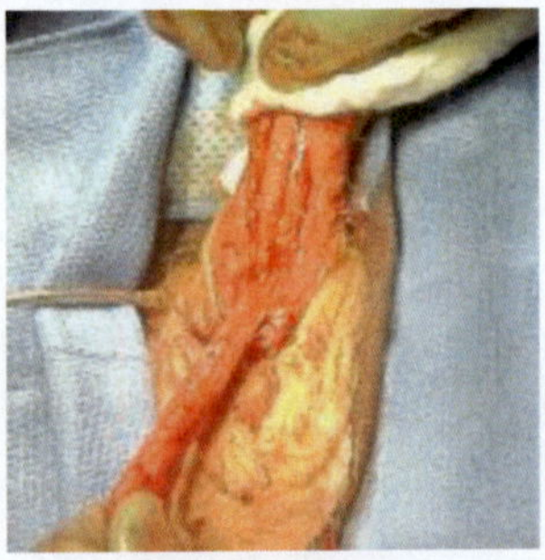

Figure 5. Urethral mobilization off the corporal bodies.

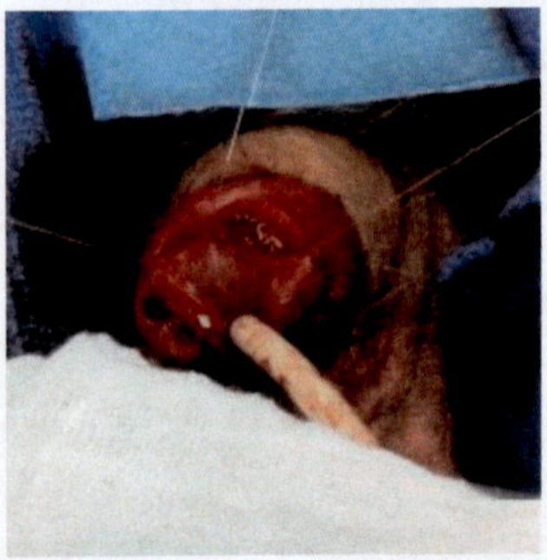

Figure 6. Urethral spatulation and advancement to cover the corporal tips.

11.4. Wide Local Excision

Wide local excision is used to excise the penile cancer in the glans or more rarely on the penile shaft. The defect can be closed by primary suturing; however, if the defect is large, STSG is used (Figure 7).

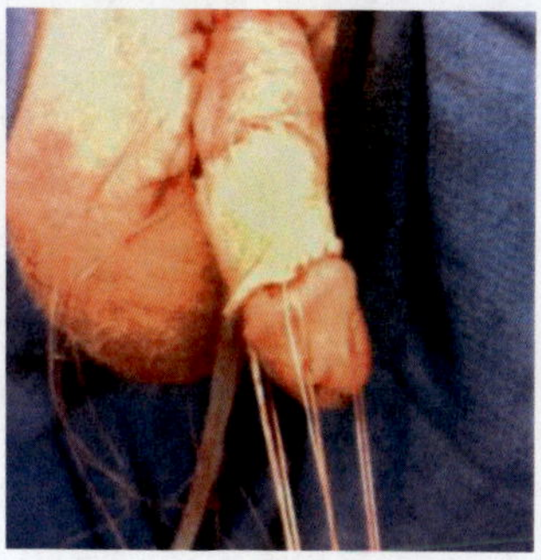

Figure 7. STSG is used to cover a defect in the penile skin.

11.5. Partial Penectomy

As mentioned previously, traditional partial penectomy involved a 2 cms safety margin which in contemporary surgical practice is no longer needed. The remaining penile stump following partial penectomy should be sufficient for forward directed urinary stream, otherwise total penectomy should be performed. Partial penectomy has a reported local recurrence rate ranging from 0-8%, sexual function is preserved in 20% of patients and the majority were able to void in the standing position [7, 32]. Patients undergoing partial penectomy should be counseled about the risks of urethral meatus stenosis (6%) and urine spraying during micturition necessitating to sit down when urinating [32].

11.5.1. Technique of Partial Penectomy

Following the application of a tourniquet at the base of the penis, a dorsal skin incision is made 1 cm proximal to the penile tumor and slanting forwards on the side. The incision is deepened to Buck's fascia. The dorsal neurovascular bundle is tied using 3-0 SAS. A scalpel is used to divide the tunica albuginea and the corporal bodies. The cut ends of the transected corporal bodies are closed using 2-0 polydioxanone in a horizontal mattress fashion incorporating the intercorporeal septum. The urethra is dissected off the corpora and divided to get an extra 1.5 cms distal to the divided corpora. The urethra is spatulated ventrally. The penile skin is advanced and anastomosed to the spatulated ends of the urethra using 3-0 SAS.

Techniques used to lengthen the penile skin includes 1) suspensory ligament division; 2) corporal mobilization from underneath the pubic arch; 3) division of the penoscrotal skin fold horizontally and suturing it vertically (Figure8); and 4) V-Y plasty at the penopubic area.

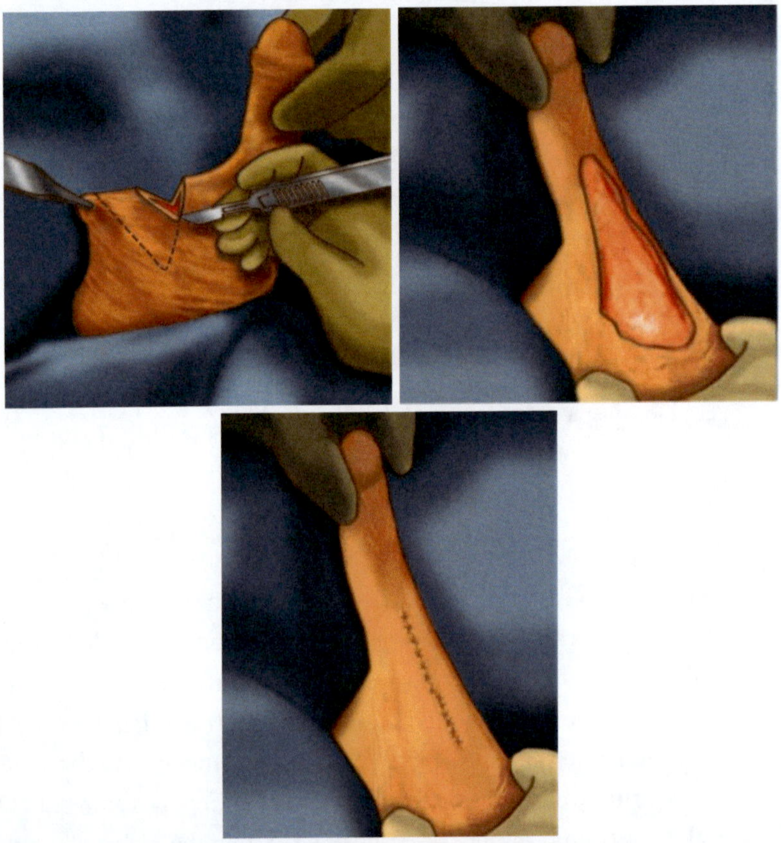

Figure 8. The penoscrotal skin fold is divided horizontally and sutured vertically to increase the length of the penile stump.

11.6. Urethra Sparing Penectomy

This technique was reported with success in few patients in whom the Pca involved the corpora cavernosa and spared the urethra. In the remaining corporal stumps, a pair of malleable penile prosthesis are placed and wrapped in vicryl mesh. A rectangular flap from the scrotal skin is created with the base at the pubis and used to wrap the penile prosthesis. The urethra can be mobilized from the perineum and brought to the tip as a neourethra (Figure 9). Bissada described this technique with success in 3 patients [33].

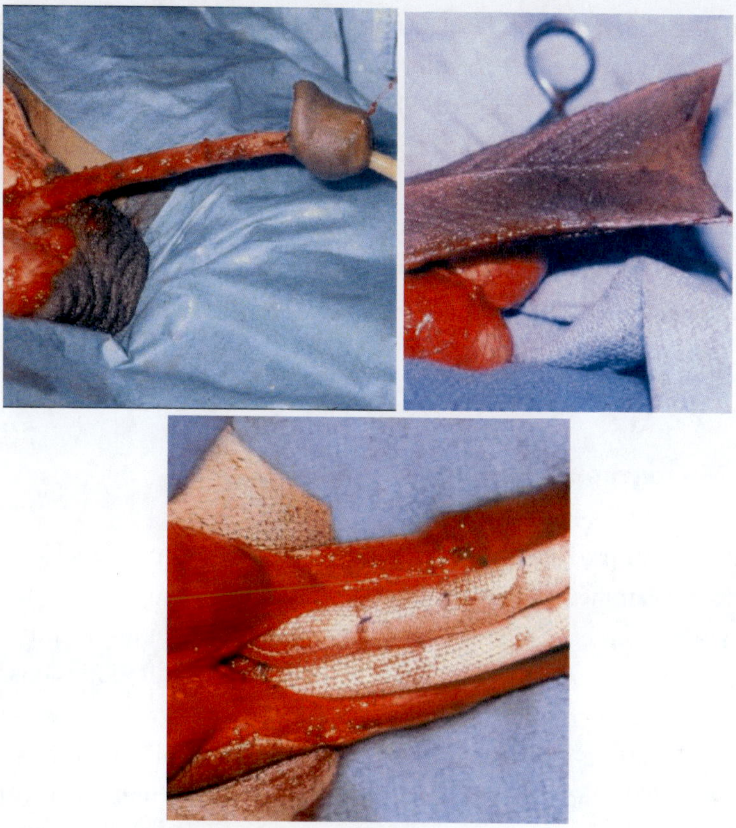

Figure 9. Technique of urethra sparing partial penectomy. Initially the urethra is spared, glans does not survive. Malleable penile prosthesis is placed at the proximal corporal stumps and rectangular scrotal skin flap with the base at the pubic bone is used to cover the prosthesis.

11.7. Laser Techniques

The 2 common types of laser used are the Carbon Dioxide (CO2) and Neodymium-doped: Yttrium Aluminium Garnet (Nd:YAG) laser. The CO2 laser does not penetrate the tissues deep; its depth of penetration is only 0.01 mm and coagulates a vessel of only 0.5mm in diameter. On the other hand, the Nd:YAG laser can penetrate tissues more deeply than the CO2 laser with a penetration depth of 3-6 mm and it can coagulate a vessel of up to 5 mm in diameter. The Nd:YAG is the more commonly used laser to treat Pca. Application of acetic acid to the penile skin 20 minutes prior to the laser procedure helps in better visualization of the penile lesion. The CO2 laser is a good cutting tool, but it does not penetrate deep enough. Therefore, it is more suitable for superficial lesions that are treated and with 5mm margin. The Nd:YAG laser is not good in cutting tissues but has deep penetration ability; so, after treating the penile lesion with the Nd:YAG laser, the treated tissue is excised, and biopsies are taken from the base.

The current indications for laser therapy are Tis, small T1 tumors or dysplastic lesions. Usually tumors selected for this type of PCS are low grade as well. Results of two post-procedure surveys reported 78% and 80% of patients enjoying satisfying cosmetic results, and 72% and 60% reported preserved erectile function [34, 35]. Laser therapy has high local recurrence rate on long term follow–up and up to 42%, without a decrease in overall survival rate [35]. Thus, long term follow-up is mandatory. The laser treatment has the limitation of no pathological evaluation of the penile tissue treated as well as complications such as risk of urethral stenosis, penile edema and adhesions between the glans and preputial skin.

11.8. Mohs Micrographic Surgery

This form of PCS provides maximum penile length. The penile lesion is removed in sections that are examined under the microscope until negative margins are achieved. Mohs Micrographic surgery (MMS) is not very popular in treating Pca. It requires much supporting staff and is costly. It is typically indicated in low grade lesions. Initial report by Mohs et al. on the oncological outcome was encouraging with a 94% five-year local cure rate and a 74% five-year overall cure rate in a study of 35 patients. This therapy failed in patients with uncontrolled metastases or extensive urethral involvement [36]. However, more contemporary literature showed the 5-year local recurrence rate to be 32% [37]. Complications of MMS include meatal stenosis for urethral involvement and disfigurement of the glans [36, 37].

CONCLUSION

Penile Conserving Surgery (PCS) is an attractive option in the management of Pca since in the appropriately selected patient the oncological outcome is comparable to penile amputation. In addition, there are obvious sexual, urinary and psychological benefits over penile amputation. The traditional 2 cm safety margin is no longer needed and a 5 mm margin is enough. Intraoperative FS helps to reduce the risk of recurrence and increase penile length. Since the reported risk of recurrence is higher than in total amputation, long term follow-up and a compliant patient are a must. Local recurrence after PCS, that is promptly treated, does not seem to adversely affect patient survival and can be managed with another PCS in select patients. There are various PCS techniques that can be used depending on the location and the tumor grade and stage as well as the comfort of the surgeon performing them.

Key Points

- PCS has obvious advantages over total amputation and should be offered to penile cancer patients whenever possible.
- The recurrence rate following PCS is higher than total amputation and consequently more rigorous follow-up is needed.
- Local recurrence following PCS does not seem to significantly affect oncological outcomes and can often be managed by another PCS.
- The 2 cm safety margin rule is abandoned. Only 5 mm is needed to achieve oncological control.
- Intraoperative frozen section is recommended to reduce the risk of positive margins.

References

[1] Maddineni, S. B., Lau, M. M., Sangar, V. K.: Identifying the needs of penile cancer sufferers: a systematic review of the quality of life, psychosexual and psychosocial literature in penile cancer. *BMC Urol*, 9: 8, 2009.

[2] Hernandez, B. Y., Barnholtz-Sloan, J., German, R. R. et al.: Burden of invasive squamous cell carcinoma of the penis in the United States, 1998-2003. *Cancer,* 113: 2883, 2008.

[3] Cubilla, A. L., Barreto, J., Caballero, C. et al.: Pathologic features of epidermoid carcinoma of the penis. A prospective study of 66 cases. *Am J Surg Pathol*, 17: 753, 1993.

[4] Opjordsmoen, S., Fossa, S. D.: Quality of life in patients treated for penile cancer. A follow-up study. *Br J Urol*, 74: 652, 1994.

[5] Johannes, C. B., Araujo, A. B., Feldman, H. A. et al.: Incidence of erectile dysfunction in men 40 to 69 years old: longitudinal results from the Massachusetts male aging study. *J Urol*, 163: 460, 2000.

[6] Pompeo, A. C., Zequi Sde, C., Pompeo, A. S.: Penile cancer: organ-sparing surgery. *Curr Opin Urol*, 25: 121, 2015.

[7] Horenblas, S., van Tinteren, H., Delemarre, J. F. et al.: Squamous cell carcinoma of the penis. II. Treatment of the primary tumor. *J Urol*, 147: 1533, 1992.

[8] Smith, Y., Hadway, P., Biedrzycki, O. et al.: Reconstructive surgery for invasive squamous carcinoma of the glans penis. *Eur Urol,* 52: 1179, 2007.

[9] Philippou, P., Shabbir, M., Malone, P. et al.: Conservative surgery for squamous cell carcinoma of the penis: resection margins and long-term oncological control. *J Urol*, 188: 803, 2012.

[10] Lont, A. P., Gallee, M. P., Meinhardt, W. et al.: Penis conserving treatment for T1 and T2 penile carcinoma: clinical implications of a local recurrence. *J Urol*, 176: 575, 2006.

[11] Bissada, N. K., Yakout, H. H., Fahmy, W. E. et al.: Multi-institutional long-term experience with conservative surgery for invasive penile carcinoma. *J Urol*, 169: 500, 2003.

[12] Minhas, S., Kayes, O., Hegarty, P. et al.: What surgical resection margins are required to achieve oncological control in men with primary penile cancer? *BJU Int,* 96: 1040, 2005.

[13] Agrawal, A., Pai, D., Ananthakrishnan, N. et al.: The histological extent of the local spread of carcinoma of the penis and its therapeutic implications. *BJU Int*, 85: 299, 2000.

[14] http://uroweb.org/wp-content/uploads/12-Penile-Cancer_LR1.pdf.

[15] Leijte, J. A., Kirrander, P., Antonini, N. et al.: Recurrence patterns of squamous cell carcinoma of the penis: recommendations for follow-up based on a two-centre analysis of 700 patients. *Eur Urol*, 54: 161, 2008.

[16] https://www.nccn.org/professionals/physician_gls/pdf/penile.pdf.

[17] Djajadiningrat, R. S., van Werkhoven, E., Meinhardt, W. et al.: Penile sparing surgery for penile cancer-does it affect survival? *J Urol*, 192: 120, 2014.

[18] Veeratterapillay, R., Sahadevan, K., Aluru, P. et al.: Organ-preserving surgery for penile cancer: description of techniques and surgical outcomes. *BJU Int,* 110: 1792, 2012.

[19] Feldman, A. S., McDougal, W. S.: Long-term outcome of excisional organ sparing surgery for carcinoma of the penis. *J Urol*, 186: 1303, 2011.

[20] Shabbir M, H. B., Swallow T, Corbishley C, Perry M, Watkin N: Management of chronic ulceration after radiotherapy for penile cancer. *J Urol*, 179 (Supplement 4): 273, 2008.

[21] Kieffer, J. M., Djajadiningrat, R. S., van Muilekom, E. A. et al.: Quality of life for patients treated for penile cancer. *J Urol*, 192: 1105, 2014.

[22] Gulino, G., Sasso, F., Palermo, G. et al.: Sexual outcomes after organ potency-sparing surgery and glans reconstruction in patients with penile carcinoma. *Indian J Urol,* 29: 119, 2013.

[23] Sansalone, S., Silvani, M., Leonardi, R. et al.: Sexual outcomes after partial penectomy for penile cancer: results from a multi-institutional study. *Asian J Androl*, 2015.

[24] Bissada, N. K., Morcos, R. R., el-Senoussi, M.: Post-circumcision carcinoma of the penis. I. Clinical aspects. *J Urol,* 135: 283, 1986.

[25] Shabbir, M., Muneer, A., Kalsi, J. et al.: Glans resurfacing for the treatment of carcinoma in situ of the penis: surgical technique and outcomes. *Eur Urol*, 59: 142, 2011.

[26] Hadway, P., Corbishley, C. M., Watkin, N. A.: Total glans resurfacing for premalignant lesions of the penis: initial outcome data. *BJU Int,* 98: 532, 2006.

[27] Ayres, B., Lam W, Al-Najjar H, Corbishley C, Perry M, Watkin N: Oncological outcomes of glans resurfacing in the treatment of selected superficially invasive penile cancers. J Urol, 187 (Supplement 4): e306, 2012

[28] Palminteri, E., Berdondini, E., Lazzeri, M. et al.: Resurfacing and reconstruction of the glans penis. *Eur Urol*, 52: 893, 2007.

[29] Parnham, A. S., Albersen, M., Sahdev, V. et al.: Glansectomy and Split-thickness Skin Graft for Penile Cancer. *Eur Urol*, 73: 284, 2018.

[30] Sedigh, O., Falcone, M., Ceruti, C. et al.: Sexual function after surgical treatment for penile cancer: Which organ-sparing approach gives the best results? *Can Urol Assoc J, 9*: E423, 2015.

[31] Hatzichristou, D. G., Tzortzis, V., Hatzimouratidis, K. et al.: Protective role of the glans penis during coitus. *Int J Impot Res*, 15: 337, 2003.

[32] Mazza, O. N., Cheliz, G. M.: Glanuloplasty with scrotal flap for partial penectomy. *J Urol*, 166: 887, 2001.

[33] Bissada, N. K.: Penile reconstruction after total penectomy or urethra-sparing total penectomy. *J Urol*, 137: 1173, 1987.

[34] Windahl, T., Andersson, S. O.: Combined laser treatment for penile carcinoma: results after long-term followup. *J Urol*, 169: 2118, 2003.

[35] Schlenker, B., Tilki, D., Seitz, M. et al.: Organ-preserving neodymium-yttrium-aluminium-garnet laser therapy for penile carcinoma: a long-term follow-up. *BJU Int*, 106: 786, 2010.

[36] Mohs, F. E., Snow, S. N., Larson, P. O.: Mohs micrographic surgery for penile tumors. *Urol Clin North Am*, 19: 291, 1992.

[37] Shindel, A. W., Mann, M. W., Lev, R. Y. et al.: Mohs micrographic surgery for penile cancer: management and long-term followup. *J Urol*, 178: 1980, 2007.

[38] Bandieramonte, G., Colecchia, M., Mariani, L. et al.: Peniscopically controlled CO2 laser excision for conservative treatment of in situ and T1 penile carcinoma: report on 224 patients. *Eur Urol*, 54: 875, 2008.

In: Penile Cancer: Challenges and Controversies
Editors: F. E. Martins and M. L. Djordjevic
ISBN: 978-1-53615-950-9

Chapter 6

SURGICAL MANAGEMENT OF LOCALLY ADVANCED DISEASE (T3-T4)

Patrick Teloken[1] and Eric Chung[1,2,*]
[1]University of Queensland, Department of Urology,
Princess Alexandra Hospital, Brisbane QLD, Australia
[2]AndroUrology Centre, Brisbane QLD, Australia

ABSTRACT

While localised penile cancer can be adequately treated with many different penile-sparing approaches associated with close surveillance, locally advanced penile cancer requires multimodal therapy due to high-risk features and poor prognosis especially in patients with more than 2 inguinal lymph node metastases. This following chapter focuses on the surgical management of the primary tumour in advanced T3-T4 penile cancer.

A Medline literature search for English language original articles, high-quality systematic reviews, evidence-based guidelines and recent narrative reviews on advanced penile cancer was performed. The management of lymph node dissection will be discussed in a separate chapter and is excluded in this book chapter.

Surgical excision with negative margin is considered the standard of care in locally advanced disease and a partial penectomy is preferred over total penectomy with an adequate residual penile stump, with or without "lengthening" techniques, to maximise patient's quality of life. Improved clinical outcomes in advanced penile cancer require an integrated multidisciplinary approach, including better identification of high-risk disease with novel technology such as dynamic sentinel lymph node identification techniques, and provision of neo-adjuvant chemotherapy in selected patients with advanced lymph node involvement or visceral metastasis.

* Corresponding Author's E-mail: ericchg@hotmail.com; Fax +617-3832 8889

Advanced penile cancer cases require a multidisciplinary collaborative approach that involves extirpative surgery to remove (or at least debulk) the primary lesion with loco-regional lymph node dissection, followed by potential neoadjuvant therapy and/or adjuvant targeted therapy for the salvage treatment of metastatic disease.

Keywords: penile cancer, locally advanced disease, management, surgical treatment, partial penectomy, total penectomy, treatment outcomes

INTRODUCTION

Penile cancer is an uncommon malignancy in the Western countries with squamous cell carcinoma (SCC) being the most common subtypes. It typically affects middle-aged to older men with less than 20% in men less than 40 years diagnosed with penile cancer [1]. Delays in health-seeking behaviour are common in patients with a penile lesion, partly attributable to psychological factors, such as physical embarrassment and denial, and perhaps related to a lack of knowledge about the potential malignant nature of such penile lesion [2]. These delays may result in disease progression and development of larger fungating or infiltrative mass within the penis with ensuing voiding dysfunction through direct compression of the urethra or invasion into urethra and prostate. In a review of epidemiology of invasive penile cancer for more than 30 years, Dillner [3] reported that phimosis, chronic inflammatory conditions (e.g., balanoposthitis and lichen sclerosis et atrophicus), treatment with psoralen and ultraviolet A photochemotherapy, history of condyloma and human papillomavirus (HPV) serotypes 16 and 18 were associated with an increased risk of in penile cancer. Recent genomic profiling studies [4] found that genomic alterations in chromosomes 3 (PPARG, gene) and 8 (DLC1 gene) were associated with worse prognostic features, including advanced pathological and clinical stages.

While penile cancer tends to spread locally or through regional lymphatics drainage, patients with advanced disease may also present with systemic symptoms, sometimes caused by paraneoplastic hypercalcaemia. The World Health Organisation (WHO) and International Society of Urological Pathology (ISUP) recently revised penile cancer classification to take into consideration the relationship between HPV and penile SCC [5].

Advanced penile cancer can be defined as SCC invasion of the corpora cavernosa with or without invasion of the urethra (T3) or invasion into adjacent structures (scrotum, prostate, bone) (T4); bulky lymph node metastases (cN2 or cN3) or failed primary lymphadenectomy leading progression to nodal metastases, matted or bulky lymphadenopathy (cN3); 2 metastatic superficial and deep inguinal lymph nodes (pN2), metastatic pelvic lymph node (N3); and distant metastases (M1) [6, 7]. While localised penile cancer can be adequately treated with various penile-sparing approaches coupled with close surveillance protocol, locally advanced penile cancer often requires more aggressive and multimodal therapy due to high-risk features and poor prognosis especially in patients with positive inguinal lymph node metastases [7, 8]. Contemporary literature supports the use of the multidisciplinary collaborative approach to providing a more standardized treatment care plan that involves extirpative surgery to remove (or at least debulk) the primary lesion with loco-regional lymph node dissection, followed by potential neoadjuvant therapy and/or adjuvant targeted therapy for the salvage treatment of metastatic disease (Figure 1).

The following chapter focuses on the surgical management of the primary tumour in advanced T3-T4 penile cancer. Description of actual surgical techniques is not covered in this chapter.

METHODS

A Medline literature search for English language original articles, high-quality systematic reviews, evidence-based guidelines and recent narrative reviews on advanced penile cancer was performed.

A detailed analysis of all relevant studies is not the goal of this review article. Because of word limitations in this publication, summarized evidence from key identified literature has been included. The management of lymph node dissection will be discussed in a separate chapter and is excluded in this chapter.

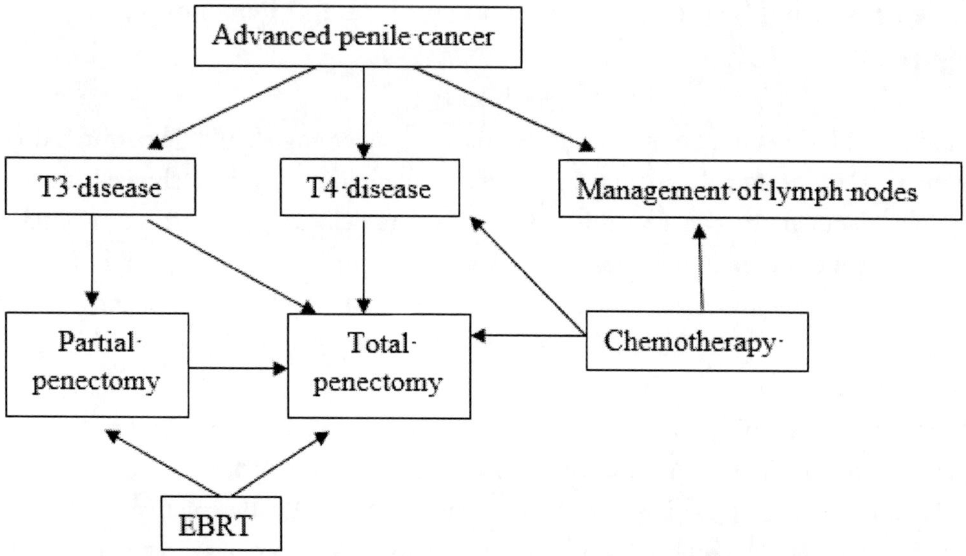

Figure 1. Proposed algorithm for surgical management of advanced penile cancer. (EBRT = external beam radiotherapy).

Discussion

Primary surgical excision remains the standard treatment for patients with locally advanced penile cancer with resectable disease who are fit for surgery [7]. Published EAU guideline reports a lack of controlled trials or large series in penile cancer management and while there is no outcome difference between local treatment modalities in superficial and T1 disease, there should be adequate margin of resection in locally advanced penile cancer [8]. Furthermore, lymph node metastases should be treated by surgery and adjuvant chemotherapy in N2/N3 disease. Recent understandings in the natural history of penile cancer have shown that local recurrence can often be treated without significant adverse impact on long-term survival provided an adequate negative surgical margin was achieved [9]. More recent studies reported that 5-year cancer-specific survivorship for pT3/4 was 54% (95% CI 25% - 76%) and that the use of neoadjuvant chemotherapy did not alter the 5-year outcome over the 16 years of study [10].

In a separate study, Chung [11] concluded that high-risk features such as tumour stage, lymph node involvement and distant metastasis carry a significantly higher risk of death and tumour recurrence in patients with penile cancer and inguinal lymph node metastasis. The Kaplan-Meier cancer-specific survival at 72 months was 64% in pT3 disease with a statistically significant difference in survival outcome in patients with local recurrence vs. systemic metastasis disease (33% vs. 17%, $p = 0.008$).

Penile Preserving Surgery (Glansectomy and Partial Penectomy) (Figure 2)

While older literature emphasized that partial penectomy should be performed with a minimum 2cm surgical margin [12, 13], contemporary series showed that good oncological outcomes can be achieved with less radical surgery and recent guidelines advocate penile preservation whenever possible to increase patient's quality of life [7, 8, 14]. While there is no clear scientific evidence on the exact requirement of minimal negative margin to prevent local cancer recurrence, a 3-5mm surgical margin has recommended on the basis of cancer grade [15].

Patients undergoing partial penectomy are more likely to report greater adverse impact in urinary and sexual functions than those undergoing less aggressive forms of penile preservation therapies for penile cancer [16]. Reconstructive surgery with intraoperative frozen section analysis (in carefully selected cases) may offer some of these patients a less radical surgery and preservation of a (longer) functional penile length.

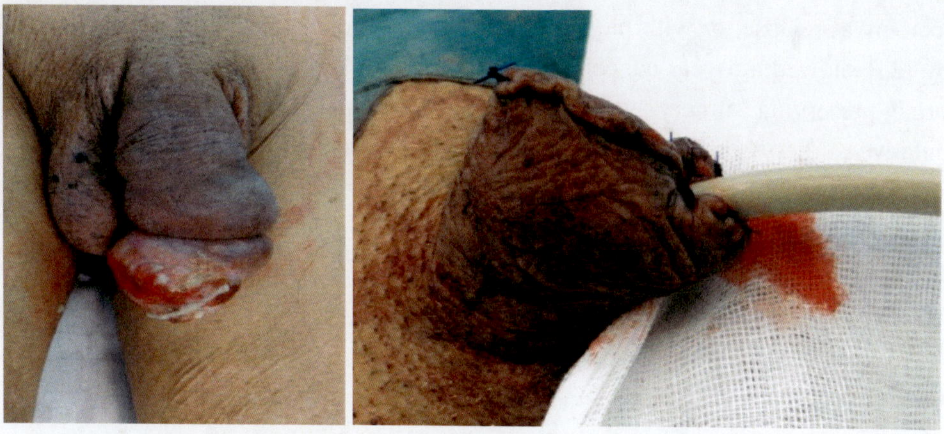

Figure 2. Locally advanced penile cancer – pre and postoperative partial penectomy.

Penile lengthening techniques such as synchronous division of dorsal suspensory ligaments or cosmetic wound closure and reconstruction to lengthen residual penile stump have been described in the literature [17, 18]. Preservation of a functional penile length whenever possible is important for several reasons. Functionally, the patient can void standing up and perhaps pursue an active sexual lifestyle. From a psychological perspective, it is well recognised that radical penectomy often leads to significant psychological distress, reduction in quality of life, and an increase in suicide risk [19]. A recent systematic review of published studies of radical treatment and sexual function in patients with penile cancer showed an adverse effect on general well-being in up to 40% of men and psychiatric conditions such as post-traumatic stress disorder is reported in approximately 50% of men [20].

Surgical complications related to partial penectomy include meatal stenosis (various urinary issues such as poor and splaying of stream, or retention) and sexual dysfunction. Meatal stenosis has been reported in up to 6% of patients and adequate urethral mobilisation and (dorsal) spatulation are important technical considerations to minimise this complication. A split-skin graft can be used for neoglans reconstruction in patients who have failed multiple meatal dilations [12]. While a significant impact on self-image, quality of life and sexual function is expected in patients who underwent partial penectomy, Sansalone found that approximately 60% of men were able to obtain erections for sexual penetration and achieve satisfactory orgasm after partial penectomy [21]. However, most patients reported a reduction in the frequency of sexual intercourse with the main reason of embarrassment related to feeling of shame due to the small penile size, and a decrease in overall sexual satisfaction.

The exact incidence of local recurrence in patients treated with partial or total penectomy is relatively low around 4%. External beam radiotherapy (EBRT) has a role in selected cases of positive surgical margin and a similar regimen to that used in primary treatment is utilised [22]. Furthermore, many patients whom initially underwent partial penectomy and subsequently developed local recurrence, can often be rescued with total penectomy at relapse, or with palliative radiotherapy for inoperable patients. One recent study [23] showed a 5-year cancer-specific survival to decrease with advancing age and in organ-preserving surgery, with local recurrence rate at 18% (compared to 4% for amputative surgery) and 94% of local recurrence occurring within 3 years of partial penectomy. In another study [24], patients with local recurrence after partial penectomy had a significantly lower cancer-specific survival compared to patients without local recurrence, highlighting an aggressive behaviour of the primary tumour.

Total Penectomy

Radical penectomy and formation of perineal urethrostomy are generally reserved for patients with cancer extending into proximal corporal bodies, or if the residual penile length is not functionally or cosmetically acceptable. In selected patients, a neophalloplasty can be offered at a later stage with the insertion of a penile prosthesis [25]. Recent data [26] showed that radical penectomy with concurrent neophallus reconstruction is associated with a higher risk of perioperative complications, including high-grade Clavien-Dindo complications. While complications such as urethral structures and fistulae, as well as penile prosthesis complications are not uncommon, these patients often require multiple revision surgeries, proper counselling and regular surgical support service.

Penile Consolidation, De-Bulking and Palliative Surgery for the Unresectable Disease

Patients with a locally advanced or bulky/unresectable disease will need a multidisciplinary team input with medical, radiation, and urologic oncologists. The preferred approach for patients with large, fixed lymphadenopathy and/or distant metastases involves the discussion of neoadjuvant cisplatin-based systemic chemotherapy [27]. Based on a patient's response to systemic chemotherapy (i.e., stable disease, partial or complete response), surgical consolidation may be considered thereafter to improve quality of life [28]. In a selected cohort of patient with metastatic penile cancer, disease stabilisation or response to chemotherapy could potentially extend survival with 5-year actuarial survival rate at 40% with a median survival of 26 months [29]. More recent studies by Pagliaro [30] reported that neoadjuvant chemotherapy with paclitaxel, ifosfamide, and cisplatin produced complete or partial responses in 50% of patients, with most patients (73.3%) subsequently undergoing surgery as planned. This finding compares favourably against historical response rates of only 30% to 35% for advanced metastatic disease.

On the other hand, Pond [31] found that concurrent chemoradiotherapy demonstrated poor clinical outcome for locally advanced penile cancer highlighting the highly aggressive tumour biology and that visceral metastasis was associated with lower overall survival rate [32]. Patients receiving cisplatin-based regimens exhibited better outcomes compared with noncisplatin-based regimens after adjusting for prognostic factors [33]. Novel agents such as epidermal growth factor receptor (EGFR)-targeted therapy such as cetuximab and panitumumab, has been used based on similar success of in squamous head and neck cancer and the expression of EGFR in penile SCC [34, 35].

Palliative and supportive care is important among patients with advanced disease. The Patients Experiences of Penile Cancer (PEPC) study group [36] reported that impact of primary surgery was interconnected with broader events of the patient's lives including urinary function, sexual function, sexual relationships, healing, recovery, masculinity, mental well-being, coping and cancer support. It is important that these men are well informed about the extent and potential consequences of their treatment as well as the need for further development and individualization of their treatment care plan [37, 38]. The goals of palliation are to alleviate pain, minimise wound complications, treat associated paraneoplastic or chemo-radiation effects, and prevent further urinary complications.

EBRT may be beneficial in improving pain from fixed inguinal masses, bony metastasis and/or spinal cord compression [39]. Emergency endovascular intervention with endoluminal vascular stents can be useful to temporarily alleviate vascular haemorrhage from tumour erosion into femoral vessels. Palliative chemotherapy in advanced cases must be adapted and weighed against the best supportive care and patient's wishes.

Adequate analgesia prescription with pain team, psychological input and hospice care are often valuable for patient and family for pain control and coordination of end of life emotional and physical issues.

CONCLUSION

Surgical excision with negative margin is considered the standard of care in locally advanced disease and a partial penectomy is preferred over total penectomy whenever the residual stump, with or without "lengthening" techniques, to maximise patient's quality of life.

Improved clinical outcomes in advanced penile cancer require an integrated multidisciplinary approach, including better identification of high-risk disease with novel technology such as dynamic sentinel lymph node identification techniques, and provision of neo-adjuvant chemotherapy in selected patients with advanced lymph node involvement or visceral metastasis.

KEY POINTS

- Primary surgical excision remains the standard treatment for patients with locally advanced penile cancer with resectable disease who are fit for surgery.
- Surgical excision with a 3 - 5mm negative margin is imperative and a partial penectomy is generally preferred over total penectomy, with or without "lengthening" techniques, to maximise patient's quality of life.
- The exact incidence of local recurrence in patients treated with partial penectomy is relatively low and can often be rescued with total penectomy (+/- radiotherapy) at relapse, or with palliative radiotherapy for inoperable patients.
- Patients with a locally advanced or bulky/unresectable disease will need a multidisciplinary team input with the preferred approach for patients with large, fixed lymphadenopathy and/or distant metastases involves the discussion of neoadjuvant cisplatin-based systemic chemotherapy.
- Palliative and supportive care is important among patients with advanced disease, with the goals of palliation to alleviate pain, minimise wound complications, treat associated paraneoplastic or chemo-radiation effects, and prevent further urinary complications.

REFERENCES

[1] Landis, S. H. Murray, T., Bolden, S. et al. Cancer statistics. *CA Cancer J. Clin.,* 1999; 49:8 - 31.

[2] Skeppner, E., Andersson, S. O., Johansson, J. E., Windahl, T. Initial symptoms and delay in patients with penile carcinoma. *Scand. J. Urol. Nephrol.,* 2012; 46(5): 315 - 25.

[3] Dillner, J., von Krogh, G., Horenblas, S. et al. Etiology of squamous cell carcinoma of the penis. *Scand. J. Urol. Nephrol. Suppl.,* 2000; 205:189 - 93.

[4] Busso-Lopes, A. F., Marchi, F. A., Kuasne, H. et al. Genomic profiling of human penile carcinoma predicts worse prognosis and survival. *Cancer Prev. Res.,* (Phila). 2015; 8(2):149 - 56.

[5] Paner, G. P., Stadler, W. M., Hansel, D. E., Montironi, R., Lin, D. W., Amin, M. B. Updates in the eighth edition of the Tumor-Node-Metastasis staging classification for urologic cancers. *Eur. Urol.,* 2018; 73(4):560 - 569.

[6] Heinlen, J. E., Buethe, D. D., Culkin, D. J. Advanced penile cancer. *Int. Urol. Nephrol.,* 2012; 44(1):139 - 48.

[7] Spiess, P. E.; National Comprehensive Cancer Network. New treatment guidelines for penile cancer. *J. Natl. Comp. Canc. Netw.,* 2013; 11(5 Suppl.):659 - 62.

[8] Hakenberg, O. W., Comperat, E. M., Minhas, S., Necchi, A., Protzel, C., Watkin, N. EAU guidelines on penile cancer: 2014 update. *Eur. Urol.,* 2015; 67(1):142 - 150.

[9] Campbell, R. A., Slopnick, E. A., Ferry, E. K., Zhu, H., Kim, S. P., Abouassaly, R. Disparity between pre-existing management of penile cancer and NCCN guidelines. *Urol. Oncol.,* 2017; 35(8):531.e9-531.e14.

[10] Moses, K. A., Winer, A., Sfakianos, J. P. et al. Contemporary management of penile cancer: greater than 15 year MSKCC experience. *Can. J. Urol.,* 2014; 21(2):7201 - 6.

[11] Chung, E., Yang, S., White, L., Wood, S., Nicol, D. Lessons learnt in the management of primary invasive penile cancer in an Australian tertiary referral centre: clinical outcomes with a minimum 48 months follow-up study. *Korean J. Urol.,* 2015; 56(2):125 - 30.

[12] Horenblas, S., van Tinteren, H., Delemarre, J. F., et al. Squamous cell carcinoma of the penis. II. Treatment of the primary tumor. *J. Urol.,* 1992; 147:1533 - 8.

[13] Hoffman, M. A., Renshaw, A. A., Loughlin, K. R. Squamous cell carcinoma of the penis and microscopic pathologic margins: How much margin is needed for local cure? *Cancer,* 1999; 85:1565 - 8.

[14] Agrawal, A., Pai, D., Ananthakrishnan, N., et al. The histological extent of the local spread of carcinoma of the penis and its therapeutic implications. *BJU Int.,* 2000; 85:299 - 301.

[15] Minhas, S., Kayes, O., Hegarty, P., Kumar, P., Freeman, A., Ralph, D. *BJU Int.,* 2005; 96:1040 - 43.

[16] Kieffer, J. M., Djajadiningrat, R. S., van Muilekom, E. A. M., Graafland, N. M., Horenblas, S., Aaronson, N. K. Quality of life for patients treated for penile cancer. *J. Urol.,* 2014; 192(4):1105 - 10.

[17] Donnellan, S. M., Webb, D. R. Management of invasive penile cancer by synchronous penile lengthening and radical tumor excision to avoid perineal urethrostomy. *Aust. NZ J. Surg.,* 1998; 68(5):369 - 70.

[18] Palminteri, E., Fusco, F., Berdondini, E., Salonia, A. Aesthetic neo-glans reconstruction after penis-sparing surgery for benign, premalignant or malignant penile lesions. *Arab. J. Urol.,* 2011; 9(2):115 - 20.

[19] D'Ancona, C. A., Botega, N. J., De Moraes, C., et al. Quality of life after partial penectomy for penile carcinoma. *Urology,* 1997; 50(4):593 - 6.

[20] Maddineni, S. B., Lau, M. M., Sangar, V. K. Identifying the needs of penile cancer sufferers: A systematic review of the quality of life, psychosexual and psychosocial literature in penile cancer. *BMC Urol.,* 2009; 8:9 - 8.

[21] Sansalone, S., Silvani, M., Leonardi, R., Vespasiani, G., Iacovelli, V. Sexual outcomes after partial penectomy for penile cancer: results from a multi-institutional study. *Asian J. Androl.,* 2017; 19(1):57 - 61.

[22] Crook, J. Radiotherapy approaches for locally advanced penile cancer: Neoadjuvant and adjuvant. *Curr. Opin. Urol.,* 2017; 27(1):62 - 67.

[23] Veeratterapillay, R., Teo, L., Asterling, S., Greene, D. Oncologic outcomes of penile cancer treatment at a UK supraregional enter. *Urology,* 2015; 85(5):1097 - 1103.

[24] Lont, A. P., Gallee, M. P., Meinhardt, W. et al. Penis conserving treatment for T1 and T2 penile carcinoma: clinical implications of a local recurrence. *J. Urol.,* 2006; 176(2):575 - 80.

[25] Garaffa, G., Raheem, A. A., Christopher, N. A., Ralph, D. J. Total phallic reconstruction after penile amputation for carcinoma. *BJU Int.,* 2009; 104(6): 852 - 6.

[26] Ottenhof, S. R., Leone, A., Djajadiningrat, R. S. et al. Surgical and oncological outcomes in patients after vascularised flap reconstruction for locoregionally advanced penile cancer. *Eur. Urol. Focus,* 2018 pii: S2405-4569(18)30026-9. doi: 10.1016/j.euf.2018.02.002.

[27] Pettaway, C. A., Pagliaro, L., Theodore, C., Haas, G. Treatment of visceral, unresectable, or bulky/unresectable regional metastases of penile cancer. *Urology,* 2010; 76(2 Suppl. 1):S58–65.

[28] Di Lorenzo, G., Buonerba, C. Federico, P., et al. Cisplatin and 5-fluorouracil in inoperable, stage IV squamous cell carcinoma of the penis. *BJU Int.,* 2012; 110(11 Pt B):E661–668.

[29] Bermejo, C., Busby, J. E., Spiess, P. E., Heller, L., Pagliaro, L. C., Pettaway, C. A. Neoadjuvant chemotherapy followed by aggressive surgical consolidation for metastatic penile squamous cell carcinoma. *J. Urol.,* 2007; 177(4):1335 - 8.

[30] Pagliaro, L. C., Williams, D. L., Daliani, D., et al. Neoadjuvant paclitaxel, ifosfamide, and cisplatin chemotherapy for metastatic penile cancer: a phase II study. *J. Clin. Oncol.,* 2010; 28:3851 - 3857.

[31] Pond, G. R., Milowsky, M. I., Kolinsky, M. P. et al. Concurrent chemotherapy for men with locally advanced penile squamous cell carcinoma. *Clin. Genitourin. Cancer,* 2014; 12(6):440 - 6.

[32] Pond, G. R., Di Lorenzo, G., Necchi, A. et al. Prognostic risk stratification derived from invidual patient level data for men with advanced penile squamous cell carcinoma receiving first-line systemic therapy. *Urol. Oncol.,* 2014; 32(4):501 - 8.

[33] Di Lorenzo, G., Federico, P., Buonerba, C., et al. Paclitaxel in pretreated metastatic penile cancer: final results of a phase 2 study. *Eur. Urol.,* 2011; 60:1280 - 1284.

[34] Necchi, A., Nicolai, N., Colecchia, M., et al. Proof of activity of antiepidermal growth factor receptor-targeted therapy for relapsed squamous cell carcinoma of the penis. *J. Clin. Oncol.,* 2011; 29:e650–e652.

[35] Carthon, B. C., Ng, C. S., Pettaway, C. A., Pagliaro, L. C. Epidermal growth factor receptor-targeted therapy in locally advanced or metastatic squamous cell carcinoma of the penis. *BJU Int.,* 2013; 113:871 - 877.

[36] Branney, P., Witty, K., Eardley, I. Patients' experiences of penile cancer. *Eur. Urol.,* 2011; 59:959 - 961.

[37] Kieffer, J. M., Djajadiningrat, R. S., van Muilekom, E. A., et al. Quality of life in patients treated for penile cancer. *J. Urol.,* 2014; 192(4):1105 - 10.

[38] Suarez-Ibarrola, R., Cortes-Telles, A., Miernik, A. health-related quality of life and sexual function in patients treated for penile cancer. *Urol. Int.,* 2018; 101(3): 351 - 57.

[39] Pettaway, C. A., Pagliaro, L., Theodore, C., Haas, G. Treatment of visceral, unresectable, or bulky/unresectable regional metastases of penile cancer. *Urology,* 2010; 76(2 Suppl. 1):S58-65.

In: Penile Cancer: Challenges and Controversies
Editors: F. E. Martins and M. L. Djordjevic
ISBN: 978-1-53615-950-9

Chapter 7

Management of Overt Inguinal Lymph Node (Regional) Disease

Grant Pollock, MD and Juan Chipollini*, MD
Department of Surgery, the University of Arizona College of Medicine, Tucson, Arizona, US

Abstract

Penile cancer is known for its aggressive nature and propensity for loco-regional metastases. It is recognized by its stepwise regional spread to the inguinal and pelvic nodes before progressing to metastatic disease. Thus, extent of lymphatic involvement remains the most important predictor of survival. For patients with clinically-node positive disease that is low-volume and resectable, inguinal node dissection (ILND) becomes an important component in management with potential for long-term survival. Several modifications have been made to reduce morbidity of ILND including limiting extent of dissection and sentinel node biopsy techniques; however, oncologic efficacy should never be compromised. Those with fixed and bulky disease will require a multidisciplinary approach and may be better served with referral to tertiary care center. Although there is limited research on the merits of systemic therapy, it can be effective in select scenarios in order to allow consolidative surgery. Due to the rarity of the disease, controversies in the management of the lymph nodes continue to this day. In this chapter, we present a summary of current recommended treatment strategies for penile cancer patients presenting with lymph node positive disease.

Keywords: inguinal lymph nodes, management, staging, regional disease, minimally invasive approach, sentinel node, predictors, prognostic factors

* Corresponding Author's E-mail: jchipollini@surgery.arizona.edu.

1. Introduction

Treatment of penile cancer (PeCa) has evolved over time with several innovative approaches for the primary tumor becoming widely adopted with no apparent detrimental impact on oncologic outcomes. However, the most important factor for survival remains involvement of the inguinal lymph nodes (LNs). Due to the rarity of PeCa, high level evidence in the management of the nodes is scarce, with treatment controversies and non-guideline care still prevalent in the United States. In this chapter, we discuss management strategies for regional LN involvement and the impact of inguinal lymph node dissection (ILND) on oncological outcomes for PeCa patients.

2. Prevalence and Pathophysiology of Lymph Node Metastases in Penile Cancer

While PeCa has several established prognostic factors, involvement of the regional LNs remains the most significant factor for survival [1]. Penile cancer is recognized by its stepwise regional spread from primary tumor to the inguinal and pelvic nodes before progression to systemic disease [2]. For patients presenting without clinical node involvement (cN0), the likelihood of micrometastatic disease approaches 25% [1]. All patients with a penile tumor require a thorough assessment of the inguinal nodes. A clinical exam should assess for palpability, size, mobility, laterality, and any degree of fixation. Imaging with Computer Tomography (CT) or Magnetic Resonance Imaging (MRI) is another option for those with difficult physical exam due to obesity or previous inguinal surgery. Those confirmed with pathologically N0 disease can expect excellent disease specific survival, approaching 100% at 3 years in one prospective study [3]. Yet even removing micro-metastatic disease significantly improves survival rather than waiting for nodal to disease to occur [4-6]. Thus, appropriate surgical management of the LNs can have a significant impact for early loco- regional control while able to cure a good proportion patients with low volume nodal disease.

Current recommendations for clinically palpable (cN+) disease includes invasive LN staging with either ILND or percutaneous biopsy if low-risk primary lesion [7]. Patients with clinically bulky disease should receive neoadjuvant chemotherapy prior to surgical consolidation (Figure 1). A course of antibiotics and reassessment of the LNs prior to ILND is no longer recommended in cases of non-infected groins. Historically, prophylactic ILND has demonstrated a survival benefit in patients with intermediate to high risk tumors (pT1b, T2-T4), as the presence of lymph node invasion has been found to be as high as 49% [8]. However, subjecting all patients to radical ILND carries considerable risk of long term complications and morbidity. Given the low incidence of

PeCa, which limits patient enrollment in prospective studies, controversies on the optimal management of the LNs continue to this day.

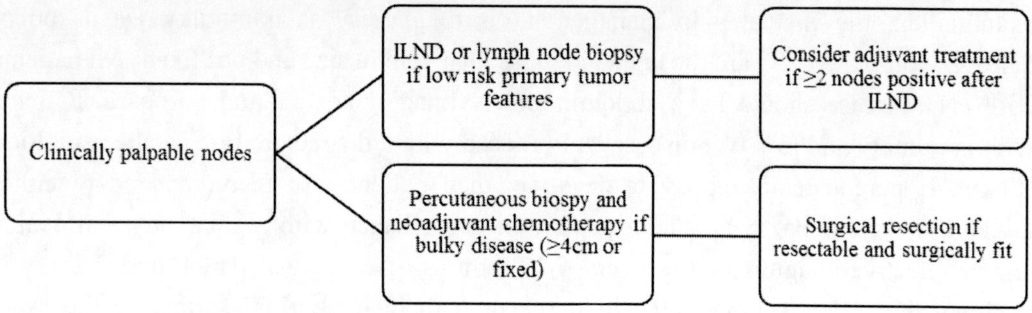

ILND: Inguinal lymph node dissection.

Figure 1. Management of palpable nodes in PeCa patients.

3. Management of Regional Disease

Following a careful physical exam, along with radiographic studies of the inguinal region, nodal disease is stratified into non-palpable and palpable disease. In patients with clinically, low-stage disease (Tis, Ta, or T1a) and no palpable adenopathy, current guidelines recommend surveillance of bilateral inguinal regions with regular physical examinations. Regular physical exams are recommended at 6 to 12 month intervals. If a patient's inguinal region is not able to be adequately assessed by physical exam due to prior surgery and/or radiation exposure, or due to obesity or body habitus, then imaging studies, either CT, MRI, or ultrasound, should be performed. One alternative in these low risk patients is to proceed to dynamic sentinel lymph node biopsy (DSNB). This treatment should only be performed in centers with appropriate surgical expertise to perform the procedure [9]. The sentinel node concept is based on the relatively consistent physiology of penile lymphatic drainage. Lymphatic drainage first passes into a sentinel node before disseminating to other nodes in the lymph node chain. A negative sentinel lymph node biopsy suggests the absence of further lymphatic spread, therefore making lymphadenectomy unnecessary [8-10]. A meta-analysis of 19 studies found 88% sensitivity and 90% specificity of the procedure [11]. Patients with intermediate to high risk disease (clinical stage T1b or higher) and negative adenopathy should proceed to bilateral modified ILND [12, 13]. If any positive nodal disease is encountered on superficial node dissection, then it is recommended to proceed to a radical procedure. It may be reasonable in the select patient with high risk disease and no palpable adenopathy to proceed with bilateral DSLNB. Regardless of the modality of treatment that is chosen, delaying lymphatic staging for greater than 3 months may be associated with worse outcomes [14].

3.1. Palpable (Non-Bulky) Nodes

Upon encountering a patient with palpable lymphadenopathy on physical examination, the first step in management is to classify as non-bulky versus bulky disease. Non-bulky LNs are those that are less than 4cm in size and not fixed. All patients with cN+ disease should have abdominopelvic imaging for staging purposes. Patients with non-bulky and low-risk disease can proceed with a diagnostic fine needle aspiration (FNA). If percutaneous biopsy is negative, then patients are recommended to either undergo an excisional lymph node biopsy or surveillance with regular physical exams and/or selective imaging studies every 6-12 months. If excisional lymph node biopsy is positive, then it is recommended to proceed to therapeutic ILND either in the same setting or shortly thereafter. Likewise if FNA is positive, then patients should undergo ipsilateral superficial and deep ILND and contralateral superficial ILND. Patients with intermediate to high risk primary lesions and palpable, bilateral adenopathy should proceed directly to bilateral superficial and deep ILND.

3.2. Bulky and/or Fixed Nodes

Bulky nodal disease is defined as greater than 4cm or a fixed nodal mass. When decided on the appropriate treatment modality in a patient with bulky disease, it is important to establish a definitive tissue diagnosis before proceeding to treatment. Upfront palliative excision can be performed in select patients that are symptomatic (pain, bleeding, skin breakdown), if deemed resectable. In more advanced stages, a multimodal approach with neoadjuvant chemotherapy (with or without radiotherapy) followed by surgery is the mainstay treatment although there is substantial lack of high-level evidence to this date.

Patients with mobile, unilateral bulky adenopathy can proceed to percutaneous LN biopsy with FNA. If FNA is negative, then an excisional biopsy should be performed. If either FNA or excisional biopsy is positive, then patients should undergo neoadjuvant chemotherapy followed by ILND. If 2 or more nodes are positive, then an ipsilateral pelvic lymph node dissection (PLND) should be performed [1, 12]. Further discussion of PLND can be found later in this chapter. Patients with fixed inguinal nodes, nodes ≥4 cm and patients with disease extending into neighboring structures like symphysis pubis and perineum should be offered systemic therapy with the goal of allowing surgical consolidation if fit to undergo surgery. Those with no evidence of response could be candidates for subsequent-line systemic or radiotherapy for local control. At the present time, no proven second-line systemic therapy exists, and patients should be considered for enrollment in clinical trials.

3.3. Chemotherapy and Radiation Therapy

Cisplatin-based chemotherapy regimens are effective first line agents for patients with positive nodal disease and advanced penile cancer. Combination therapy with paclitaxel, ifosfamide, and cisplatin (TIP) is the first line treatment regimen with reportedly significant response rates. TIP is generally well-tolerated and is the only regimen evaluated in a prospective study [15]. Objective response rate is approximately 50% with 73% of men able to undergo lymph node dissection following neoadjuvant treatment. Cisplatin and 5-fluorouracil had historically been used in the treatment of metastatic penile cancer and can be considered as an alternative to TIP [16]. This regimen does appear to be effective for some patients, although the toxicities may be limiting and may require dose reductions. Bleomycin containing regimens are associated with unacceptable toxicity and are no longer recommended [17]. There are no standard second-line therapy options for advanced PeCa although single-agent paclitaxel has shown moderate response in this setting [18]. Unfortunately, due to the low incidence of penile cancer, no large studies have been reported concerning chemotherapy in the metastatic setting. Alternatively, radiation therapy can be considered in patients with bulky nodal disease. It has been shown beneficial as neoadjuvant, adjuvant, or palliative therapy while improving loco-regional control [19].

Due to the rarity of the disease, studies are few for patients with loco-regional PeCa. No randomized studies exist on current merits of both neoadjuvant and adjuvant systemic therapies. In order to garner more evidence, the International Rare Cancer Initiative has recently opened the International Penile Advanced Cancer Trial (InPACT) (NCT02305654). InPACT is a multinational, multidisciplinary collaboration which plans on recruiting 400 patients (200 from the UK and 200 from USA and Europe) with locally-advanced disease over a five year period [20]. Patients will be randomized in three arms: 1. ILND with no neoadjuvant treatment, 2. neoadjuvant chemotherapy followed by ILND, or 3. neoadjuvant chemoradiotherapy followed by ILND. Additionally, the study will examine whether prophylactic PLND can improve outcomes in men at high risk of recurrence. Results from InPACT will address some of the current controversies in regional lymph node surgery for PeCa, along with clarifying the optimal timing for systemic therapies in the neoadjuvant or adjuvant settings.

4. Surgical Management of the Inguinal Lymph Nodes

ILND has traditionally been known as a technically demanding procedure with high complication rates. However, there is evidence to support cure in patients with limited inguinal metastasis. Although the timing of ILND is controversial, most contemporary series demonstrate improved outcomes for early versus delayed surgical intervention

[5, 21]. Awaiting for antibiotic therapy to reassess the groins is no longer recommended unless evidence of infection is present in which culture-specific treatment should precede ILND.

4.1. Surgical Approach

Methods to minimize complications have included limiting dissection techniques. In 1988, Catalona introduced the modified LND by reducing dissection lateral to the femoral vessels and caudal to the fossa ovalis while preserving the saphenous veins [13]. Over time, other modifications have added a shorter incision and avoidance of Sartorius muscle transposition [22]. Although this dissection is appealing for cN0 patients in which the risks of surgery may outweigh the benefits, a radical ILND is still recommended in the presence of inguinal disease.

The most common types of incisions reported in the literature have been the horizontal versus "S" or "T"-type incisions, although the former has been the most commonly used by centers of excellence due to its lower risk of skin necrosis [3, 22]. There is little reported on the ideal number of LNs removed at the time of ILND although a registry study reported a yield >15 as an independent predictor of survival [23]. Nonetheless, a good understanding of the surgical anatomy is necessary and referral to centers with experience with inguinal surgery is recommended.

Typically, patients are placed in the frog-leg position and prophylactic antibiotic coverage is given within 30 minutes prior to incision. A 10-cm parallel incision below the inguinal ligament is enough to gain exposure to the superficial inguinal nodes. The skin flaps should not be too thin and should have a good amount of subcutaneous tissues above Camper's fascia to keep vascularization of the flaps and minimize risks of wound ischemia and dehiscence [12, 24]. Skin hooks can also be used to handle the flaps with minimal disturbance of subcutaneous tissues. Careful ligation is necessary to decrease risk of leaks and seroma. Metallic clips should be used throughout dissection to control perforating blood vessels and lymphatic channels. Self-sustaining retractors can be used to maintain exposure to the surgical field.

Dissection should be carried to the level of the external oblique fascia and external ring, and proceed superiorly to the edge of the skin flaps as well as distally to the edge of the template. Intraoperative frozen section has been shown to have diagnostic value in determining the need to proceed to a radical dissection [25]. It may be time-saving to proceed to the contralateral dissection while awaiting frozen section results. To harvest the deep nodes, the fascia lata is entered at the level of the fossa ovalis. The deep nodes are typically no more than 3 to 5 LNs contained within the femoral sheath. The node of Cloquet is the most proximal and considered the margin between the inguinal and pelvic LNs.

4.2. Post-Operative Care

If a myocutanenous flap is needed for coverage of the femoral vessels after radical ILND, a period of rest is advisable 48-72hr [12]. Compressive devices have been studied in other cancer types for lymphedema reduction although no studies have been performed specifically for PeCa patients. At the minimum, sequential compressive devices may help with early lymphedema and decreased the risk of thromboembolic complications. Perioperative low-dose heparin for can also be used, although it might increase lymphatic leakage [24]. Closed suction drains are left until drainage is 30 to 50 mL per day [26]. By doing so, fluid accumulation can be prevented and result in early adhesions between skin flaps and underlying fascia and muscle [27].

4.3. Complications

The majority of the ILND-related complications are secondary to infections, wound healing, and lymphedema, with the latter two shown to be decreasing over time [12, 28]. With hopes of decreasing complications, trends in operative management have resulted in more limited dissection. Surgical morbidity remains a significant concern for those requiring more extensive dissections and some of these complications can result in long-term disability. Table 1 contains a list of common complications from contemporary series of patients undergoing ILND. Meticulous technique, avoidance of infection, and inguinal reconstruction with myocutaneous flaps for coverage of larger defects can help with tissue vascularization and wound healing in most cases.

Table 1. Contemporary reports of post-operative morbidity after ILND

First author	Year	Country	Number of patients	Complication rate	Most common complications
Gopman, et al. [29]	2015	United States, Netherlands, China, Germany	327	55.4%	Infection, seroma, dehiscence, lymphocele, necrosis, scrotal edema
Koifman, et al. [28]	2013	Brazil	170	10.3%	Lymphedema, seroma
Stuvier, et al. [30]	2013	Netherlands	163	58%	Infection, seroma, necrosis
Yao, et al. [31]	2010	China	75	24.7%	Infection, necrosis, lymphedema, seroma, lymphocele
Spiess, et al. [12]	2008	United States	43	49%	Lymphedema, wound dehiscence, infection

4.4. Pelvic Lymph Node Dissection

Prophylactic PLND is indicated if 2 or more LNs are found to be positive and can be performed either in the same setting as ILND or in a delayed fashion [32]. PLND can be also be performed in the presence of inguinal LN metastasis of greater than 3cm in diameter or extranodal extension [32, 33]. A bilateral dissection could be considered if 4 or more inguinal LNs are found to harbor disease (Figure 2) [34]. One study of 102 patients found those with 1 or 2 positive LNs without extracapsular growth and no poorly differentiated tumors had a low risk for pelvic nodal involvement with 5 year survival rates at approximately 90% [35].

In cases of pelvic adenopathy on imaging studies; patients could have percutaneous biopsy to evaluate if metastasis is indeed present before proceeding with any definitive management. If biopsy is negative, then the provider should proceed with management of the inguinal nodes as outlined previously in the chapter. If percutaneous biopsy is positive, and nodes are potentially resectable, then the patient should undergo a course of neoadjuvant chemotherapy followed by repeat imaging. If stable disease or clinical response, then PLND should be performed. In patients who are not surgical candidates, or patients who have evidence of disease progression following neoadjuvant therapy, second-line systemic with or without radiation therapy and/or a clinical trial should be considered.

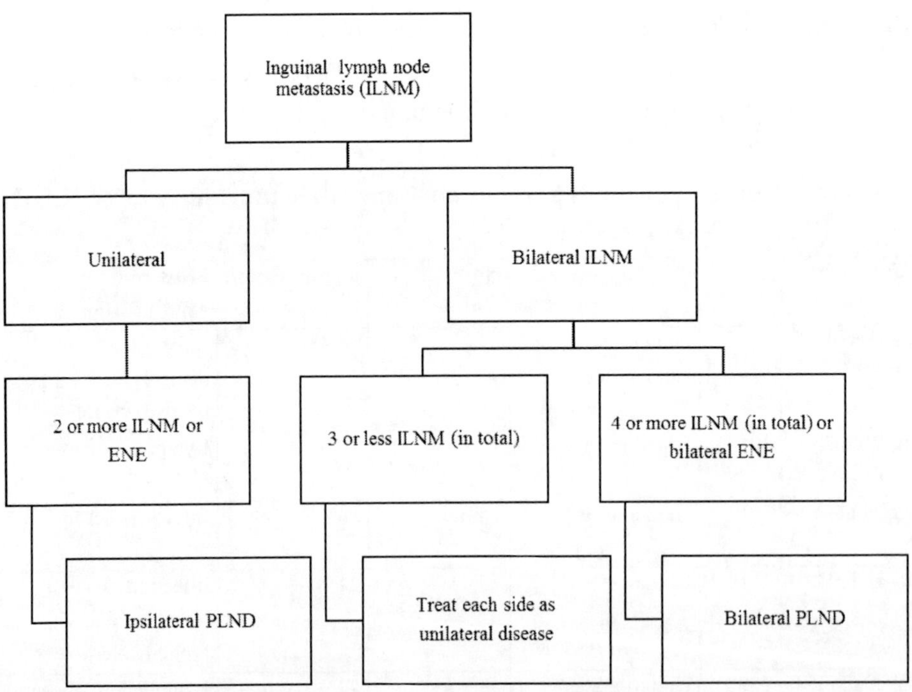

ENE: Extranodal extension; PLND: Pelvic lymph node dissection.

Figure 2. Algorithm for inguinal lymph node metastasis.

CONCLUSION

Penile cancer is an aggressive disease with a paucity of data limiting evidence-based recommendations. Prompt and meticulous lymphadenectomy can be curative in patients with low-volume regional disease. In higher-volume or locally-advanced cases, a multidisciplinary approach can optimize outcomes; thus, referral to centers of experience with penile cancer is highly recommended. Patient enrollment in prospective studies continues to be a priority for this rare malignancy.

KEY POINTS

- A complete and thorough evaluation of the inguinal lymph nodes is fundamental for penile cancer survival.
- Inguinal lymph node dissection (ILND) is a significant component is treatment strategies with potential for long-term survival.
- Traditionally, ILND has carried significant patient morbidity but various modifications and techniques have been described in the literature in order to improve post-operative outcomes.
- Current recommendations are for systemic therapy for men with advanced nodal disease prior to consolidative surgery, if clinical response.
- Multidisciplinary approaches can be effective in select clinical scenarios, but few therapeutic options exist for chemotherapy-resistant disease.

REFERENCES

[1] Hakenberg OW, Comperat EM, Minhas S, et al. EAU guidelines on penile cancer: 2014 update. *Eur Urol* 67:142-50, 2015.

[2] Zhu Y, Ye DW: Lymph node metastases and prognosis in penile cancer. *Chin J Cancer Res* 24:90-6, 2012.

[3] Hegarty PK, Dinney CP, Pettaway CA: Controversies in ilioinguinal lymphadenectomy. *Urol Clin North Am* 37:421-34, 2010.

[4] McDougal WS: Carcinoma of the penis: improved survival by early regional lymphadenectomy based on the histological grade and depth of invasion of the primary lesion. *J Urol* 154:1364-6, 1995.

[5] Kroon BK, Horenblas S, Lont AP, et al. Patients with penile carcinoma benefit from immediate resection of clinically occult lymph node metastases. *J Urol* 173:816-9, 2005.

[6] Lont AP, Horenblas S, Tanis PJ, et al. Management of clinically node negative penile carcinoma: improved survival after the introduction of dynamic sentinel node biopsy. *J Urol* 170:783-6, 2003.

[7] Clark PE, Spiess PE, Agarwal N, et al. Penile cancer: Clinical Practice Guidelines in Oncology. *J Natl Compr Canc Netw* 11:594-615, 2013.

[8] O'Brien JS, Perera M, Manning T, et al. Penile Cancer: Contemporary Lymph Node Management. *J Urol* 197:1387-1395, 2017.

[9] Leijte JA, Kroon BK, Valdes Olmos RA, et al. Reliability and safety of current dynamic sentinel node biopsy for penile carcinoma. *Eur Urol* 52:170-7, 2007.

[10] Leijte JA, Hughes B, Graafland NM, et al. Two-center evaluation of dynamic sentinel node biopsy for squamous cell carcinoma of the penis. *J Clin Oncol* 27:3325-9, 2009.

[11] Sadeghi R, Gholami H, Zakavi SR, et al. Accuracy of sentinel lymph node biopsy for inguinal lymph node staging of penile squamous cell carcinoma: systematic review and meta-analysis of the literature. *J Urol* 187:25-31, 2012.

[12] Spiess PE, Hernandez MS, Pettaway CA: Contemporary inguinal lymph node dissection: minimizing complications. *World J Urol* 27:205-12, 2009.

[13] Catalona WJ: Modified inguinal lymphadenectomy for carcinoma of the penis with preservation of saphenous veins: technique and preliminary results. *J Urol* 140:306-10, 1988.

[14] Chipollini J, Tang DH, Gilbert SM, et al. Delay to Inguinal Lymph Node Dissection Greater than 3 Months Predicts Poorer Recurrence-Free Survival for Patients with Penile Cancer. *J Urol* 198:1346-1352, 2017.

[15] Pagliaro LC, Williams DL, Daliani D, et al. Neoadjuvant paclitaxel, ifosfamide, and cisplatin chemotherapy for metastatic penile cancer: a phase II study. *J Clin Oncol* 28:3851-7, 2010.

[16] Di Lorenzo G, Buonerba C, Federico P, et al. Cisplatin and 5-fluorouracil in inoperable, stage IV squamous cell carcinoma of the penis. *BJU Int* 110:E661-6, 2012.

[17] Haas GP, Blumenstein BA, Gagliano RG, et al. Cisplatin, methotrexate and bleomycin for the treatment of carcinoma of the penis: a Southwest Oncology Group study. *J Urol* 161:1823-5, 1999.

[18] Di Lorenzo G, Federico P, Buonerba C, et al. Paclitaxel in pretreated metastatic penile cancer: final results of a phase 2 study. *Eur Urol* 60:1280-4, 2011.

[19] Ravi R, Chaturvedi HK, Sastry DV: Role of radiation therapy in the treatment of carcinoma of the penis. *Br J Urol* 74:646-51, 1994.

[20] *The Institute of Cancer Research*. https://www.icr.ac.uk/our-research/centres-and-collaborations/ centres-at-the-icr/ clinical-trials-and-statistics-unit/ clinical-trials/ inpact. Accessed 02/20/2019.

[21] Leijte JA, Kirrander P, Antonini N, et al. Recurrence patterns of squamous cell carcinoma of the penis: recommendations for follow-up based on a two-centre analysis of 700 patients. *Eur Urol* 54:161-8, 2008.

[22] Leone A, Diorio GJ, Pettaway C, et al. Contemporary management of patients with penile cancer and lymph node metastasis. *Nature Reviews Urology* 14:335, 2017.

[23] Soodana-Prakash N, Koru-Sengul T, Miao F, et al. Lymph node yield as a predictor of overall survival following inguinal lymphadenectomy for penile cancer. *Urol Oncol* 36:471.e19-471.e27, 2018.

[24] Heyns CF, Fleshner N, Sangar V, et al. Management of the lymph nodes in penile cancer. *Urology* 76:S43-57, 2010.

[25] Chipollini J, Tang DH, Manimala N, et al. Evaluating the accuracy of intraoperative frozen section during inguinal lymph node dissection in penile cancer. *Urol Oncol* 36:14.e1-14.e5, 2018.

[26] Chipollini J, Garcia-Castaneda J, Rosa AH, et al. Important surgical concepts and techniques in inguinal lymph node dissection. *Curr Opin Urol*, 2019.

[27] Azizi M, Chipollini J, Peyton CC, et al. Current controversies and developments on the role of lymphadenectomy for penile cancer. *Urol Oncol*, 2018.

[28] Koifman L, Hampl D, Koifman N, et al. Radical open inguinal lymphadenectomy for penile carcinoma: surgical technique, early complications and late outcomes. *J Urol* 190:2086-92, 2013.

[29] Gopman JM, Djajadiningrat RS, Baumgarten AS, et al. Predicting postoperative complications of inguinal lymph node dissection for penile cancer in an international multicentre cohort. *BJU Int 116*:196-201, 2015.

[30] Stuiver MM, Djajadiningrat RS, Graafland NM, et al. Early wound complications after inguinal lymphadenectomy in penile cancer: a historical cohort study and risk-factor analysis. *Eur Urol 64*:486-92, 2013.

[31] Yao K, Tu H, Li YH, et al. Modified technique of radical inguinal lymphadenectomy for penile carcinoma: morbidity and outcome. *J Urol* 184:546-52, 2010.

[32] Djajadiningrat RS, van Werkhoven E, Horenblas S: Prophylactic pelvic lymph node dissection in patients with penile cancer. *J Urol* 193:1976-80, 2015.

[33] Lughezzani G, Catanzaro M, Torelli T, et al. The relationship between characteristics of inguinal lymph nodes and pelvic lymph node involvement in penile squamous cell carcinoma: a single institution experience. *J Urol* 191:977-82, 2014.

[34] Zargar-Shoshtari K, Djajadiningrat R, Sharma P, et al. Establishing Criteria for Bilateral Pelvic Lymph Node Dissection in the Management of Penile Cancer: Lessons Learned from an International Multicenter Collaboration. *J Urol* 194:696-701, 2015.

[35] Lont AP, Kroon BK, Gallee MP, et al. Pelvic lymph node dissection for penile carcinoma: extent of inguinal lymph node involvement as an indicator for pelvic lymph node involvement and survival. *J Urol* 177:947-52; discussion 952, 2007.

Section C. Non-Surgical Management of Penile Cancer

In: Penile Cancer: Challenges and Controversies
Editors: F. E. Martins and M. L. Djordjevic ISBN: 978-1-53615-950-9

Chapter 8

ROLE OF RADIOTHERAPY FOR PENILE CANCER

Marina Marban, MD and Juanita Crook*, MD
Department of Radiation Oncology, University of British Columbia,
BC Cancer Center for the Southern Interior, Kelowna, BC, Canada

ABSTRACT

The most common malignancy diagnosed in the penis is Squamous Cell Cancer (SCC), which is both radiosensitive and radiocurable. Other SCC sites such as cervix, head and neck, vulva and anal canal demonstrate excellent results with either radiotherapy alone or combined with sensitizing chemotherapy such as cisplatinum. Radiotherapy can thus have an important role in all stages and presentations of penile cancer. In localized disease, radiotherapy, either in the form of brachytherapy or external beam provides potentially curative treatment while preserving penile morphology and function. Penile preservation rates at 10 years after brachytherapy are in the neighbourhood of 70%. In loco-regionally advanced cases, external radiotherapy can be part of a (neo)adjuvant treatment approach with or without chemotherapy, especially in management of malignant adenopathy. Optimal sequencing with surgery is under investigation. In metastatic disease, a short course of palliative radiotherapy can help to manage symptoms such as pain or bleeding.

Keywords: penile cancer, radiotherapy, brachytherapy

* Corresponding Author's E-mail: jcrook@bccancer.bc.ca.

1. INTRODUCTION

The most common malignancy diagnosed in the penis is Squamous Cell Cancer (SCC), which is radiosensitive and radiocurable. Other SCC sites such as cancer of the cervix, head and neck, vulva and anal canal demonstrate excellent results with either radiotherapy alone or combined with sensitizing chemotherapy such as cisplatinum. Radiotherapy potentially can thus have an important role in all stages and presentations of penile cancer, as a radical/curative approach for localized disease, definitively in locally advanced cases, and can be part of a (neo)adjuvant treatment approach with or without chemotherapy.

In metastatic disease, radiotherapy can help to manage symptoms such as pain or bleeding.

2. RADIOTHERAPY FOR LOCALIZED DISEASE

Radiation treatment can be delivered as either traditional external beam radiation (EBRT) or from within the tumor as brachytherapy (BT). One of the main advantages of radiotherapy is the possibility of a definitive penile-sparing approach with manageable acute side effects. Late side effects can be kept to an acceptable level by experienced practitioners using optimal technique, as several series reveal. Penile cancer and its treatment are notorious for their impact on quality of life and sexual identity, leading even to an increased suicide risk associated with penectomy [1-3].

Localized disease includes tumors staged I or IIA [4]:

Stage I: T1a N0 M0

- T1a: Tumor invades subepithelial connective tissue without lymphovascular invasion or perineural invasion and is not high grade (G3 or sarcomatoid)

Stage IIA: T1b and T2 N0 M0

- T1b: Tumor invades subepithelial connective tissue and has lymphovascular invasion and/or perineural invasion or is high grade (G3 or sarcomatoid)
- T2: Tumor invades into corpus spongiosum (either glans or ventral shaft) with or without urethral invasion

According to the NCCN staging (2018) and TNM 8th edition, invasion of the corpora cavernosum is considered T3 and invasion of adjacent structures, T4. Involved lymph nodes are the strongest negative prognostic indicator and their presence dictates a much more aggressive approach but this does not necessarily preclude penile sparing in cases with a low volume primary tumour.

2.1. External Beam Radiotherapy (EBRT)

2.1.1. Indications

EBRT is normally considered when brachytherapy is not available, is not appropriate as in the very elderly or debilitated patient, or in case of locoregionally advanced disease where pelvic nodes will be also treated. EBRT has the advantage of being widely available and does not require any special expertise beyond that expected of a Radiation Oncologist.

2.1.2. Positioning

Patients positioned for EBRT for penile cancer will generally lie supine with arms on the chest. The penis must be positioned such that it can be accessed by the radiation beam while adjacent normal tissue is avoided. This can be challenging, given the anatomy and the fact that SCC originates on the skin, and full dose has to be delivered to the skin surface.

The recommended approach involves using a bivalved block of tissue-equivalent material with a central cylindrical cavity to position the penis vertically. Tissue-equivalent material provides the required electron build-up for mega voltage beams to deliver full dose to the skin while the lead sheet protects adjacent tissues from scattered radiation. If additional testicular protection is required, commercially available lead "clam shell" testicular shields can be used.

Although wax was used in the past to fabricate the block, verification of the penile position through the opaque wax was problematic. Transparent Plexiglas or Lucite are preferred materials which ensure visualization and reproducibility of set-up. 3D printers can also be used to design custom moulds. Different size blocks should be available in the radiotherapy department to accommodate a change in target volume in case of tumor shrinkage or penile edema. It is also important to ensure that the air space within the block beyond the glans is filled with tissue-equivalent material (bolus) to ensure adequate dose at the tip of the penis.

2.1.3. Volume Delimitation and Planning

The Gross Tumor Volume (GTV) is the clinically identifiable disease by physical examination and imaging. The Clinical Target Volume (CTV) adds a 1-cm margin for uncertainty in clinical exam and possibility of microscopic spread. The Planning Target Volume (PTV) adds a further 1-cm margin to the CTV (or 2 cm to the GTV) to account for set-up error and beam penumbra. However, the whole penile shaft may need to be included in the treatment volume in cases with difficult set up or short penile length.

Usually 4-6MV photons arranged as parallel-opposed fields are used. For tumor in situ (Tis), electrons can be considered, using 6MeV energy. In that case the treatment volume will include GTV plus a 2-cm margin circumferential margin, and the required depth will be covered by the 90% isodose line with 100% at the skin surface by using a layer of bolus material such as Superflab. SCC-in situ can also be treated by alternative modalities such as laser surgery or topical 5-FU or Imiquimod [5, 6].

2.1.4. Dose and Fractionation

When mega voltage beams are used and the full thickness of the penis is treated, a total dose of 66 to 70 Gy to CTV, using a standard fractionation of 2 Gy/fraction is recommended. If the set-up is secure, a 2 cm margin is sufficient but non-affected shaft can be treated to a lower dose of 45-50.4 Gy [7, 8].

Sarin et al. [1] performed a subset analysis of 44 patients with T1 SCC of the penis treated with EBRT. They reported a relationship between lower biological equivalent dose (BED < 60 Gy), fraction size < 2Gy and treatment time over 45 days, all associated with increased risk of local recurrence, statistically significant in the case of BED ($p = 0.05$) even with the relatively small patient numbers.

For Tis treated with superficial electron treatment, 35 Gy in 5 Gy fractions can be prescribed (9).

2.1.5. Results

Average local control and penile preservation rate with EBRT for T1–T2 tumors at 5-years is 62% (41-70%) and for T3–T4 tumors is lower at 40%. Most isolated local failures can be salvaged surgically with either partial or total penectomy. For this reason continued close follow up is necessary.

Patients with locally advanced T3-T4 disease are often elderly at presentation with comorbidities and superimposed infection and may be served better by an amputation rather than a prolonged course of radiotherapy, which may require hospitalization. If their condition warrants more aggressive treatment, chemoradiotherapy to the primary and the nodes will not only give excellent palliation but is potentially curative.

Results from selected studies are shown in Table 1 [1,7–14].

2.1.6. Side Effects

Local skin reaction will appear during the second or third week of external beam treatment, healing gradually over the subsequent 3-6 weeks. Frequent soaks in baking soda and water ensure cleanliness, and flamazine will prevent infection. Healing takes longer in diabetics and the elderly, or if there is co-existing infection. Meatal stenosis is reported in up to 29% (median 14%) and necrosis rarely (1%-8%).

Table 1. Selected series for external beam radiotherapy:

Author, year	N	F/U (mo)	Dose (Gy)	Fractions	CSS (%)	LC (%)	Toxicity	Penile preservation %
Neave et al(10), 1993	20	36+	50-55	20-22	58	70	stenosis 10%	-
McLean et al(9), 1993	26	116	35 or 60	10 or 25	69	62	27% (un specified)	100
Ravi et al(11), 1994	128	83	50-60	-	-	65	necrosis 6% stenosis 34%	-
Sarin et at(1), 1997	59	62	50-60	-	66	59	necrosis 3% stenosis 14%	55
Gotsadze et al(12), 2000	155	40	40-60	-	88	65	necrosis 1% stenosis 7%	65
Zouhair et al(7), 2001	23	70	45-74	25-37	-	57	stenosis 10%	36
Ozsahin et al(13), 2006	33	62	52	-	53	44	stenosis 10%	52
Azrif et al(14), 2006	41	54	50-52	16	96	62	necrosis 8% stenosis 29%	62
Mistry et al(8), 2007	18	62	50 or 55	20 or 16	85	63	necrosis11% stenosis 6%	66

N, number of patients included in study cohort; F/U, follow-up; mo, months; Gy, Gray; CSS, cause specific survival; LC, local control

2.2. Brachytherapy

Brachytherapy is a form of radiation applied as either a surface applicator or interstitially from within the tumor, lowering the dose to adjacent tissue and achieving a higher internal dose compared to EBRT. Given its location and anatomy, penile cancer is ideally suited to brachytherapy. There are 3 different forms of interstitial brachytherapy, differentiated by their dose rate, which depends on the activity of the radioactive source. Low Dose Rate (LDR) Brachytherapy is given as a continuous treatment over 4-6 days. Pulsed Dose Rate (PDR) Brachytherapy uses a high-activity source to deliver an equivalent dose in interrupted hourly fractions over the same overall time interval in order to imitate LDR radiobiology. Finally High Dose Rate (HDR) Brachytherapy is administered in larger fractions, usually twice daily, separated by at least 6-8 hours, using a high activity source that steps through a scaffolding of catheters in the target area. Both the dwell time and dwell positions of the source can be modified to achieve the desired dose distribution.

2.2.1. Indications

Given the impact on quality of life that mutilating surgery can have, treatment options that offer an opportunity for organ preservation should be discussed.

Brachytherapy is indicated in T1 or T2 tumors, less than 4 cm in diameter and confined to the glans. Those patients presenting with tumor extension across the coronal sulcus may still be candidates for brachytherapy if the volume can be well covered with a single additional plane of needles (15).Larger lesions can be treated, but entail a higher risk of local side effects. Tumor volume is not predictive for local failure (LF) after brachytherapy (16,17) although larger lesions (≥T2, $\geq 22cm^3$) are associated with a higher risk of post treatment ulceration and necrosis [15,16,18]. T3 tumors with extension into the penile urethra won't usually be candidates for brachytherapy. If urethroscopy confirms absence of mucosal disruption they may still be treated successfully, albeit with an increased risk of urethral stenosis.

Tumor grade is not an exclusion factor for brachytherapy as demonstrated by Crook et al. [19], although it does determine management of the inguinal nodes [20]. The combination of brachytherapy for the primary tumor and groin staging by inguinal node dissection or sentinel lymph node evaluation is a reasonable option. The risk of micrometastases reaches 25% even in some cN0 patients with high grade tumors.

It is mandatory to perform a nodal evaluation for high grade T1, and for stage T2 or higher, and when there are clinically suspicious nodes on examination or imaging. Ficarra et al. [21] examined a cohort of 175 patients who underwent total penectomy. 18% were T1 or Tis, 59% T2, and 22% T3-4. 115 patients were cN0 and 60 cN+. Eighty-one patients received groin treatment (72 lymphadenectomy). They proposed two different predictive models, one based on the pathological features of the primary and the groin clinical staging, and the other considering also the nodal pathology. Clinical node staging was borderline predictive of 5-year cause specific survival (CSS) ($p = 0.08$) whereas in the second model the pathological staging was the strongest predictive factor ($p = 0.003$). 94 patients didn´t undergo lymphadenectomy. Of those, 85 were cN0 of which 18 had nodal progression within 24 months of the penectomy.

Correa et al. [22] also looked at the importance of nodal status and analyzed a cohort of 2224 patients from the National Cancer Database, 606 of whom underwent inguinal lymphadenectomy. Predictive factors for decreased overall survival included pN1 and high grade disease (HR 1.5), pT3 (HR 1.2) and pT4 (HR 2.3). All parameters were statistically significant at $p < 0.001$.

Delayed lymphadenectomy has also been associated with poorer survival [23]. Chipollini et al. [24] reported on a cohort of 84 consecutive patients who had a 5-year-RFS of 77% and a 5-year CSS of 64% if they underwent early dissection versus 38% and 40% respectively when it was delayed 3 months or more. The European Association of Urologistst (EAU) and National Comprehensive Cancer Network (NCCN) recommend inguinal node dissection for intermediate (T1b G1-2) and high risk (T2 or G3-4) tumors, and recommend pelvic node dissection if 2 or more inguinal nodes are involved [5].

All patients must undergo circumcision prior to any type of radiotherapy. This ensures optimal visualization of the tumor, avoids the risk of subsequent ulceration/

necrosis of the prepuce and also may debulk the tumor. Radiation can begin within 10 days to 2 weeks.

2.2.2. Low Dose and Pulsed Dose Rate Brachytherapy (LDR and PDR)

2.2.2.1. Implant Technique

LDR and PDR brachytherapy are considered together since the radiobiology, technique and duration of treatment are the same. The procedure is performed under general or local anesthesia with sedation. In experienced hands it takes 45 minutes to 1 hour. An indwelling Foley catheter is placed at the beginning of the procedure and remains until the implant is removed. Having a urethral catheter while placing the needles helps to localize the urethra by palpation and avoid transfixing it with the needles.

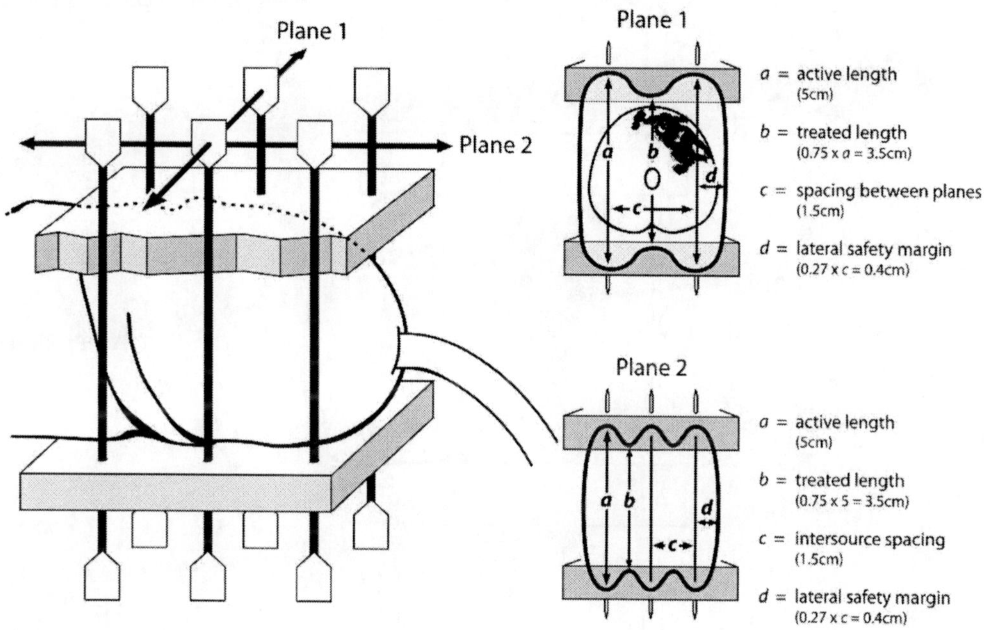

Figure 1. Schematic of a 2-plane, 6-needle implant following the Paris system of dosimetry. With permission from [15].

The tumor (GTV) is defined by inspection and palpation, and a margin of 10 mm in all directions is added to establish the CTV. This is necessary because of the challenge of accurately establishing the depth of invasion. The tumor volume will determine the geometry of the implant, including the number of needles (19.5 gauge for LDR and 17.5 gauge for PDR), their spacing, and the orientation of the planes. Usually 2-3 parallel planes are needed, avoiding the urethra. A single plane implant is not recommended. An appropriate template is chosen with spacing such that the needles cover the disease and avoid the urethra. It is helpful to have an array of 6-hole (2 planes of 3 needles), 9-hole (3 planes of 3 needles) and 12 hole (3 planes of 4 needles) clear Lucite templates to choose from.

Ideal spacing for an LDR implant is 14 to 16 mm, although a range of 12-18 mm is acceptable (15). The Paris system of implant geometry and prescription should be followed, placing the needles parallel and equidistant [25] (Figure 1).

Source strength must be uniform and identical. The lateral margin will be determined by the distance between the needles and is approximately 1/3 of the separation. It is important to be aware of the lateral margin so as not to place needles too deeply (surface will be under dosed) or too shallow (leads to linear ulceration and scarring). In the case of a superficial or asymmetric tumor, an extra plane can be added external to the penis, equidistant from the other planes (Figure 2). A tissue-equivalent material such as Superflab is added between the needles and the skin/tumor for a satisfactory coverage.

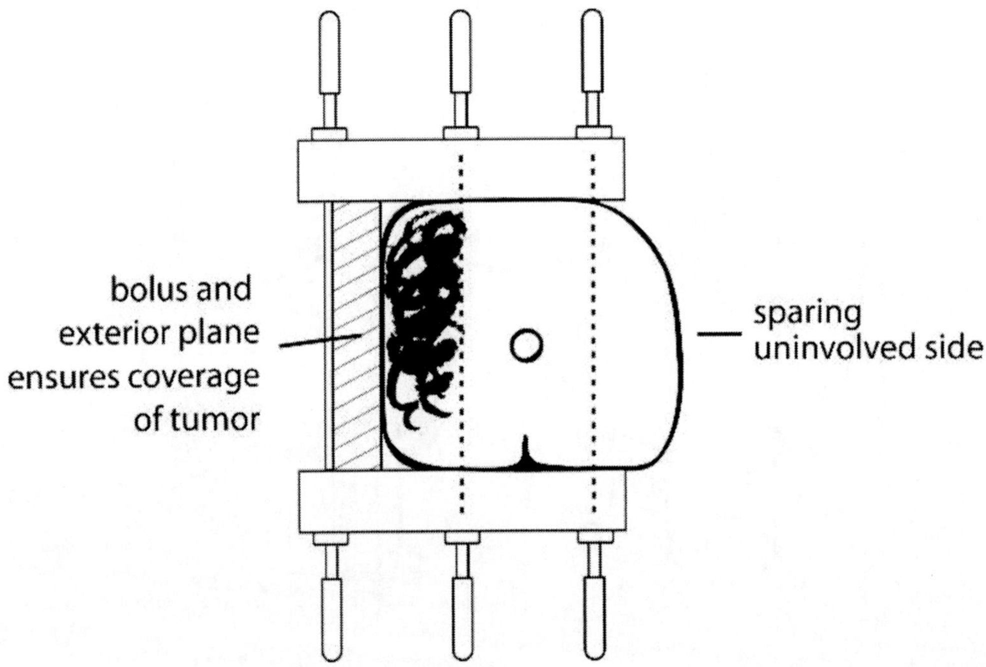

Figure 2. Schematic of implant for unilateral tumor which allows an asymmetric implant with contralateral sparing. With permission from [26].

After securing the implant by tightening the lock nuts on each needle on the external surface of each template, it will be stable during the duration of the treatment. The patient will be able to walk within the room if desired. The dosimetry can be performed based on either computer tomography (CT) imaging or direct measurements of the geometry and spacing of the planes and needles.

The patient is admitted and remains in an isolated room during the 5 days of the treatment. The penis, with the implant in place, will be positioned in a sponge or Styrofoam collar to separate it from the rest of the body. If further reproductive capacity is desired, a thin layer of lead can be placed in the collar. Medication after the implant and during the admission includes analgesia and antithrombotic prophylaxis with low-dose heparin (5000 U every 12 hours) or low-molecular-weight heparin. The penile implant is usually well tolerated but analgesic requirements vary amongst individuals, from plain acetaminophen to regular parenteral morphine. Patients receiving PDR can have their treatment catheters disconnected once a day between the hourly fractions in order to ambulate about the room.

Removal of the implant can take place either in the operating room under sedation or at the bedside with adequate premedication. Bleeding is minimal and can be easily controlled with light compression. The patient is discharged the same day. Post-implant instructions include frequent soaks using baking soda and water. Tolerance is very good, and analgesia is not required. Polysporin or flamazine can be prescribed, At 3 weeks resolution of the tumor will leave a crater corresponding to the depth of invasion which will gradually re-epithelialize over 6-8 weeks. Follow up should be every 4 weeks until healing is complete, then every 3 months for 2 years, every 6 months to 5 years and then annually. 20% of local recurrences can occur after 5 years and the patient should be informed to report any changes promptly.

2.2.2.2. Dose and Fractionation

For LDR brachytherapy, Iridium 192 wire is used with an activity of 1.5 mCi/cm to deliver a total dose of 60-65 Gy at a dose rate of 40-75 cGy/hour over about 5 days. The dose is prescribed at 85% of the basal dose rate as recommended by the Paris system [25] Figure 1. A dose rate higher than 0.6 Gy/h and larger volume implants are related to increased late toxicity [26].

Total dose ≥62Gy is associated with better local control in N0 patients as described by Escande et al. [18] in a cohort of 201 patients.

When a PDR afterloader is used with a high-activity Iridium 192 source, the prescribed dose is the same, 60-65 Gy, with an hourly fraction size of 50-60 cGy/h.

2.2.2.3. Results

There are two series reporting results on LDR brachytherapy with significant numbers and mature follow up. De Crevoisier [16] analysed a cohort of 144 patients with a median follow up of 5.7 years (0.5-29). They reported a penile preservation rate of 72% at 10 years, and local failure rate of 20% at 8 years. Failures were treated with salvage surgery, achieving second complete remission in 86%. 10-year cause-specific survival (CSS) was 92%. This highlights the importance of continued follow up beyond 5 years as local recurrence after brachytherapy can be rescued with salvage surgery, impacting little on overall survival (OS).

Crook et al. [19] reported results on 67 patients treated in two Canadian centers. Median follow-up was 4 years (0.2-16.2). Local control (LC) at 5 years was 87%, and at

10 years 72%. Penile preservation was 88% at 5 years, and 67% at 10 years. 10-year actuarial cause specific survival was 84%.

Hasan et al. (27) performed a meta-analysis of 20 retrospective studies, including 2,178 patients, of whom 1,505 were treated surgically and 673 with brachytherapy. Outcomes were comparable in terms of 5-year OS (76% with surgery, 73% with LDR, $p = 0.128$). Penile preservation rate with brachytherapy was 74%, and 5-year local control rate was 84%. Subset analysis by stage revealed 5-year OS 80% and LC 86% for stage I/II tumours. For stage III/IV, penile preservation rate for brachytherapy was maintained at 74%, with no difference in OS compared to surgery.

The results of selected LDR studies are summarized in Table 2.

Table 2. Results for LDR brachytherapy

Author, year	N	F/U (mo)	Dose (Gy)	CSS	LC	Penile Preservation	Necrosis N (%)	Stenosis N (%)
Mazeron et al.(28), 1984	50	36-96	60-70	79%	78%	74%	3 (6%)	8 (19%)
Delannes et al.(29), 1992	51	12-144	50-65	85%	86%	75%	9 (23%)	21 (45%)
Rozan et al. (30), 1995	184	139	59	88% (10 y)	85% (10y)	76%	21%	45%
Soria et al.(31), 1997	102	11	61-70	66% (10y)	42% (10y)	68%	1	1
Chaudhary et al. (32), 1999	23	24	40-60	-	70%	70%	0	2 (9%)
Kiltie et al. (33), 2000	31	62	64	85%	81%	75%	1 (8%)	11 (44%)
De Crevoisier et al. (16), 2009	144	3-348	65	92% (10y)	80% (10y)	70% (10 yr)	26% (10y)	29% (10 yr)
Crook et al. (19), 2009	67	44-194	60	84%	72% (10y)	67% (10 yr)	16%	12%
Pimenta et al. (34), 2015	25	0-228	60-65	91%	-	86%	0	43%

N, number of patients included in study cohort; F/U, follow-up mean and range; mo, months; Gy, Gray; CSS, cause specific survival; LC, local control; yr, years; OS, overall survival

2.2.2.4. Side Effects

Moist desquamation appears within 2 weeks and can take up to 3-4 months to heal, longer in smokers and diabetics. Management centers on good hygiene including frequent soaks in warm saline or baking soda and water, non-occlusive, non-stick dressings (such as Telfa) that prevent friction, and topical treatments including antibiotics, Flamazine, hydrocortisone and vitamin E. When intercourse is resumed, water-based lubricant is recommended to minimize trauma to the healing area. Long-term cosmesis is generally very good but patchy hypo or hyperpigmentation or telangiectasia can occur. As the disease involutes, the true depth of invasion can be seen in the form of an ulcer 3-4 weeks after the procedure.

The main bothersome long-term side effects include soft tissue ulceration (0-23%), and meatal stenosis (9-45%), depending on the proximity of the tumor to the meatus. Self-dilatation with a meatal dilator is recommended if there is any evidence of early meatal adhesions. Late toxicity increases with doses over 65Gy. Hyperbaric oxygen has been beneficial in those cases where healing is not achieved with other conservative measures [35].

Sexual function is usually maintained, given that the radiation is limited to the glans and does not include the penile shaft. Delaunay et al. [3] reported a series of 21 T1-2 patients treated with exclusive LDR brachytherapy who were offered to complete a sexuality questionnaire. Of the 19 patients that participated (ages 44-89 years), 17 were sexually active before BT and 10 remained so, although all 17 reported erectile function and 13 considered that function to be good.. One patient reported PDE-5 use. 10 patients reported no change in sensitivity of the glans. It's important to note again that the cases for brachytherapy are selected for early disease limited to the glans.

The tolerance and results have been excellent also in an elderly population as analyzed recently by Escande et al. [36]. In this subgroup of patients the rate of meatal stenosis was 22%, pain or ulceration 13%, pain and ulceration 4%, and focal necrosis needing surgery 6%. 5-year OS and local relapse free survival were 75% and 91% respectively.

2.2.3. High Dose Rate Brachytherapy (HDR)

HDR is widely available because of its versatility and advantages in radioprotection. HDR brachytherapy can be used for multiple treatment sites including cervix, breast, skin and prostate. A high intensity (10 Ci) Iridium-192 source is programmed to step through the appropriate applicator (s) delivering the required dose over a few minutes. When used for penile cancer, the treatment is fractionated twice daily. Nursing care between fractions is not an issue as there is no radioactivity present. Data on the use of HDR in penile cancer have been recently emerging. The series are generally small and the follow up relatively short, but the results are promising.

The reported fractionation schemes include 36-54 Gy with twice-daily fractions of 3-3.5 Gray generally over 7 to 9 days. Late toxicities in the form of necrosis or meatal stenosis are reported in 0-9%, and penile preservation in 80-100% (Table 3).

The implant procedure is similar to LDR. Needles or plastic catheters can be used, but must be spaced more closely (range 9-12mm) to minimize inhomogeneity. It is suggested that in order to minimize necrosis or skin ulceration, the skin dose should be limited to 125% of the prescription, and homogeneity parameters strictly observed such that the $V125 < 40\%$, $V150 < 20\%$ and $V200 < 5\%$. Spacing between needles can be varied as necessary, for needles bracketing the urethra up to 12 mm and 9-10 mm elsewhere (Figure 3). If the spacing is close enough, optimization through adjustment of dwell times should not be difficult. Planning is done through CT imaging and contouring of the GTV. The recommended CTV margin is 1cm.

Table 3. Results for HDR brachytherapy

Author, year	N	F/U (range mo)	Dose Gy	Fractio-nation	CSS	LC	OS	Penile preservation	Late toxicity
Petera et al. (37), 2011	10	20 (3-91)	51	BID, 3Gy/fr	100%	100%	100%	100%	Necrosis 0 Stenosis 0
Sharma et al. (38), 2014	14	22 (6-40)	42-45	BID, 3Gy/fr	83%	86%	83% (3yr)	93%	Fibrosis 29% pigmen-tation 14%
Rouscoff et al. (39), 2014	12	27 (5-83)	36- 39	6Gy+ 2x 3.75 OR 7Gy+2 X 4Gy	100%	92%	78%	92%	telangiectasia 33% Fibrosis 9% Necrosis 9% Stenosis 9%
Kellas-Sleczka et al. (40), 2015	55	59 (8-152)	30-54	BID, 3-3.5 Gy/fr	-	84% (5yr) 63% 10 yr	77% 5 yr 57% 10 yr	80%	telangiectasia 21% Necrosis 3% Stenosis 1%
Pohkanova et al. (41), 2019	26	85(7-200)	51	BID 3 Gy/fr	100%	77% crude	92%	73%	Necrosis 4%

N, number of patients included in study cohort; F/U, follow-up mean and range; mo, months; Gy, Gray; BID, twice a day; CSS, cause specific survival; LC, local control; yr, years; OS, overall survival

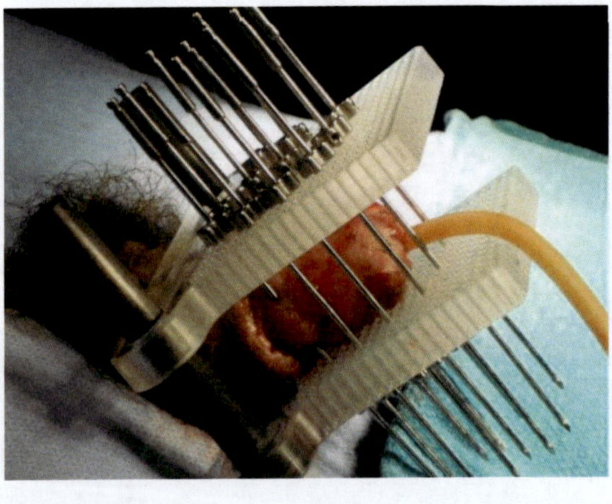

Figure 3. HDR template with treatment needles in place

2.3. Plesiotherapy

Plesiotherapy ("plesio" means "close" in Greek) is a technique consisting of applying radiation to a surface area. A mold containing the radiation sources or plastic catheters for delivery of Iridium-192 (for HDR or PDR) encloses the penis and is in contact with the tumor (Figure 4a-d). An approach similar to that used in other skin carcinomas can be employed. HDR mold treatment should only be used for superficial penile cancers (Tis; T1a and b, < 2-3 mm thick) to guarantee sufficient coverage at a depth.

Although the initial response to LDR Plesiotherapy was reported decades ago [10], inability to deliver a sufficient dose at a depth resulted in a high rate of relapses and the technique was essentially abandoned.

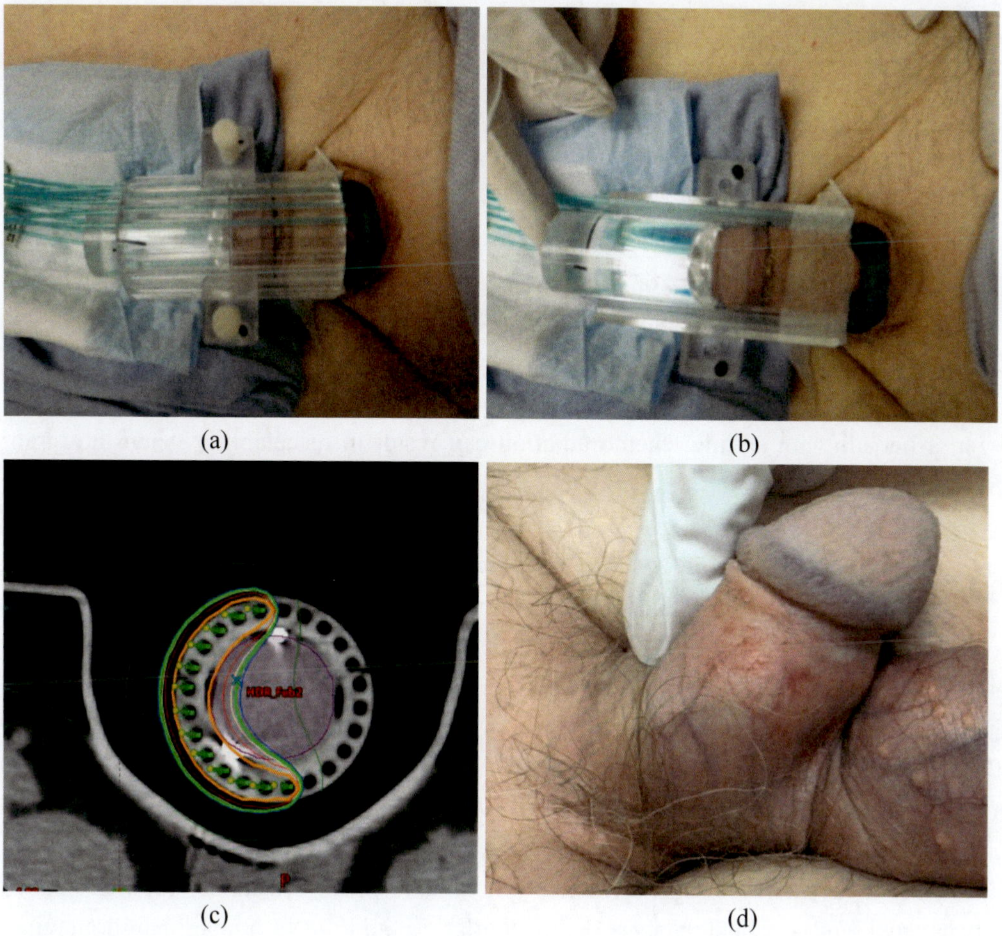

(a) (b) (c) (d)

Figure 4. Cylindrical applicator enclosing the penis with longitudinal catheters embedded for HDR treatment. In (b) the top of the applicator is removed to show 5 mm of superflab filling the airspace where the glans tapers. A blue retraction ring holds back redundant skin at the base of the penis. Dosimetry shown in (c). Appearance at 2 years (d).

For HDR mold brachytherapy, standard applicators based on penile diameter can be used. Lately, stereolithographic-individualized applicators (3D-printed molds) have been reported by Helou et al. [42] with catheters embedded as based on the physical anatomy. An optimized plan delivers 40Gy in 10 fractions over 5 days. As for interstitial HDR, mold plesiotherapy can deliver a very high dose to the tumor with rapid fall-off through adjacent healthy tissues. The treatment catheters are embedded in the mold such that they are separated 5mm from the skin surface. This prevents linear overdose in the skin from contact with the source, which would result in telangiectasia and scarring. Full dose can be delivered to the skin surface and 90% at 5-10mm, providing some central (urethral) sparing.

The reaction peaks at about 2-3 weeks after treatment and heals in 6-8 weeks. Local care is the same as for interstitial treatment.

3. Radiotherapy for Locoregional Disease

3.1. Neoadjuvant and Radical Radiotherapy

Radiotherapy can be used as definitive treatment if the patient is not a surgical candidate or refuses surgery, or when the tumor is not resectable. Nodal staging is essential; therefore if the patient is not suitable for surgical staging, nodal imaging with CT, ultrasound (US) and fine needle aspiration cytology (FNAC) and/or positron emission tomography PET-CT is highly recommended.

In a neoadjuvant setting, chemoradiation can result in resectability when the tumor response is good.

3.1.1. Rationale for Neoadjuvant/Radical Radiotherapy

There is no level I evidence for definitive chemo-radiation in SCC of the penis because of the low incidence in developed nations, which precludes completion of randomized prospective studies. A recent review by Robinson et al. [43] found only 7 retrospective small series analysing the role of adjuvant radiotherapy. The heterogeneity of those series made recommendations impossible as the reported recurrence rate ranged from 10-92%. Currently, the cooperative InPACT trial (International Penile Advanced Cancer Trial: discussed later) is recruiting. In the meantime, the recommendations for other SCC sites where stronger evidence is available provide a model for SCC penis. Vulvar, anal and cervical cancers have similar radiobiology, human papillomavirus (HPV) etiology, and nodal drainage, so a similar behaviour would be expected. Experience from HPV-induced oropharyngeal carcinoma could also be considered.

3.1.1.2. Vulvar Studies

The benefit of combined chemo-radiation for vulvar cancer was established by the Gynecologic Oncology Group (GOG) 101 trial [44]. 96 patients with stage IVA N2/N3 vulvar cancer were treated with split-course radiation (2 courses of 23.8 Gy) combined with cisplatin and 5-FU chemotherapy, followed by resection of the residual tumor and bilateral inguinal lymph node dissection. For patients with N2 or N3 lymphadenopathy (n = 41), 95% became resectable and of these patients, 41% had a complete pathological response.

A later GOG trial [45] used standard fractionation of 1.8 Gy daily to a total dose of 57.6 Gy combined with weekly cisplatin (40 mg/m2) and followed by surgery. 58 women with T3-T4N0-3 vulvar SCC were treated, 47% of whom were over the age of 60 and 24% over the age of 70. These results were even more encouraging with complete clinical response seen in 64% (n = 37).

3.1.1.2. Anal SCC

Neoadjuvant chemo-radiation is favoured in this site to maximize the possibilities of sphincter preservation. Two European trials have established the standard of care for chemo-RT. An advantage was found in both response rate and local control (HR 0.46, $P<0.001$) on the ACT 1 trial by the UK Coordinating Committee on Cancer Research where 585 patients of any stage were randomized to have RT alone (45 Gy to the pelvis with a 15–35 Gy boost to the primary) or chemo-RT with 5-FU and mitomycin C. Complete response was found to be significantly better with the combination (39% vs. 30%, $P = 0.08$) and LC (54% vs. 30%).

Similar results were seen in the EORTC trial that analysed 110 patients with locally advanced anal canal SCC randomized to chemo-radiation or radiotherapy alone. The addition of chemotherapy to radiotherapy increased the complete response rate from 54% to 80% (96% if patients salvaged by surgery are included). The improvement in loco regional control was 18% at 5 years ($p = 0.02$) and in colostomy free survival was 32% ($p = 0.002$). Forty-six percent of the studied population were over age 60.

3.1.1.3. Cervical Cancer

Chemo-radiation was established as the gold standard after the GOG 123 trial reported an adjusted hazard ratio for death of 0.63 (95% CI: 0.43–0.91, $P < 0.015$), favouring chemoradiotherapy. They analysed 374 patients with bulky cervical cancer (>4 cm) randomized to RT alone (45 Gy in 1.8–2 Gy fractions and a boost of 30 Gy LDR brachytherapy prescribed to point A) or RT combined with cisplatin 40 mg/m2. After 72 months, DFS in the combination arm was 71% versus 60% for RT alone.

3.1.2. DOSE

The gross primary disease should receive 66 to 70 Gy, 2 Gy/fraction. Inguinal and pelvic nodes are prescribed 45Gy at 1.8Gy/fraction, boosting areas of known extracapsular disease post resection to 54 Gy and enlarged nodes on imaging to 57 Gy. Based on vulvar and cervical evidence, concomitant cisplatinum at a dose of 40mg/m2/week can be prescribed if renal function is adequate.

3.2. Radiotherapy as Adjuvant Treatment

Nodal disease is one of the most potent predictors of OS and relapse free survival (RFS) [46] in penile cancer. Tumor stage T2 or higher, or high grade (G3) T1, should have surgical nodal examination as part of the initial management.

Nodal management [47]:

1. High risk disease: dynamic sentinel node biopsy (DSNB) or superficial/modified inguinal lymph node dissection (ILND)
   a. If negative: follow up.
   b. If positive
      i. 1 node without extracapsular extension (ECE): complete ipsilateral ILND
      ii. 2 nodes or ECE: ipsilateral ILND and uni/bilateral pelvic nodal dissection
2. cN+ 1 node bigger than 4cm: fine needle aspiration (FNA)
   c. If positive: superficial and deep ILND
   d. If negative: excisional biopsy OR superficial ILND and as 1.

The appropriate approach for the node negative patient has been established but the approach for those patients who are clinically node positive is less clear. Unfortunately, we lack prospective randomized studies specific to penile cancer to establish guidelines for adjuvant treatment. Until such evidence is available, guidelines are extrapolated from other SCC sites such as vulvar cancer [48].

3.2.1. Rationale for Adjuvant Radiotherapy on Vulvar SCC

In 1986 the GOG 37 protocol [49] established the standard for adjuvant radiotherapy in addition to nodal dissection for vulvar SCC for patients with a high risk groin (two or more nodes involved or extracapsular disease). They randomized 114 patients with positive inguinal nodes at groin dissection to receive either pelvic lymph node dissection (PLND) alone (n = 55), or adjuvant radiotherapy to pelvis and inguinal regions (n = 59). The dose delivered was 45–50.4 Gy using conventional fractionation and a simple 2 parallel beam arrangement. The vulva was not included in treatment. Radiotherapy was found to decrease groin recurrence (5% vs. 24%, p = 0.02) and improve 2-year overall survival (68% vs. 54%, p=0.03). On multivariate analysis, the number and size of lymph nodes did not impact outcome. Those results were updated in 2009 [50]. At 6-year follow up, the survival benefit persisted (OS of post-operative RT was 51% vs. 41% for PLND alone). Similar late toxicities rates were reported in both groups.

After lymph node dissection, radiotherapy is recommended for patients with those factors most predictive of local recurrence.

- positive or close margins
- multiple node involvement
- single node involvement with extra capsular extension (ECE)

The EBRT dose administered to the inguinal region will be 45Gy in 25 fractions, adding a boost to a total of 54-57 Gy to areas of ECE or gross residual. Pelvic nodal areas can be spared if they are confirmed to be negative. If pelvic nodes were involved or the status of the pelvic nodes is unknown, the pelvis should be treated following the same scheme. An intensity modulated beam arrangement (IMRT) is recommended to spare dose to central pelvic organs and improve tolerance (Figure 5).

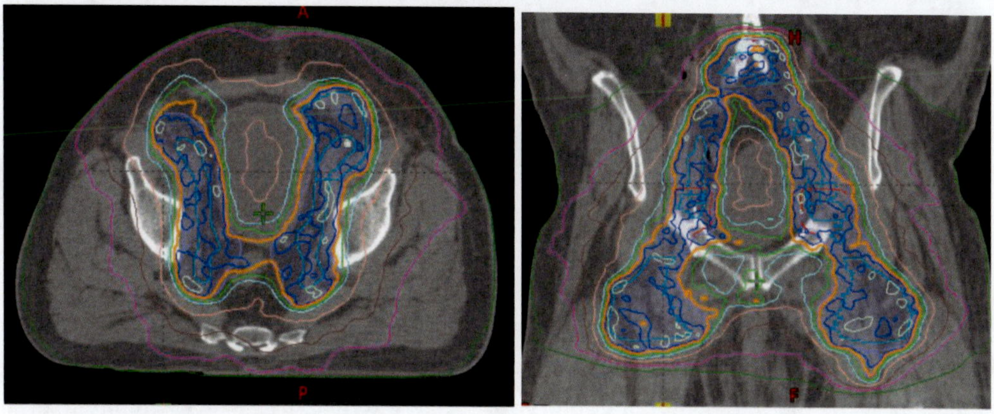

Figure 5. Volumetric modulated arc therapy (VMAT) for irradiation of nodal volumes while sparing central organs. A) axial and b) coronal.

3.3. Future Directions

The next step in penile cancer is now focused on determining the optimal combination and sequencing of surgery, chemotherapy and chemoradiotherapy in node positive penile cancer. The InPACT trial (International Penile Advanced Cancer Trial) (REF: https://clinicaltrials.gov/ct2/show/NCT02305654) was started in May 2017 and will recruit 400 patients from Europe and the Americas. The primary aim is to compare overall survival between 3 randomized groups: standard Inguinal Lymph Node Dissection (ILND), neoadjuvant chemotherapy followed by ILND, and neoadjuvant chemoradiotherapy followed by ILND.

After ILND, those patients at high risk of relapse according to the inguinal node pathology will be randomized a second time into receiving either prophylactic pelvic node dissection or chemoradiation to the pelvis.

Secondary objectives will include disease specific and disease free survival, Quality of Life, toxicity, nodal response to treatment and feasibility measured as operability and on-schedule delivery of treatments. The results will provide level I evidence for development of international guidelines to determine the optimal role and sequence of surgery, radiation and chemotherapy for node positive disease.

4. Palliative Treatment

EBRT can be used with palliative intent in advanced cases to help control symptoms such as bleeding and pain produced by the primary, nodal masses or metastasis, improving quality of life.

As for other epidermoid tumors, the response is expected to be quick and significant, although less so in case of bulky nodes. Indicated schemas include 30 Gy in 10 fractions (30/10), 20/5, or 8/1. To optimize the response, concurrent chemotherapy with platinum can be considered but requires a standard fractionation of 1.8-2.0 Gy/day.

Conclusion

Penile cancer is a radiosensitive and radiocurable tumor. Although surgery has been the standard of care and has proven to be a good radical treatment, detriment in quality of life encouraged the medical community to seek alternatives. Brachytherapy is an effective organ-sparing curative treatment for T1 and T2 tumors, and carefully selected T3 cases.

External beam radiation can not only improve quality of life in palliative patients but also has a crucial role in loco-regionally advanced disease. As part of a neoadjuvant approach in combination with chemotherapy, unresectable disease can be rendered operable. Adjuvant radiotherapy or chemoradiotherapy should be considered for those patients with multiple nodal involvement or extracapsular disease. Those indications are extrapolated from other SCC sites such as vulvar cancer, until results from the InPACT trial become available to formulate guidelines based on Level One evidence.

Key Points

- Penile Cancer is most commonly a squamous cell cancer, often of HPV origin, and is radiosensitive and radiocurable.
- Radiotherapy, especially in the form of brachytherapy, is a penile-conserving approach for localized disease (confined to the glans, < 4 cm) associated with penile preservation rates of ~85% at 5 years.

- For penile brachytherapy, high dose rate treatments are supplanting the previously common low dose rate applications, and can be given as either interstitial implants or as a surface mold for more superficial tumors. The dose is generally in the neighbourhood of 40 Gy in twice daily fractions over 5-6 days.
- Regional node involvement is the most important prognostic factor for disease specific survival.
- Surgical nodal staging is indicated for high grade T1 cancers or stage T2 or higher.
- Based on vulvar SCC literature, post-operative adjuvant radiotherapy is indicated for cases with multiple positive lymph nodes or evidence of extracapsular spread.
- In cases where nodes are unresectable, neoadjuvant radiotherapy or combined chemo-radiotherapy (40 mg/m2 cisplatinum weekly) can render them operable or can be continued with definitive intent although dose must be titrated appropriately for the bulk of disease.
- The ongoing InPACT trial (International Penile Advanced Cancer Trial) is exploring the optimal sequencing of surgery, radiation and chemotherapy for node positive patients.

REFERENCES

[1] Sarin R, Norman AR, Steel GG, Horwich A. Treatment results and prognostic factors in 101 men treated for squamous carcinoma of the penis. *Int J Radiat Oncol Biol Phys*. 1997 Jul 1;38(4):713–22.

[2] Audenet F, Sfakianos JP. Psychosocial impact of penile carcinoma. *Transl Androl Urol.* 2017;6(5):874–8.

[3] Delaunay B, Soh PN, Delannes M, Riou O, Malavaud B, Moreno F, et al. Brachytherapy for penile cancer: Efficacy and impact on sexual function. *Brachytherapy*. 2014;13(4):380–7.

[4] National Comprehensive Cancer Network. *Penile Cancer* (Version 2.2018). https://www.nccn.org/professionals/physician_gls/pdf/penile.pdf Accessed July 10, 2018.

[5] Hakenberg OW, Comperat EM, Minhas S, Necchi A, Protzel C, Watkin N, et al. EAU guidelines on penile cancer: 2014 update. *Eur Urol.* 2015;67(1):142–50.

[6] Manjunath A, Brenton T, Wylie S, Corbishley CM, Watkin NA. Topical Therapy for non-invasive penile cancer (Tis)—updated results and toxicity. *Transl Androl Urol.* 2017;6(5):803–8.

[7] Zouhair A, Coucke PA, Jeanneret W, Douglas P, Do HP, Jichlinski P, et al. Radiation therapy alone or combined surgery and radiation therapy in squamous-

cell carcinoma of the penis? *Eur J Cancer.* 2001;37(2):198–203.

[8] Mistry T, Jones RWA, Dannatt E, Prasad KK, Stockdale AD. A 10-year retrospective audit of penile cancer management in the UK. *BJU Int.* 2007 Dec;100(6):1277–81.

[9] Mclean M, Akl AM, Wards P, Bissett R, Panzarella T, Gospodarowicz M. The results of primary radiation therapy in the management of squamous cell carcinoma of the penis. *Int J Radiat Oncol.* 1993;25(4):623–8.

[10] Neave F, Neal AJ, Hoskin PJ, Hope-Stone HF. Carcinoma of the penis: A retrospective review of treatment with iridium mould and external beam irradiation. *Clin Oncol.* 1993 Jan 1;5(4):207–10.

[11] Ravi R, Chaturvedi HK, Sastry D. V. L. N. Role of radiation therapy in the treatment of carcinoma of the penis. *Br J Urol.* 1994 Nov;74(5):646–51.

[12] Gotsadze D, Matveev B, Zak B, Mamaladze V. Is Conservative Organ–Sparing Treatment of Penile Carcinoma Justified? *Eur Urol.* 2000;38(3):306–12.

[13] Ozsahin M, Jichlinski P, Weber DC, Azria D, Zimmermann M, Guillou L, et al. Treatment of penile carcinoma: To cut or not to cut? *Int J Radiat Oncol.* 2006;66(3):674–9.

[14] Azrif M, Logue JP, Swindell R, Cowan RA, Wylie JP, Livsey JE. External-beam Radiotherapy in T1-2 N0 Penile Carcinoma. *Clin Oncol.* 2006;18(4):320–5.

[15] Crook JM, Haie-Meder C, Demanes DJ, Mazeron JJ, Martinez AA, Rivard MJ. American Brachytherapy Society-Groupe Européen de Curiethérapie-European Society of Therapeutic Radiation Oncology (ABS-GEC-ESTRO) consensus statement for penile brachytherapy. *Brachytherapy.* 2013;12(3):191–8.

[16] de Crevoisier R, Slimane K, Sanfilippo N, Bossi A, Albano M, Dumas I, et al. Long-Term Results of Brachytherapy for Carcinoma of the Penis Confined to the Glans (N- or NX). *Int J Radiat Oncol Biol Phys*. 2009;74(4):1150–6.

[17] Crook JM, Jezioranski J, Grimard L, Esche B, Pond G. Penile brachytherapy: Results for 49 patients. *Int J Radiat Oncol Biol Phys*. 2005;62(2):460–7.

[18] Escande A, Haie-Meder C, Mazeron R, Maroun P, Cavalcanti A, de Crevoisier R, et al. Brachytherapy for Conservative Treatment of Invasive Penile Carcinoma: Prognostic Factors and Long-Term Analysis of Outcome. *Int J Radiat Oncol Biol Phys.* 2017;99(3):563–70.

[19] Crook J, Ma C, Grimard L. Radiation therapy in the management of the primary penile tumor: An update. *World J Urol.* 2009;27(2):189–96.

[20] Solsona E, Iborra I, Rubio J, Casanova JL, Ricós J V, Calabuig C. Prospective validation of the association of local tumor stage and grade as a predictive factor for occult lymph node micrometastasis in patients with penile carcinoma and clinically negative inguinal lymph nodes. *J Urol.* 2001 May;165(5):1506–9.

[21] Kattan MW, Ficarra V, Artibani W, Cunico SC, Fandella A, Martignoni G, et al. Nomogram Predictive of Cancer Specific Survival in Patients Undergoing Partial

or Total Amputation for Squamous Cell Carcinoma of the Penis. *J Urol.* 2006;175(6):2103–8.

[22] Correa AF, Handorf E, Joshi SS, Geynisman DM, Kutikov A, Chen DY, et al. Differences in Survival Associated with Performance of Lymph Node Dissection in Patients with Invasive Penile Cancer: Results from the National Cancer Database. *J Urol.* 2018;199(5):1238–44.

[23] Ornellas AA, Kinchin EW, Nóbrega BLB, Wisnescky A, Koifman N, Quirino R. Surgical treatment of invasive squamous cell carcinoma of the penis: Brazilian National Cancer Institute long-term experience. *J Surg Oncol*. 2008;97(6):487–95.

[24] Chipollini J, Tang DH, Gilbert SM, Poch MA, Pow-Sang JM, Sexton WJ, et al. Delay to Inguinal Lymph Node Dissection Greater than 3 Months Predicts Poorer Recurrence-Free Survival for Patients with Penile Cancer. *J Urol.* 2017 Dec;198(6):1346–52.

[25] Pierquin B, Dutreix A, Paine CH, Chassagne D, Marinello G, Ash D. The Paris System in Interstitial Radiation Therapy. *Acta Radiol Oncol Radiat Phys Biol.* 1978 Jan 8;17(1):33–48.

[26] Crook J, Jezioranski J, Cygler JE. Penile brachytherapy: Technical aspects and postimplant issues. *Brachytherapy.* 2010;9(2):151–8.

[27] Hasan S, Francis A, Hagenauer A, Hirsh A, Kaminsky D, Traughber B, et al. The role of brachytherapy in organ preservation for penile cancer: A meta-analysis and review of the literature. *Brachytherapy*. 2015;14(4):517–24.

[28] Mazeron JJ, Langlois D, Lobo PA, Huart JA, Calitchi E, Lusinchi A, et al. Interstitial radiation therapy for carcinoma of the penis using iridium 192 wires: the Henri Mondor experience (1970-1979). *Int J Radiat Oncol Biol Phys.* 1984 Oct;10(10):1891–5.

[29] Delannes M, Malavaud B, Douchez J, Bonnet J, Daly NJ. Iridium-192 interstitial therapy for squamous cell carcinoma of the penis. *Int J Radiat Oncol Biol Phys.* 1992;24(3):479–83.

[30] Rozan R, Albuisson E, Giraud B, Donnarieix D, Delannes M, Pigneux J, et al. Interstitial brachytherapy for penile carcinoma: a multicentric survey (259 patients). *Radiother Oncol*. 1995;36(2):83–93.

[31] Soria J-C, Fizazi K, Piron D, Kramar A, Gerbaulet A, Haie-Meder C, et al. Squamous cell carcinoma of the penis: Multivariate analysis of prognostic factors and natural history in a monocentric study with a conservative policy. *Ann Oncol.* 1997 Nov 1;8(11):1089–98.

[32] Chaudhary AJ, Ghosh S, Bhalavat RL, Kulkarni JN, Sequeira BVE. Interstitial brachytherapy in carcinoma of the penis. *Strahlentherapie und Onkol*. 1999 Apr 1;175(1):17–20.

[33] Kiltie AE, Elwell C, Close HJ, Ash D V. Iridium-192 Implantation for Node-Negative Carcinoma of the Penis: The Cookridge Hospital Experience. *Clin*

Oncol. 2000;12(1):25–31.

[34] Pimenta A, Gutierrez C, Mosquera D, Pera J, Martínez E, Londres B, et al. Penile brachytherapy—Retrospective review of a single institution. *Brachytherapy.* 2015;14(4):525–30.

[35] Gomez-Iturriaga A, Crook J, Evans W, Saibishkumar EP, Jezioranski J. The efficacy of hyperbaric oxygen therapy in the treatment of medically refractory soft tissue necrosis after penile brachytherapy. *Brachytherapy*. 2011 Nov;10(6):491–7.

[36] Escande A, Maroun P, Dumas I, Schernberg A, Bossi A, De Crevoisier R, et al. Brachytherapy for conservative treatment of invasive penile carcinoma in older patients: Single institution experience. *J Geriatr Oncol.* 2018;9(3):275–8.

[37] Petera J, Sirák I, Kašaová L, Mačingová Z, Paluska P, Zouhar M, et al. High dose rate brachytherapy in the treatment of penile carcinoma - First experience. *Brachytherapy*. 2011 Mar 1;10(2):136–40.

[38] Sharma DN, Joshi NP, Gandhi AK, Haresh KP, Gupta S, Julka PK, et al. High-dose-rate interstitial brachytherapy for T1–T2-stage penile carcinoma: Short-term results. *Brachytherapy.* 2014 Sep;13(5):481–7.

[39] Rouscoff Y, Falk AT, Durand M, Gal J, Chand M-E, Gautier M, et al. High-dose rate brachytherapy in localized penile cancer: short-term clinical outcome analysis. *Radiat Oncol*. 2014 Jun 19;9(1):142.

[40] Kellas-Sleczka S, Bialas B, Fijalkowski M, Wojcieszek P, Szlag M, Cholewka A, et al. Interstitial HDR Brachytherapy for Penile Cancer: A Thirteen-Year Follow Up of 55 Patients. B*rachytherapy*. 2015 May;14(2015):S33.

[41] Pohanková D, Sirák I, Kašaová L, Grepl J, Paluska P, Louda M, et al. High-Dose Rate Brachytherapy in the Treatment of Early Stages of Penile Carcinoma. *Klin Onkol*. 2019;32(1):52–7.

[42] Helou J, Morton G, Easton H, Jurincic L, D'Alimonte L, Ravi A. Customized penile plesiobrachytherapy using latest stereolithography techniques. *Brachytherapy.* 2015; 14(1):S99-S100.

[43] Robinson R, Marconi L, MacPepple E, Hakenberg OW, Watkin N, Yuan Y, et al. Risks and Benefits of Adjuvant Radiotherapy After Inguinal Lymphadenectomy in Node-positive Penile Cancer: A Systematic Review by the European Association of Urology Penile Cancer Guidelines Panel. *Eur Urol.* 2018;74(1):76–83.

[44] Montana GS, Thomas GM, Moore DH, Saxer A, Mangan CE, Lentz SS, et al. Preoperative chemo-radiation for carcinoma of the vulva with N2/N3 nodes: a gynecologic oncology group study. *Int J Radiat Oncol Biol Phys.* 2000 Nov 1;48(4):1007–13.

[45] Landrum LM, Skaggs V, Gould N, Walker JL, McMeekin DS. Comparison of outcome measures in patients with advanced squamous cell carcinoma of the vulva treated with surgery or primary chemoradiation. *Gynecol Oncol.* 2008

Mar;108(3):584–90.

[46] Reddy JP, Pettaway CA, Levy LB, Pagliaro LC, Tamboli P, Rao P, et al. Factors associated with regional recurrence after lymph node dissection for penile squamous cell carcinoma. *BJU Int.* 2017;119(4):591–7.

[47] Engelsgjerd JS, LaGrange CA. *Cancer, Penile*. StatPearls. 2018.

[48] Heaps JM, Fu YS, Montz FJ, Hacker NF, Berek JS. Surgical-pathologic variables predictive of local recurrence in squamous cell carcinoma of the vulva. *Gynecol Oncol*. 1990;38(3):309–14.

[49] Homesley HD, Bundy BN, Sedlis A, Adcock L. Radiation therapy versus pelvic node resection for carcinoma of the vulva with positive groin nodes. O*bstet Gynecol.* 1986 Dec;68(6):733–40.

[50] Kunos C, Simpkins F, Gibbons H, Tian C, Homesley H. Radiation therapy compared with pelvic node resection for node-positive vulvar cancer: a randomized controlled trial. *Obstet Gynecol*. 2009 Sep;114(3):537–46.

In: Penile Cancer: Challenges and Controversies
Editors: F. E. Martins and M. L. Djordjevic
ISBN: 978-1-53615-950-9

Chapter 9

Management of Metastatic Penile Cancer: The Role of Chemotherapy, Multimodal Therapy and Novel Systemic Therapies

Jad Chahoud*
Department of Cancer Medicine, The University of Texas MD Anderson Cancer Center, Houston, Texas, US

Abstract

This chapter will discuss the multidisciplinary approach for the management of locally advanced and metastatic penile squamous cell carcinoma (PSCC) focusing on the role of systemic therapies. We will review the major studies that evaluated different chemotherapy regimens in the neoadjuvant, adjuvant and palliative settings for the treatment of advanced PSCC. We will also summarize the available data and ongoing clinical trials evaluating targeted therapies, immunotherapies, and Human papillomavirus (HPV) directed therapies for PSCC.

Keywords: penile cancer, penile squamous cell carcinoma, human papillomavirus, HPV, chemotherapy, targeted therapy, immunotherapy, clinical trials

Introduction

In patients with regional lymph node involvement or distant metastases of penile squamous cell carcinoma (PSCC), the optimal timing for chemotherapy administration with respect to lymph node dissection has been debated, as data supporting the current

* Corresponding Author's E-mail: jchahoud@mdanderson.org.

treatment paradigm is limited to non-randomized trials [1–3]. Relapsed disease after first line chemotherapy is associated with poor survival and limited treatment options are available [4]. In this chapter, we will review the literature of available evidence on systemic therapy options, focus on the immense gaps in the current recommendations for an optimal approach to the management of this disease and discuss the current clinical trials in PSCC.

The Role of Neoadjuvant Chemotherapy in Locally Advanced PSCC

Regional lymph node involvement remains the most important predictor of survival outcomes in patients with penile cancer. This population is heterogeneous, with disease-specific survival rates for pN 0, 1, 2, 3 categories of 96%, 80%, 66% and 37%, respectively ($p < 0.001$) [5]. We also know that current imaging modalities cannot accurately predict the lymph node status of patients with early presentation. In fact, CT imaging misses 20% of micrometastasis, while it has a high false positive rate with 70% of lymph node positivity on imaging having pN0 disease at the time of inguinal nodal staging [6, 7].

Therefore, regional lymph node involvement represents a major dilemma in the clinical care of patients with PSCC, as it is the most frequent clinical presentation in comparison to the rare occurrence of distant metastases [8–10]. The management of patients with suspected clinical lymphadenopathy is usually multidisciplinary to first confirm nodal disease and then determine the extent of disease involvement with the clinical exam, imaging, and percutaneous biopsy. In fact, only a small proportion of patients with bulky, fixed or bilateral inguinal lymphadenopathy will benefit from upfront surgery as a standalone therapeutic option [11]. Neoadjuvant systemic therapy in these patients is currently recommended as the preferred strategy by the National Comprehensive Cancer Network (NCCN) and the European Association of Urology (EAU) guidelines [2, 3]. There are multiple benefits to neoadjuvant chemotherapy as it allows timely delivery of systemic chemotherapy, results in volume reduction for enlarged lymphadenopathies, provides prognostic information, and facilitates subsequent surgical consolidation [12, 13]. The important factors to select a chemotherapy regimen when considering such an approach include (1) the tolerability of the chemotherapy regimen; (2) the overall response rates to the chemotherapy regimen; (3) the percentage of patients proceeding with consolidation surgery; and (4) the complete pathological response rates as it is the strongest predictor of survival for patients with locally advanced PSCC. We reviewed the currently available data and summarized the above factors per chemotherapy regimen in Table 1 [1, 14–17]. Unfortunately, there are currently no clinical or pathological factors that can accurately predict the benefit from neoadjuvant chemo-therapy [18–20]. The only strong predictor of better survival after neoadjuvant chemotherapy is achievement of a pathological complete response (pCR) at the time of consolidative surgery [1]. Limited molecular or imaging biomarkers have been proven useful for early assessment of the benefit during neoadjuvant chemotherapy, but scarce data is available regarding the possible role of [^{18}F]-fluorodeoxyglucose positron emission tomography for assessing interim response to neoadjuvant therapy [21, 22].

There has not been any major development in the past decade, in regards to the approved systemic therapies for PSCC. The study that established the approach of neoadjuvant chemotherapy followed by surgery as the standard of care, was a prospective, single center, non-randomized, phase II clinical trial [1]. This study's objective was determining the response rate, time to progression (TTP), and overall survival (OS) among patients with bulky adenopathy receiving neoadjuvant chemotherapy with the following combinations: paclitaxel 175 mg/m^2 administered over 3 hours on day 1; ifosfamide 1,200 mg/m^2 on days 1 to 3; and cisplatin 25 mg/m^2 on days 1 to 3 every 3 weeks (TIP) with the goal of completing a total of four cycles prior to proceeding with consolidation surgery. Thirty men received chemotherapy, 23 patients (76.7%) completed the planned four courses of chemotherapy. The other seven patients discontinued chemotherapy after one to three courses; the reasons were rapid tumor progression (three patients), hypersensitivity to paclitaxel (one patient), cardiac event (one patient), and patient's decision not to receive further treatment (two patients). The study reported that 15 patients (50.0%) had an objective response with three CRs, 12 PRs achieved, and 22 patients (73.3%) subsequently underwent consolidation surgery. Three patients (10%) had a complete pathological response. Nine patients (30.0%) remained alive and free of recurrence at the time of last follow up (median follow-up, 34 months; range, 14-59 months), and two patients died of other causes without recurrence. The estimated median TTP was 8.1 months (95% CI, 5.4 to 50 months) and median OS of 17.1 months (95% CI, 10.3 to 60 months) [1]. It was noted that an improved TTP and OS were significantly associated with a response to chemotherapy ($P < .001$ and $P = .001$, respectively), absence of bilateral residual tumor ($P = .002$ and $P = .017$, respectively), and absence of extranodal extension ($P = .001$ and $P = .004$, respectively) or skin involvement ($P = .009$ and $P = .012$, respectively). Grade 3 infections (in 16.7% of patients) was the only adverse event experienced by more than one patient during the chemotherapy phase. This was the first prospective study with sufficient study sample size to reliably estimate the outcomes of multimodality therapy for advanced penile carcinoma and established neoadjuvant chemotherapy with TIP followed by consolidation surgery as the preferred treatment option for patients with bulky lymphadenopathy.

Table 1. Summary of reported studies of neoadjuvant chemotherapy for advanced PSCC

Regimen	Authors	Study design	No. Patients Evaluable	No. operated	ORR/ CPR	G3-4 Toxicities	Median PFS/OS
Cisplatin	Gagliano et al. 1989	Phase II	26	NA	15%/0%	NA	2 months/ 4.7 months
5-FU + Cisplatin	Di Lorenzo et al. 2012	Retrospective	25	NA	32%/0%	20% neutropenia	5 months/8 months
Irinotecan + Cisplatin	Theodore et al., 2008	Phase II	26	NA	31%/ 11.5%	40% neutropenia	NA
Paclitaxel Ifosfamide Cisplatin (TIP)	Pagliaro et al., 2010	Phase II	30	22	50%/ 10%	3.3% neutropenia	7.1 months/ 13.9 months
Docetaxel, cisplatin and 5-flurouracil (TPF)	Nicholson, 2013	Phase II	26	5	38.5%/ 7.7%	- 46.4 neutropenia - 68% any G3/G4	7.1 month/ 13.9 months

Another neoadjuvant chemotherapy regimen using three agents that has been evaluated by multiple studies, but has shown to be more toxic and less efficacious is the combination of docetaxel, cisplatin, and 5-fluorouracil (TPF). In a single arm phase II clinical trial, 26 patients with locally advanced and metastatic PSCC received TPF, including 7 patients with visceral metastasis [17]. The combination reported an objective response rate (ORR) with 38.5%, an estimated median progression-free survival (PFS) of 7.1 months, and an estimated median OS of 13.9 months. However, it appeared to be very toxic, with more than two thirds of patients having grade 3–4 toxicities and 40% having grade 3-4 neutropenia. This high rate of toxicities is very limiting especially in a neoadjuvant approach. These findings were also confirmed in two retrospective studies evaluating the use of TPF combination. The first study from the Italian group, that included 28 patients treated with TPF, with an ORR of 42.8% and pCR of 14.3% [23]. The second study included 26 patients, with an ORR of 60% and pCR of 4% but was shown to be very toxic [24]. A major limitation from these retrospective studies is to reproduce toxicity results, but interestingly, the comparison of the three agents chemotherapy with TPF and the two agents chemotherapy PF, in a retrospective study did not show significant differences in the estimated PFS and OS [25]. It is important to look at the results from this multicenter retrospective study with caution, as it has all the inherent biases of retrospectively collected data, in addition to the limited number of patients in each group.

As we summarized in Table 1, multiple retrospective studies and phase II clinical trials using various chemotherapeutic agents reported ORRs ranging between 30 - 50% and pCRs between 0 - 15% among patients who underwent consolidative lymph node dissection [1, 14–17, 24]. Older Retrospective studies with limited numbers of patients had also evaluated the combination of bleomycin, methotrexate, and cisplatin (BMP) [26, 27]. This combination, or any other one that includes bleomycin, should not be considered in clinical practice for the management of PSCC due to the major toxicity and limited activity of bleomycin reported in this patient population.

In conclusion, the current standard of care is founded on limited data but remains to be neoadjuvant chemotherapy with TIP as the preferred regimen, followed by surgery [1]. The care of patients with locally advanced and metastatic PSCC remains best provided at centers of excellence and under the care of an experienced multidisciplinary team. We encourage all oncologists and urologists to enroll patients on clinical trials when available. Until recently, it was not possible to conduct randomized controlled trials in penile cancer to answer the basic management questions before the design of the International Penile Advanced Cancer Trial (InPACT). InPACT is a 400-patient trial to be conducted in the United Kingdom, United States, Columbia and Canada, and employs a Bayesian design to randomize treatment of patients with inguinal lymph node metastases from PSCC. The study has two independent randomizations to answer two main questions. The first being, the role of neoadjuvant therapy prior to standard surgery, by randomizing to chemotherapy, chemoradiotherapy, or no neoadjuvant therapy. This will answer whether there is any benefit for neoadjuvant chemotherapy or chemoradiation. The second question is on the role of prophylactic pelvic lymph node dissection following the standard surgery with therapeutic inguinal lymph node dissection, in patients with high pathological risk factors after receiving chemoradiotherapy. The primary outcome measure of the InPACT study is overall survival. The study schema is described in Figure 1. In addition, an immense need exists for innovative clinical trials in the neoadjuvant setting to improve on the current accepted standard of care chemotherapy regimen.

The Role of Adjuvant Chemotherapy in Locally Advanced PSCC

There are no prospective data on adjuvant chemotherapy; only small retrospective studies have been reported, as well as large retrospective and multicenter case series. The NCCN guidelines recommend for adjuvant chemotherapy, with level 2A evidence for patients with high pathological risk features (pathological N2, N3 or ECE) [3]. The guidelines state that there is no conclusive evidence to support this use, but based on extrapolation from the neoadjuvant chemotherapy evidence they recommend 4 cycles of TIP adjuvant chemotherapy. As an alternative adjuvant regimen they suggest 5-FU with cisplatin to be considered for patients that cannot receive ifosfamide [3]. Similarly there is level 2B evidence for adjuvant chemotherapy in the current EAU guidelines, and this should be regarded as a treatment option for patients with pathological N2 or N3 disease after lymphadenectomy [2]. As for patients with pathological N1 disease, the EAU guidelines recommend adjuvant therapy only in the setting of clinical trials [2].

Historically, a single institution retrospective study showed long-term disease-free survival occurred in 84% of 25 consecutive node-positive patients treated with adjuvant vincristine with bleomycin and methotrexate. This study has the major limitation of all retrospective trials, toxicity was not reported and it remains a major concern with the use of bleomycin in this specific population [28]. More recently, a large multicenter retrospective study assessed 141 patients with more advanced pathological pelvic lymph node involvement showing a median OS improvement with the use of adjuvant chemotherapy [29]. It is important to know that this study is hampered by the limitations of a retrospective study and the incomplete information on the specific chemotherapy combinations used but it highlights the potential benefit of adjuvant chemotherapy in patients with pelvic lymphadenopathy and did not receive neoadjuvant chemotherapy.

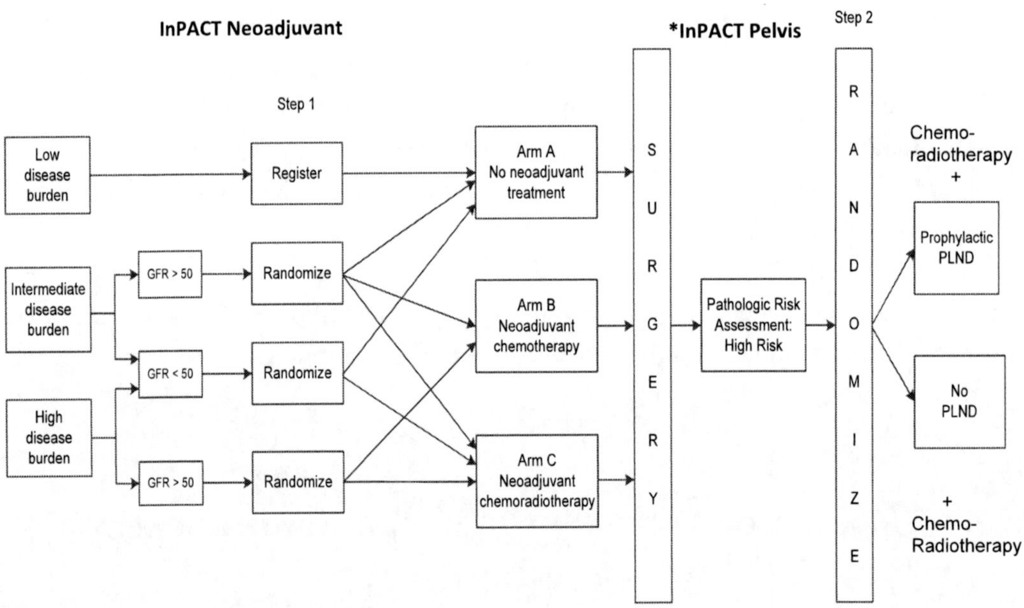

Neo adjuvant chemotherapy- 4 cycles paclitaxel, ifosfamide, cis-platin
Neo adjuvant chemoradiotherapy 45 Gy, 25 fractions + weekly cisplatin
Postoperative chemoradiotherapy 54 Gy 25 fractions + weekly cisplatin
* Step 2- InPACT Pelvis- High Risk Patients must have been registered/treated at Step 1- No patients can enter Step 2 independent of Step 1

Figure 1. InPACT study schema.

The Role of Chemotherapy for Metastatic Disease and Relapsed Disease

As we discussed, there is limited evidence to guide the preferred chemotherapy regimen in the first-line setting to be used in clinical practice. The same applies to patients with distant metastatic disease, and the outcomes are dismal especially in patients with visceral metastasis [4]. With the palliative goal in mind, single-agent regimens have been tested with cisplatin alone, but unfortunately it displayed modest activity, with an ORR of 15% when evaluated among 26 patients and an estimated median overall survival of only 4.7 mo with limited toxicity data available [14]. Thereafter, a two-agent regimen was tested by Theodore et al., in a prospective phase II non-randomized clinical trial with the European Organization for the Research and Treatment of Cancer (EORTC 30992). The trial used cisplatin with irinotecan in 26 patients; both as neoadjuvant therapy for four cycles followed by surgery for locally advanced, and a total of 8 cycles for more advanced disease [15]. The study reported an ORR of 30.8%, and was associated with significant grade 3-4 neutropenia and diarrhea [15]. The study did not report on the survival estimates and this is a major limitation for informing clinical practice. The Current NCCN guidelines recommend TIP chemotherapy at similar doses as in the neoadjuvant setting for first line therapy of metastatic PSCC [3]. For patients that are not eligible to receive TIP, the recommended alternative by the NCCN, is cisplatin plus continuous infusion of 5-FU, that was used for palliative purposes in a retrospective study with a homogenous sample of 25 patients with advanced PSCC [16]. This study reported partial responses and stable disease in 8 (32%) and 10 (40%) patients, respectively, with a median PFS of 5 months and a median OS of 8 months. The toxicity profile appeared to be acceptable, with grade 3-4 neutropenia as the most significant side effect observed, occurring in 20% of patients [16].

We summarized all available options that have been considered for the first line and subsequent lines of therapies in the management of metastatic PSCC in Table 2 [1, 16, 17, 30–34]. Recently, a single-agent phase II clinical trial using vinflunine, a third-generation compound with less toxicity than older vinca alkaloids, was reported to meet its primary endpoint. The reported clinical benefit rate was 45% and the objective response rate at 27% was comparable to two chemotherapy combination regimens tested in other phase II trials in PSCC [31]. Patients received vinflunine at 320 mg/m^2 every 3 weeks for 4 cycles, in 26 patients, 24 had stage IV disease and two patients had stage IIIb disease. The study reported 10 patients had an objective response or stable disease, for a clinical benefit rate of 45.5%. The median PFS was 2.9 months, and median OS was 8.4 months. Pre-specified adverse events that occurred in at least 10% of patients included constipation (64%, grade 3) and neutropenia (32%, grade 3 or higher) [31]. Another phase II trial evaluated Dacomitinib in 28 patients with treatment naïve PSCC with an

ORR of 32%. We will further discuss this clinical trial in the below paragraph for targeted therapies [32].

As for relapsed disease, the evidence for therapies after platinum-based therapy is very limited. Outcomes are dismal with estimated median overall survival of 5 months and clinical trial enrollment is the preferred treatment options [4]. Even though every effort should be made to enroll patients with relapsed disease on clinical trial, paclitaxel monotherapy reported an initial response rate under 30% with minimal toxicity. Therefore, this may be a possible option to be discussed with patients in the palliative setting [15]. Microsatellite instability (MSI) testing could also be considered, with the possibility to offer the FDA-approved pembrolizumab for microsatellite instability- high (MSI- H) relapsed cancers, even though the rate of MSI-H PSCC are thought to be very low [35]. Best supportive care should be considered in patients with relapsed PSCC, who do not have the capacity to be enrolled in clinical trials and cannot tolerate further systemic therapy due to deteriorating performance status or major comorbidities.

Table 2. Summary of studies of systemic therapy in metastatic or relapsed PSCC

Regimen	Authors	Study design	No. Patients Evaluable	ORR/CPR	G3-4 Toxicities	Median PFS/OS
Paclitaxel	Di Lorenzo et al. 2011	Phase II in pretreated	25	20%/0	28% neutropenia	2.75 months/5.75 months
5-FU + Cisplatin	Di Lorenzo et al. 2012	Retrospective first line stage 3/4	25	32%/0%	20% neutropenia	5 months/8 months
Paclitaxel Ifosfamide Cisplatin (TIP)	Pagliaro et al., 2010	Phase II first line therapy in locally advanced	30	50%/10%	3.3% neutropenia	7.1 months/13.9 months
Docetaxel, cisplatin and 5-flurouracil (TPF)	Nicholson, 2013	Phase II first line therapy stage 3/4	26	38.5%/7.7%	- 46.4% neutropenia - 68% any G3/G4	7.1 month/13.9 months
Vinflunine	Pickering et al. 2018	Phase II first line therapy for stage 3/4	26	27%/0%	- 32% nuetropenia - 64% constipation	2.9 months/8.4 months
Dacomintinib	Necchi et al. 2018	Phase II first line therapy stage 3/4	28	32.1%/3.5%	- 10% skin rash	4.1 months/13.7 months
Nimotusumab	Huang et al. 2019	Pilot study in pretreated advanced disease	6	33%/16%	NA	4.8 months/9.2 months
Cabozantinib and Nivolumab	Apolo et al. 2018	Phase I in pretreated advanced GU squamous tumors	4	25%/0%	NA	NA

THE POTENTIAL ROLE OF TARGETED THERAPIES

The ability to personalize therapy for patients with PSCC and potentially improve treatment outcomes has been hindered by a limited understanding of the molecular drivers of disease. Previous profiling efforts identified recurrent alterations in PSSC including mutations in TP53, CDKN2A and PIK3CA. We summarized the published studies evaluating molecular alterations in PSCC (Table 3) [35–39]. Until this year, these studies have been limited by sample size, number of HPV cases and variability in molecular testing methods with only one study using whole exome sequencing. While these studies have increased our understanding of the molecular pathology of PSSC, their impact on personalized treatment strategies is still unclear. The recent study by Jacob et al., evaluated 78 cases with metastatic PSCC with potential targeted therapy opportunities in more than 32% of mPSCC. This included alterations in MTOR pathway (*NF1* GA in 7% and *PTEN* GA in 4%), DNA repair pathway (*BRCA2* and *ATM* GA, each in 7%) and tyrosine kinase (*EGFR* GA in 6%; *FGFR3* and *ERBB2* GA each in 4%) [35]. Our group, also performed the largest whole exome sequencing analysis in PSCC with 34 patients composing the study cohort that appear to be representative of the broader population of individuals with PSCC [39]. These individuals had a median age of 61, and the majority had known penile cancer risk factors (e.g., uncircumcised, tobacco use, and phimosis). Three-quarters of patients (74%) presented with intermediate- or high-grade tumors, 64% had primary tumors staged as T2 or greater, and 36% had lymph node involvement at the time of nodal surgical staging. HPV positivity was identified for 30% of patients. This whole exome sequencing data uncovered several notable findings. First, there was a negligible difference in the tumor mutational burden between HPV-negative and HPV-positive PSCC, suggesting that HPV etiology bears little influence on this factor, which is in concordance with previously published work in head and neck cancers. Second, the tumor mutational burden of PSCC was similar to that for other SCCs, more specifically, tumors of the head and neck, esophagus, cervix, bladder, and lung, for which immune checkpoint inhibitors are approved as part of the paradigm of systemic treatment. The most common mutations identified in the PSCC cases occurred in *TP53* (35%), *NOTCH1* (35%), *CDKN2A* (23%), *PIK3CA* (21%), and *CASP8* (21%). The frequency of most mutations was similar between HPV-negative and HPV-positive cases, except for mutations in *TP53*, *FAT1*, *CASP8*, and *FBXW7*, which were much more common in HPV-negative cases. A comparison of PSCC with SCCs, using the TCGA data, from other anatomic sites demonstrated convergence among the mutations, with frequent alterations observed in *TP53*, *NOTCH1*, *CDKN2A*, *PIK3CA*, *CASP8*, and *FAT1*. The *PIK3CA* mutations identified in the PSCC cases appeared to be similar to those in head and neck SCC and included some of the same oncogenic hotspot mutations. As for *NOTCH1*, which encodes a tumor suppressor protein, it appears to be mutated at higher rates in PSCC at 35% compared with head and neck and other SCCs. However, similar to head and neck SCCs, the mutations in *NOTCH1* in PSCCs are loss-of-function mutations, which may render the cancer cells vulnerable to PI3K/mTOR inhibition [40]. Therefore, this could constitute a potential treatment option for clinical trial evaluation in patients with penile cancer and *NOTCH1* mutations.

The HER/PTEN/Akt pathway also appeared to be disrupted in PSCC and with available targeted treatment options [41, 42]. Dacomintinib has been recently approved for the treatment of patients with metastatic non-small cell lung cancer (NSCLC) with epidermal growth factor receptor (EGFR) exon 19 deletion or exon 21 L858R substitution mutations [43]. Recently, a phase II study by Necchi et al., used the second-generation, pan-HER tyrosine kinase inhibitor dacomitinib in 28 chemotherapy-naïve patients with locally advanced or metastatic PSCC [32]. The ORR for dacomitinib was 32.1% with median PFS of 4.1 months and OS of 13.7 months. The treatment was relatively well tolerated with only 10% grade 3-4 skin rash as the major toxicity [32]. This trial enrolled patients irrespective of their mutational status, interestingly the translational results from this study highlighted the need for patient selection in the use of such targeted therapy as mutations of downstream effectors of HER receptors, as well as *TERT* mutations, seemed to be associated with the clinical benefit of dacomitinib [32]. This could constitute a therapeutic option for patients who have relapsed on chemotherapy, if clinical trials are not available.

Table 3. Summary of studies assessing the genomic alterations in PSCC

Author/year	Center/Country	Study population/HPV Status	Type of molecular testing	Findings
Mcdaniel et al. 2015	Single center USA	N = 43 5 HPV	• Next Generation Sequencing	TP53: 45% CDKN2A: 54% PIK3CA: 20%
S. Ali et al. 2016	Multi center USA	N = 20 3 HPV+	• Next Generation Sequencing	TP53: 65% CDKN2A: 40% NOTCH1: 25% PIK3CA: 25%
Feber et al. 2016	Multi center UK	N = 27 5 HPV +	• Whole-exome sequencing	TP53: 15% FAT1: 15% CSN1: 11%
Chahoud et al. 2019	Single center USA	N = 34 10 HPV+	• Whole exome sequencing	TP53: 35% CDKN2A: 23% NOTCH1: 35% PIK3CA: 21% TMB > 10 = 21%
Jacob et al. 2019	Multicenter USA	N = 78 22 HPV+	• Next Generation Sequencing	TP53: 58% CDKN2A: 47% NOTCH1: 22% TMB > 10 = 18%

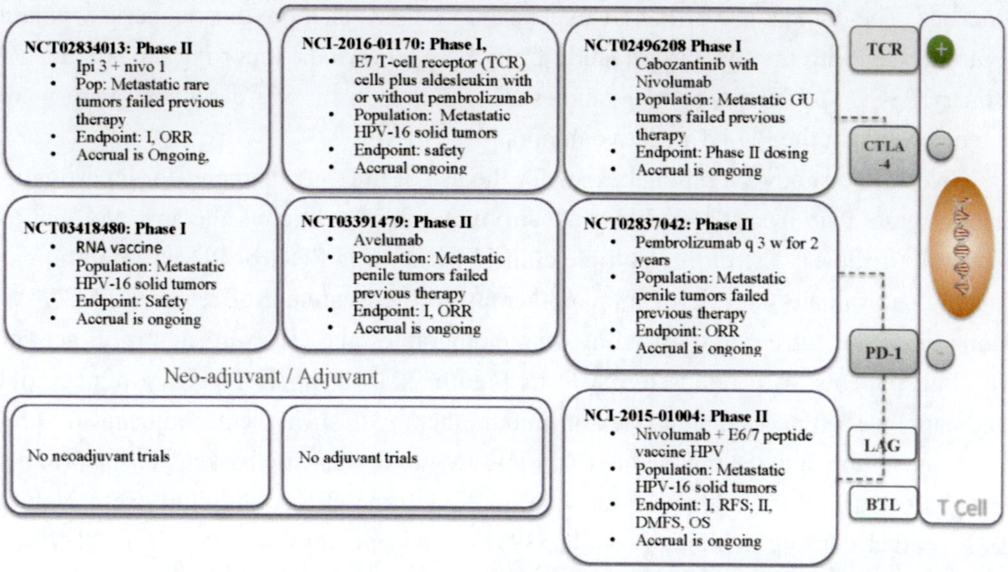

Figure 2. Immunotherapy clinical trial landscape in PSCC.

Finally, cabozantinib is a multi-targeted tyrosine kinase inhibitor and was recently shown to block PI3K signaling in MDSCs to enable efficacy from ICB in metastatic castration-resistant prostate cancer models [44]. It is important to highlight the interim results from a phase I study with the combination of cabozantinib and nivolumab that showed objective responses in genitourinary tumors with squamous cell histology, including PSCC [34]. Further follow up on the results of this combination for the subsequent stages of development in PSCC would be of interest.

The Potential Role of Immunotherapy

Pembrolizumab, recently received the first FDA tumor agnostic approval for patients with advanced solid cancers and DNA mismatch repair- deficient tumors, or microsatellite instability- high (MSI- H). This study with pembrolizumab reported an ORR of 71% across any tumor type. Limited data are available regarding the prevalence of MSI-H in PSCC, but the studies that assessed it have shown low rates of MSI-H PSCC [35], which would limit the use of pembrolizumab outside of clinical trials. Another predictive marker of response to combination immunotherapy can be a tumor mutational burden of $\geq$ 10 mutations per Mb, this has been shown in lung cancer [45], our group reported that 21% of PSCC specimens were found to have $\geq$ 10 mutations per Mb [39]. On the other hand, multiple studies have shown that 48 - 60% of PSCCs are also positive for PD-L1 expression on infiltrating immune cells in PSCC [46–50], PD-L1 expression has been used in other types of cancers to predict the activity of immune checkpoint blockade. The clinical use of PD-L1 expression in PSCC as a prognostic marker remains controversial, with the two largest study from the Netherlands, reporting on 213 and 220 primary PSCC specimens, in both studies PD-L1 expression was associated with worse outcomes than in the PD-L1 negative tumors [49, 50].

Given all the above, a rational exists for the use of immune therapies for investigation in a disease that has reported dismal survival with traditional therapy and limited approved therapies. Therefore, multiple clinical trials using PD-1 or PD-L1 inhibition are ongoing to evaluate the role of immunotherapy in the treatment of relapsed PSCC. We summarized the current trial assessing immunotherapies and HPV-directed trials actively enrolling patients with relapsed PSCC in Figure 2. In a quick overview of the trials landscape, we can notice (1) the lack of immunotherapy trials in the neoadjuvant first line treatment setting, and (2) the majority of trials are tumor agnostic basket trials. Currently, two phase II trials are evaluating the role of PD-L1 and PD-1 inhibition exclusively in PSCC patients, using avelumab (NCT03391479) and pembrolizumab (NCT02837042), respectively, both with the primary endpoint as overall response rate (ORR) (Figure 2). Other combination trials that are available for patients with relapsed advanced PSCC, are nivolumab with ipilimumab at the approved dosing for advanced renal cell carcinoma and nivolumab with cabozantinib both in the relapsed setting with advanced PSCC.

The Potential Role of HPV Directed Therapies

HPV infection is responsible for approximately 50% of PSCC cases worldwide [51], a major part of the advancement in our molecular understanding of PSCC carcinogenesis is the molecular divergence between HPV and non HPV-related cases [52]. The HPV proteins E6 and E7 have key roles in HPV-mediated carcinogenesis and in the pathogenesis of PSCC. Thus, the increased interest in targeting the HPV pathway with adoptive T-cell therapy selected for E6 and E7 reactivity with lymphocytedepltion and aldesleukin treatment are being tested in HPV related cancers in combination with PD-L1 inhibition. This approach is the basis for two ongoing phase I/II trials (NCT02379520) and (NCI-2016-01170) in all HPV-related malignancies, including PSCC, that will evaluate therapy with HPV-specific T cells in combination with the antiprogrammed cell death 1 (PD-1) antibody nivolumab and pembrolizumab respectively (Figure 2). As other squamous cell carcinomas appear to be genomically and immunologically similar to PSCC, where patients with head and neck, bladder and lung squamous cell carcinomas have shown improved survival outcomes with PD-1 and PD-L1 checkpoint inhibitors, these therapies are now part of the approved systemic therapies for these cancers. On the other hand, a trial using therapeutic vaccines with synthetic plasmids targeting the HPV12 and HPV18 E6 and E7 proteins as single agent are being conducted in patients with advanced HPV- related cancers, including PSCC (NCT03418480) (Figure 2); early results are showing a favorable safety profile for this approach. In the era of immunotherapy, continued investigation of chemotherapy and immune targeting therapy combinations in the neoadjuvant setting is justified and should be the interest of future clinical trials.

CONCLUSION

Neoadjuvant chemotherapy with TIP followed by consolidation surgery is the preferred treatment approach in patients with locally advanced PSCC today. This approach is being compared to neoadjuvant chemoradiation in a large prospective international study (InPACT, NCT02305654) currently enrolling patients worldwide. The evidence for adjuvant chemotherapy for patient with N2 or higher PSCC that did not receive neoadjuvant chemotherapy is limited but remains recommended. Referral to clinical trials should be a priority in these patients when available. Unfortunately, survival outcomes remain modest in locally advanced PSCC treated using the current multimodal management that combines systemic chemotherapy with surgery and is primarily dependent on the extent of lymph node involvement. There should be an increasing effort for clinical research to improve on the current neoadjuvant systemic therapies offered through global collaboration efforts among centers of excellence for PSCC clinical care and innovation in combination systemic therapies. Given the major challenges facing clinical trials development in PSCC, collaborative efforts between centers of excellence worldwide to evaluate the tumor biology and innovation in the combination of systemic therapy in the first line setting, should guide the strategy to make future therapeutic advances in this rare and fatal disease.

KEY POINTS

- Neoadjuvant chemotherapy followed by consolidation surgery is the recommended approach for locally advanced PSCC.
- Combination chemotherapy with TIP is the recommended regimen for first line therapy of PSCC.
- Clinical trial enrollment and collaborative international efforts should be a priority for this rare disease.
- The InPACT trial is the first international randomized clinical trial currently open for accrual with the objective to determine the best treatment approach for the management of locally advanced PSCC.

- Further understanding of the molecular alterations involved in PSCC progression is needed to direct the development of clinical trial design for targeted therapies.
- Relapsed PSCC after first line therapy lacks approved systemic therapies; immunotherapy and HPV directed clinical trials are ongoing in this setting.

References

[1] Pagliaro, LC; Williams, DL; Daliani, D; et al. Neoadjuvant Paclitaxel, Ifosfamide, and Cisplatin Chemotherapy for Metastatic Penile Cancer: A Phase II Study. *J Clin Oncol.*, 2010, 28(24), 3851-3857. doi:10.1200/JCO.2010.29.5477.

[2] Hakenberg, OW; Compérat, EM; Minhas, S; Necchi, A; Protzel, C; Watkin, N. EAU Guidelines on Penile Cancer: 2014 Update. *Eur Urol.*, 2015, 67(1), 142-150. doi:10.1016/j.eururo.2014.10.017.

[3] Clark, PE; Spiess, PE; Agarwal, N; et al. Penile cancer: Clinical Practice Guidelines in Oncology. *J Natl Compr Canc Netw.*, 2013, 11(5), 594-615. http://www.ncbi.nlm.nih.gov/pubmed/23667209. Accessed February 27, 2019.

[4] Wang, J; Pettaway, CA; Pagliaro, LC. Treatment for Metastatic Penile Cancer After First-line Chemotherapy Failure: Analysis of Response and Survival Outcomes. *Urology.*, 2015, 85(5), 1104-1110.

[5] Djajadiningrat, RS; Graafland, NM; van Werkhoven, E; et al. Contemporary Management of Regional Nodes in Penile Cancer—Improvement of Survival? *J Urol.*, 2014, 191(1), 68-73. doi:10.1016/J.JURO.2013.07.088.

[6] Heyns, CF; Mendoza-Valdés, A; Pompeo, ACL. Diagnosis and Staging of Penile Cancer. *Urology.*, 2010, 76(2), S15-S23. doi:10.1016/j.urology.2010.03.002.

[7] Hughes, B; Leijte, J; Shabbir, M; Watkin, N; Horenblas, S. Non-invasive and minimally invasive staging of regional lymph nodes in penile cancer. *World J Urol.*, 2009, 27(2), 197-203. doi:10.1007/s00345-008-0288-6.

[8] Siegel, RL; Miller, KD; Jemal, A. Cancer statistics, 2018. *CA Cancer J Clin.*, 2018, 68(1), 7-30. doi:10.3322/caac.21442.

[9] Pham, MN; Deal, AM; Ferguson, JE; et al. Contemporary survival trends in penile cancer: Results from the National Cancer Database. *Urol Oncol Semin Orig Investig.*, 2017, 35(12), 674.e1-674.e9. doi:10.1016/j.urolonc.2017.08.009.

[10] Burt, LM; Shrieve, DC; Tward, JD. Stage Presentation, Care Patterns, and Treatment Outcomes for Squamous Cell Carcinoma of the Penis. *Int J Radiat Oncol.*, 2014, 88(1), 94-100. doi:10.1016/j.ijrobp.2013.08.013.

[11] Tward, J. The case for nonsurgical therapy of nonmetastatic penile cancer. *Nat Rev Urol.*, 2018, 15(9), 574-584.

[12] Protzel, C; Hakenberg, OW. Chemotherapy in Penile Cancer. *Textb Penile Cancer.*, 2017, 235-243.

[13] Necchi, A. Systemic Therapy for Penile Cancer. *Eur Urol Suppl.*, 2018, 17(6), 160-163.

[14] Gagliano, RG; Blumenstein, BA; Crawford, ED; Stephens, RL; Coltman, CA; Costanzi, JJ. cis-Diamminedichloroplatinum in the treatment of advanced epidermoid carcinoma of the penis: a Southwest Oncology Group Study. *J Urol.*, 1989, 141(1), 66-67. http://www.ncbi.nlm.nih.gov/pubmed/2642312. Accessed February 27, 2019.

[15] Theodore, C; Skoneczna, I; Bodrogi, I; et al. A phase II multicentre study of irinotecan (CPT 11) in combination with cisplatin (CDDP) in metastatic or locally advanced penile carcinoma (EORTC PROTOCOL 30992). *Ann Oncol.*, 2008, 19(7), 1304-1307. doi:10.1093/annonc/mdn149.

[16] Di Lorenzo, G; Buonerba, C; Federico, P; et al. Cisplatin and 5-fluorouracil in inoperable, stage IV squamous cell carcinoma of the penis. *BJU Int.*, 2012, 110(11b), E661-E666. doi:10.1111/j.1464-410X.2012.11453.x.

[17] Nicholson, S; Hall, E; Harland, SJ; et al. Phase II trial of docetaxel, cisplatin and 5FU chemotherapy in locally advanced and metastatic penis cancer (CRUK/09/001). *Br J Cancer.*, 2013, 109(10), 2554-2559.

[18] Dickstein, RJ; Munsell, MF; Pagliaro, LC; Pettaway, CA. Prognostic factors influencing survival from regionally advanced squamous cell carcinoma of the penis after preoperative chemotherapy. *BJU Int.*, 2016, 117(1), 118-125. doi:10.1111/bju.12946.

[19] Reddy, JP; Pettaway, CA; Levy, LB; et al. Factors associated with regional recurrence after lymph node dissection for penile squamous cell carcinoma. *BJU Int.*, 2017, 119(4), 591-597. doi:10.1111/bju.13686.

[20] Rieken, M; Djajadiningrat, RS; Kluth, LA; et al. Predictors of Cancer-specific Mortality After Disease Recurrence in Patients with Squamous Cell Carcinoma of the Penis. *Eur Urol.*, 2014, 66(5), 811-814. doi:10.1016/j.eururo.2014.05.032.

[21] Ottenhof, SR; Vegt, E. The role of PET/CT imaging in penile cancer. *Transl Androl Urol.*, 2017, 6(5), 833. doi:10.21037/TAU.2017.04.36.

[22] Salazar, A; Júnior, EP; Salles, PGO; Silva-Filho, R; Reis, EA; Mamede, M. 18F-FDG PET/CT as a prognostic factor in penile cancer. *Eur J Nucl Med Mol Imaging.*, August 2018. doi:10.1007/s00259-018-4128-7.

[23] Nicolai, N; Sangalli, LM; Necchi, A; et al. A Combination of Cisplatin and 5-Fluorouracil With a Taxane in Patients Who Underwent Lymph Node Dissection for Nodal Metastases From Squamous Cell Carcinoma of the Penis: Treatment Outcome and Survival Analyses in Neoadjuvant and Adjuvant Settings. *Clin Genitourin Cancer.*, 2016, 14(4), 323-330. doi:10.1016/j.clgc.2015.07.009.

[24] Djajadiningrat, RS; Bergman, AM; van Werkhoven, E; Vegt, E; Horenblas, S. Neoadjuvant Taxane-Based Combination Chemotherapy in Patients with Advanced

Penile Cancer. *Clin Genitourin Cancer.*, 2015, 13(1), 44-49. doi:10.1016/ j.clgc.2014.06.005.

[25] Necchi, A; Pond, GR; Raggi, D; et al. Clinical Outcomes of Perioperative Chemotherapy in Patients With Locally Advanced Penile Squamous-Cell Carcinoma: Results of a Multicenter Analysis. *Clin Genitourin Cancer.*, 2017, 15(5), 548-555.e3. doi:10.1016/j.clgc.2017.02.002.

[26] Dexeus, FH; Logothetis, CJ; Sella, A; et al. Combination chemotherapy with methotrexate; bleomycin and cisplatin for advanced squamous cell carcinoma of the male genital tract. *J Urol.*, 1991, 146(5), 1284-1287. http://www.ncbi.nlm.nih.gov/ pubmed/1719241. Accessed February 28, 2019.

[27] Hakenberg, OW; Nippgen, JBW; Froehner, M; Zastrow, S; Wirth, MP. Cisplatin, methotrexate and bleomycin for treating advanced penile carcinoma. *BJU Int.*, 2006, 98(6), 1225-1227. doi:10.1111/j.1464-410X.2006.06496.x.

[28] Pizzocaro, G; Piva, L. Adjuvant and neoadjuvant vincristine, bleomycin, and methotrexate for inguinal metastases from squamous cell carcinoma of the penis. *Acta Oncol.*, 1988, 27(6b), 823-824. http://www.ncbi.nlm.nih.gov/pubmed/ 2466471. Accessed February 28, 2019.

[29] Sharma, P; Djajadiningrat, R; Zargar-Shoshtari, K; et al. Adjuvant chemotherapy is associated with improved overall survival in pelvic node–positive penile cancer after lymph node dissection: A multi-institutional study. *Urol Oncol Semin Orig Investig.*, 2015, 33(11), 496.e17-496.e23. doi:10.1016/j.urolonc.2015.05.008.

[30] Di Lorenzo, G; Federico, P; Buonerba, C; et al. Paclitaxel in Pretreated Metastatic Penile Cancer: Final Results of a Phase 2 Study. *Eur Urol.*, 2011, 60(6), 1280-1284. doi:10.1016/j.eururo.2011.08.028.

[31] Pickering, LM; Tovey, H; Elliott, T; et al. VinCaP: A phase II trial of vinflunine chemotherapy in locally-advanced and metastatic carcinoma of the penis (CRUK/12/021). *J Clin Oncol.*, 2018, 36(15_suppl), 4514-4514. doi:10.1200/ JCO.2018.36.15_suppl.4514.

[32] Necchi, A; Lo Vullo, S; Perrone, F; et al. First-line therapy with dacomitinib, an orally available pan-HER tyrosine kinase inhibitor, for locally advanced or metastatic penile squamous cell carcinoma: results of an open-label, single-arm, single-centre, phase 2 study. *BJU Int.*, 2018, 121(3), 348-356. doi:10.1111/ bju.14013.

[33] Huang, K; Liu, R; Peng, Q; et al. EGFR mono-antibody salvage therapy for locally advanced and distant metastatic penile cancer: Clinical outcomes and genetic analysis. *Urol Oncol Semin Orig Investig.*, 2019, 37(1), 71-77. doi:10.1016/ J.UROLONC.2018.10.016.

[34] Apolo, AB; Mortazavi, A; Stein, MN; et al. A phase I study of cabozantinib plus nivolumab (CaboNivo) and ipilimumab (CaboNivoIpi) in patients (pts) with refractory metastatic urothelial carcinoma (mUC) and other genitourinary (GU)

tumors. *J Clin Oncol.*, 2017, 35(6_suppl), 293-293. doi:10.1200/JCO.2017.35.6_suppl.293.

[35] Jacob, JM; Ferry, EK; Gay, LM; et al. Comparative Genomic Profiling of Refractory and Metastatic Penile and Nonpenile Cutaneous Squamous Cell Carcinoma: Implications for Selection of Systemic Therapy. *J Urol.*, 2018, 201(3), 541-548.

[36] McDaniel, AS; Hovelson, DH; Cani, AK; et al. Genomic Profiling of Penile Squamous Cell Carcinoma Reveals New Opportunities for Targeted Therapy. *Cancer Res.*, 2015, 75(24), 5219-5227. doi:10.1158/0008-5472.CAN-15-1004.

[37] Feber, A; Worth, DC; Chakravarthy, A; et al. CSN1 somatic mutations in penile squamous cell carcinoma. *Cancer Res.*, 2016, 76(16):4720-4727. doi:10.1158/0008-5472.CAN-15-3134.

[38] Ali, SM; Pal, SK; Wang, K; et al. Comprehensive Genomic Profiling of Advanced Penile Carcinoma Suggests a High Frequency of Clinically Relevant Genomic Alterations. *Oncologist.*, 2016, 21(1), 33-39. doi:10.1634/theoncologist.2015-0241.

[39] Jad, Chahoud; Barrett, Z. McCormick; Frederico, Netto; Priya, Rao; Curtis, R; Pickering, CAP. Penile squamous cell carcinoma is genomically similar to other HPV-driven tumors. In: *GU ASCO Symposium.*, 2019, meetinglibrary.asco.org/record/170199/abstract.

[40] Sambandam, V; Frederick, MJ; Shen, L; et al. PDK1 mediates NOTCH1-mutated head and neck squamous carcinoma vulnerability to therapeutic PI3K/mTOR inhibition. *Clin Cancer Res.*, February 2019, clincanres.3276.2018. doi:10.1158/1078-0432.CCR-18-3276.

[41] Hsieh, AC; Moasser, MM. Targeting HER proteins in cancer therapy and the role of the non-target HER3. *Br J Cancer.*, 2007, 97(4), 453-457. doi:10.1038/sj.bjc.6603910.

[42] Hassan, B; Akcakanat, A; Holder, AM; Meric-Bernstam, F. Targeting the PI3-kinase/Akt/mTOR signaling pathway. *Surg Oncol Clin N Am.*, 2013, 22(4), 641-664. doi:10.1016/j.soc.2013.06.008.

[43] Mok, TS; Cheng, Y; Zhou, X; et al. Improvement in Overall Survival in a Randomized Study That Compared Dacomitinib With Gefitinib in Patients With Advanced Non-Small-Cell Lung Cancer and EGFR-Activating Mutations. *J Clin Oncol.*, 2018, 36(22), 2244-2250. doi:10.1200/JCO.2018.78.7994.

[44] Lu, X; Horner, JW; Paul, E; et al. Effective combinatorial immunotherapy for castration-resistant prostate cancer. *Nature.*, 2017, 543(7647), 728-732. doi:10.1038/nature21676.

[45] Hellmann, MD; Ciuleanu, TE; Pluzanski, A; et al. Nivolumab plus Ipilimumab in Lung Cancer with a High Tumor Mutational Burden. *N Engl J Med.*, 2018, 378(22), 2093-2104. doi:10.1056/NEJMoa1801946.

[46] Udager, AM; Liu, TY; Skala, SL; et al. Frequent PD-L1 expression in primary and metastatic penile squamous cell carcinoma: potential opportunities for immunotherapeutic approaches. *Ann Oncol.*, 2016, 27(9), 1706-1712. doi:10.1093/annonc/mdw216.

[47] Cocks, M; Taheri, D; Ball, MW; et al. Immune-checkpoint status in penile squamous cell carcinoma: a North American cohort. *Hum Pathol.*, 2017, 59, 55-61. doi:10.1016/j.humpath.2016.09.003.

[48] Deng, C; Li, Z; Guo, S; et al. Tumor PD-L1 expression is correlated with increased TILs and poor prognosis in penile squamous cell carcinoma. *Oncoimmunology.*, 2017, 6(2), e1269047. doi:10.1080/2162402X.2016.1269047.

[49] Ottenhof, SR; Djajadiningrat, RS; de Jong, J; Thygesen, HH; Horenblas, S; Jordanova, ES. Expression of Programmed Death Ligand 1 in Penile Cancer is of Prognostic Value and Associated with HPV Status. *J Urol.*, 2017, 197(3 Part 1), 690-697. doi:10.1016/j.juro.2016.09.088.

[50] Davidsson, S; Carlsson, J; Giunchi, F; et al. PD-L1 Expression in Men with Penile Cancer and its Association with Clinical Outcomes. *Eur Urol Oncol.*, 2018, 0(0). doi:10.1016/j.euo.2018.07.010.

[51] Olesen, TB; Sand, FL; Rasmussen, CL; et al. Prevalence of human papillomavirus DNA and p16INK4a in penile cancer and penile intraepithelial neoplasia: a systematic review and meta-analysis. *Lancet Oncol.*, 2019, 20(1), 145-158. doi:10.1016/S1470-2045(18)30682-X.

[52] Spiess, PE; Dhillon, J; Baumgarten, AS; Johnstone, PA; Giuliano, AR. Pathophysiological Basis of Human Papillomavirus in Penile Cancer: Key to Prevention and Delivery of More Effective Therapies Pathophysiological Basis of Human Papillomavirus in Penile Cancer : Key to Prevention and Delivery of More Effective Therapies. *CA Cancer J Clin.*, 2016, 66(6), 481-495. doi:10.3322/caac.21354.

In: Penile Cancer: Challenges and Controversies ISBN: 978-1-53615-950-9
Editors: F. E. Martins and M. L. Djordjevic

Chapter 10

Follow-Up of Penile Cancer: Contemporary Recommendations for Primary Disease and Inguinal Lymph Nodes

Lona Vyas and Oliver Kayes*
Leeds Teaching Hospitals NHS Trust, Leeds, United Kingdom

Abstract

Penile cancer is a rare malignancy, but favorable overall survival outcomes are achievable. However, the physical and psychological trauma of penile amputation and high morbidity associated with traditional inguinal lymphadenectomy have encouraged surgeons to adopt more minimally invasive and tissue sparing approaches. However, this should not be at the expense of primary oncological control. Evidenced-based approaches have helped to develop surveillance strategies that are effective in detecting disease recurrence early in order to allow second/third line therapy. Likewise, close follow up of the highest risks groups for disease progression is mandated to permit timely and efficacious intervention. Finally, long-term survivorship and quality of life remain realistic and important goals for these patients. The collective experience of treating men with a rare genital cancer highlights the benefits of centralized care and follow up in high volume centres with dedicated skills and infrastructure.

Keywords: penile cancer, follow-up, primary disease, regional inguinal nodes, recommendations, penile cancer surveillance

* Corresponding Author's E-mail: o.kayes@nhs.net.

Introduction

The management of penile cancer has changed with the evolution of penile preserving surgery and improvements in diagnosis. The primary aim for penile cancer treatment is to eradicate disease with minimal morbidity. The secondary goals are to reduce the risk of recurrence, optimize survival rates whilst protecting the patient's body image and overall wellbeing. Therefore, appropriate follow up of patients is a crucial step in the management of penile cancer patients. Often these men are self-conscious and exhibit psychological dysfunction1 which can impact on effective surveillance [1]. The aims of follow up should incorporate early detection of disease recurrence or progression and assess any complications of surgery alongside continual patient education and ongoing psychosexual support.

It is useful to define what is understood by the terms: cancer recurrence and/or cancer progression. Generally, penile cancer identified after treatment is completed, and after a period of time when the cancer could not be detected, is typically called a cancer recurrence. Usually, penile cancer can recur at a local site associated with the primary tumour (i.e. penile stump), the locoregional lymph nodes (i.e. groin or pelvic mass) or it might return somewhere else in the body (i.e. subcutaneous or distant metastases). Cancer progression is a term that describes a disease that is progressing or worsening. With cancer, progressive disease can be defined as increased size of the tumour (tumour burden) or spread of the tumour since the beginning of treatment. Both terms do not necessarily equate to treatment failure and may share similarities regarding the patterns of disease observed. Men can be risk stratified using several parameters namely: stage, grade, histological risk factors and lymph node involvement to aid surveillance planning; particularly with respect to the frequency and type of clinical and/or radiological review utilized. Current guidelines suggest that men are followed up for a minimum of five years and discharged if there has been no recurrence or ongoing functional or cosmetic issues. This chapter discusses how to optimally manage the follow up for men treated with penile cancer.

Rates and Patterns of Disease Recurrence

In one study, looking at 700 patients, 29.3% (n=205) had a cancer recurrence; consisting of 18.6% local, 9.3% regional, and 1.4% distant recurrences [2]. Of the recurrences, 92.2% occurred within five years after primary treatment. All regional and distant recurrences occurred within 50 and 16 months respectively. The local recurrence rate was 27.7% after penile-preserving therapy and 5.3% after amputation. The regional recurrence rate was 2.3% in patients staged as pN0, 19.1% in patients staged as pN+, and

9.1% in patients undergoing a wait-and-see policy. The 5-yr disease-specific survival was 92% after a local recurrence and 32.7% after a regional recurrence. All patients with a distant recurrence died within 22 months. This forms the basis for the rationale for more intensive follow up in the first two years with typically a reduction in frequency of consultations over the subsequent years. Follow up regimens have not changed despite evolving surgical technique moving towards organ sparing surgery, with a recent study reporting further organ sparing surgery for local recurrence, when feasible [3].

Individual recurrence rates are dependent on several important factors:

- Higher primary tumour stage (pTNM)
- Worse tumour differentiation (Grade) [4,5]
- Presence of high risk human papilloma virus (hrHPV) [6]
- Presence of lymphovascular or perineural invasion [7,8]
- Presence of lymph node or distant metastases

When considering an appropriate surveillance strategy one should consider the above prognostic factors alongside the nature of the primary surgical treatments undertaken. The advent of penile preserving surgery and sentinel lymph node biopsy techniques pertain to an acknowledged increased risk of disease relapse mandating a more intensive surveillance protocol. Conversely, men treated with radical intent and with lower risk disease (≤pT2 and/or pN0) can be spared extensive clinical and radiological follow up. Recurrence is often categorized into local, regional or distant disease.

Premalignant Lesions

Men treated with topical therapies or penile preserving procedures for premalignant lesions (pTis) usually have a clinical review every three months for two years. Subsequently, six monthly visits for a further three years. At five years the patient can be discharged with advice to self-examine. The association with other skin dermatoses (e.g. lichen sclerosus) can be effectively managed through the above strategy and patients potentially discharged earlier if their clinical response is absolute [9]. Disease progression from penile intraepithelial neoplasia (PeIN) to invasive squamous cell carcinoma is reported to occur in upto 35% of higher risk undifferentiated lesions; often typified by disease persistence or early recurrence despite adequate topical therapy.

Local Recurrence

The reported incidence of local recurrence following partial or total penectomy is low (0-7%). This can increase to 50% for patients treated more conservatively [10-14]. However, there is very little difference in cancer specific survival (CSS) between penile preservation and partial penectomy [15]. More importantly, if local recurrence is detected early, the cancer specific survival may be unaffected [16]. Conversely nodal disease significantly increases the risk of disease specific mortality.

Therefore, clinical assessment is aimed at early detection involving the: primary site (penis/scrotum), locoregional sites (inguinal) and distant sites (chest, abdomen and pelvis). Excellent oncological control can be achieved using penile preserving surgery, with excision margins of few millimetres, and has led to the routine implementation of these techniques internationally over the last 10 years. However, vigilant clinical examination during follow up is paramount to detect locally recurrent or de novo primary tumours [1]. Penile cancers (<5%) have been detected beyond the typical five-year surveillance period and probably represent true, new tumours rather than standard recurrent disease. Therefore, some experts still advocate surveillance over longer periods in excess of 10 years or even for life. This may be unnecessary with appropriate patient education and counselling.

Estimated five-year cancer survival for lesions pT1a or greater is 81% with an overall survival for all penile cancer patients of 66% [17]. Conversely, lymph node involvement is associated with poorer prognostic outcomes. If local recurrence does occur, salvage surgery can be used without negatively impacting on long-term survival [15,18,19]. Human factors play a vital role in this strategy, as a commitment to frequent follow up is required to ensure prompt detection and treatment. Risk stratification is also required as different treatments have different recurrence rates. Repeat examination, nodal staging and optimal salvage treatment is paramount if recurrence occurs.

Nodal Disease and Locoregional Recurrence

Approach to initial staging of nodal disease depends on the presence of palpable inguinal lymph nodes plus the pathological stage (pT) and grade of the primary tumour [20-22] and is covered elsewhere this textbook. Men with a low risk for metastatic disease, such as Tis and Ta disease, can be managed conservatively. However, following initial treatment, men at higher risk of locoregional recurrence will require further imaging for early detection [23].

For men presenting initially with impalpable inguinal lymph nodes, the main diagnostic procedure for nodal disease in Europe is dynamic sentinel node biopsy

(DSNB) and the technique is outlined in chapter 4. The role of DSNB as part of the standard assessment of men who develop local tumour recurrence during follow up remains controversial. However, DSNB should be considered in all men who develop local recurrence in the absence of clinical or radiological suspicious lymphadenopathy [24]. The risk of developing locoregional relapse (i.e., recurrence) in men with initial negative DSNB (i.e., false negative) is between 4 to 15%. This mandates routine surveillance in all men with negative DSNB for a minimum of two years to detect the small proportion who will relapse or progress early due to a potential technical issue or error.

In men with non-visualization or technical difficulties during DSNB, it may be appropriate to perform a second, immediate DSNB [24]. Alternatively, a modified template inguinal lymph node dissection (ILND) is a reasonable alternative to increase diagnostic accuracy against balancing potential morbidity concerns in such higher risk patients. Conversely, some clinicians may opt for clinical and radiological observation [25]. Following modified ILND, up to 15% patients can suffer disease recurrence or progression; usually occurring within two years.

A poorer cancer specific survival is reported for node positive disease [26] and therefore long-term surveillance is recommended for high risk patients with a combination of image modalities. In the era of DSNB, and despite changes in the TNM staging system leading directly to more precise evaluation of disease states with superior prognostic value compared to previous classification systems [27, 28]; the survival rates in contemporary series for cN0, cN1, cN2 and cN3 disease is static reported as: 96%, 80%, 66%, 37% respectively [2]. This phenomenon is likely underpinned by a lack of improvement in (neo)adjuvant treatments for node positive patients. Therefore, men developing locoregional recurrence currently will continue to face poorer overall survival outcomes.

Regional recurrence rates are more complex and are determined by:

I. Development of local recurrence with new lymphatic spread and concurrent regional recurrence.
II. Initial nodal treatment option (close surveillance, DSNB or lymphadenectomy).
III. Pathological nodal status and presence of extranodal disease.

Pathological nodal disease differs slightly from the clinical stage with pN0 disease reporting regional recurrence rates ranging between 0-10%. Conversely, up to 45% of node positive disease (pN+) [29, 30] cases can recur. Overall 10-20% chance of recurrence for patients with node negative disease on surveillance. Thus, early detection of nodal metastasis is crucial [31, 32].

Most experts and guidelines advocate a similar follow up regimen to mirror primary surveillance with close follow up for the first 2 years and less frequent 6 monthly thereafter (see below). Salvage treatment is reported as effective despite regional recurrence having a negative prognostic effect [33].

Distant Recurrence

Distant recurrence is incurable and palliative chemoradiotherapy is used in certain cases. Therefore, whilst self-examination and clinical locoregional surveillance is important, the role of imaging or surgical assessment is critical. Pelvic node disease can be present in 20-30% of men with positive inguinal nodes [34, 35].

As discussed, Lont et al found that the number of positive inguinal nodes and/or extranodal extension directly relates to the likelihood of pelvic node disease [31]. Concurrently, if there is one affected lymph node with no adverse prognostic factors, these affected men have less risk of distant recurrence. If either, at first presentation or if recurrent disease is beyond the groins, this can be difficult to treat, especially in cases where large fungating masses protrude from the groin. Aggressive resection and reconstruction with tissue flaps and adjuvant radiotherapy may provide a survival advantage for some men with a true localized recurrent nodal mass; whilst for almost all, it allows optimization of quality of life issues (i.e., pain, wound care, bleeding, mobility) and end of life planning. However, as alluded to previously, the disease specific survival is often poor in men with distant or subcutaneous metastases, with limited benefit from conventional therapy. Additionally, these men often have a poor performance status on presentation and therefore often do not qualify for a trial of treatment. Palliation (chemoradiation and/or surgery) and best supportive care remain the most appropriate management option in the vast majority of similar cases.

Surveillance and Management

The aim of follow up is clearly designed to detect disease recurrence or progression at the earliest opportunity to allow an appropriate intervention that will improve longer term outcomes for these patients. Follow up guidelines, based on level 1 evidence, recommend a maximum of five years follow up in patients without any observed recurrence.

The advent of increasing levels of penile preserving surgery suggests that a focus has been developed to detect recurrences at the primary site amendable to further penile preserving surgery or limited partial penectomy. Likewise, the ability to assess patients regularly allows for higher risk disease to be investigated and treated appropriately. This may be through partial or total amputation in the case of high-risk local recurrence or multimodal therapy if disease recurrence or progression is at the level of (or beyond) the inguinal region is suspected.

The different American and European advisory groups offer similar follow up strategies based on increased frequency during the first two years when most recurrences or treatment failures will present. Self-examination should be explained to all patients. For penile preserving surgery patients 3 monthly follow up for the first 2 years is recommended. More radical techniques including, penile amputation, require 6 monthly consultations.

For regional lymph nodes, close surveillance is advised especially following minimally invasive techniques such as DSNB. The consensus for detection of regional recurrence is that it should be clinically driven through examination in the clinic. Clinical findings can be further augmented with USS +/- FNAC or cross-sectional imaging such as CT or MRI. Imaging is otherwise not routinely advocated by the EAU or ESMO groups but the NCCN (36) suggest its validity in the long-term surveillance of advanced disease patients who are at the highest risk of relapse over the initial two-year period. All groups advise a minimum five year follow up period but acknowledge the presence of unusual cases developing disease progression or relapse many years after the initial diagnosis.

Predictive and prognostic nomograms have been developed to help risk stratify patients. However, the clear message from the EAU and ESMO guidelines is that they are unreliable and lack accuracy for clinical practice. Interestingly, the institute for the Study of Urological Disease (ISUD) have posted these nomograms on their website (http://www.imop.gr/en/urotools-nomograms-penile-cancer). Thuret et al has shown that the AJCC staging system combined with tumour grade was the simplest and most accurate method available; reflected across all guidelines (LE 3; Grade C) [37]. External validation using a different patient population has corroborated these conclusions. The nomogram consisting of TNM classification and tumour grading was shown to have better performance for predicting cancer-specific mortality in penile cancer patients who underwent definitive surgery.

Management of Recurrent Disease

Men with recurrent disease are broadly assessed and treated in a similar manner as previously described. Most guidelines acknowledge that recurrent disease involving the penile corpora or the inguinal region carries a significantly worse prognosis. Therefore, all groups advocate partial or total penile amputation for oncological control of significant local recurrence and implement multimodal therapy using a combination of surgery and chemoradiation to treat inguinal recurrence in these clinical settings.

Otherwise men can be treated as per the standard guidance for treating primary penile cancer.

The approach to patients with advanced local, regional or distant disease is mostly based on small, retrospective, case series. Historically, the favoured approach has been with combinations of chemotherapy, although the evidence base for the most optimal regime and timing of treatment (adjuvant vs neoadjuvant) is not strong. It is unusual for men to be cured using one treatment modality alone. Therefore, this guidance cannot exceed a level of evidence 3 or grade C recommendation. Only limited recommendation on the use of precision medicine or targeted therapy is outlined in the EAU guidance and remains a core area for development in the future.

Quality of Life (QoL): Role of Follow up

Only the EAU guidelines attempt to consolidate the sparse data in this area and provide a summary of recommendations. It has long since been acknowledged that men suffering from penile cancer, who subsequently undergoing potentially mutilating surgery, are at high risk of suffering the negative psychological and functional consequences of the illness. Whilst oncological cure remains paramount, long term cancer survivorship plays an important role in men treated for penile cancer. Current data on sexual function and QoL is sparse and limited by the retrospective nature of the studies, lack of control groups and the use of non-validated questionnaires. The clearest message from the guideline states that nearly 80% of men will be cured of their disease and live in the longer-term with the consequences of their illness and/or treatment. Partial penectomy has a negative impact on patient self-esteem and sexual function. Increasing experience with penile preserving surgery allows for better QoL and sexual function and should be offered whenever feasible. Referral to centres with experience is recommended and psychological support is very important for penile cancer patients.

Conclusion

Recurrence for penile cancer occurs mainly in the first 2 years with almost all recurrence within the first 5 years. Therefore, more intensive follow up occurs in the initial two years following treatment. Provided there is adequate surveillance there is no impact on overall survival. Imaging can be used as an adjunct to history and examination to detect regional and distant metastases. Further studies are required to assess the role of PET/CT, molecular markers and psychological intervention in follow up protocols of the future.

7.1.4. ***Guidelines for follow-up in penile cancer***

	Interval of follow-up		**Examinations and investigations**	**Minimum duration of follow-up**	**Strength rating**
	Years one to two	Years three to five			
Recommendations for follow-up of the primary tumour					
Penile-preserving treatment	Three months	Six months	Regular physician or self-examination. Repeat biopsy after topical or laser treatment for penile intraepithelial neoplasia.	Five years	Strong
Amputation	Three months	One year	Regular physician or self-examination.	Five years	Strong
Recommendations for follow-up of the inguinal lymph nodes					
Surveillance	Three months	Six months	Regular physician or self-examination.	Five years	Strong
pN0 at initial treatment	Three months	One year	Regular physician or self-examination. Ultrasound with fine-needle aspiration biopsy optional.	Five years	Strong
pN+ at initial treatment	Three months	Six months	Regular physician or self-examination. Ultrasound with fine-needle aspiration cytology optional, computed tomography/magnetic resonance imaging optional.	Five years	Strong

Figure 1. Example of Good Practice: European Guidelines.

KEY POINTS

- Follow up protocols focus on the possible chance of cancer recurrence at the local or regional sites.
- Most recurrences occur within 2 years and nearly all recurrences occur within 5 years.
- Men can be risk stratified for interval surveillance based on the nature of their primary surgery (penile preserving versus radical amputation), node staging investigations and adverse prognostic features.

- Early detection of recurrence can be treated with curative intent and similar cancer specific survival rates.
- Men living with the consequences of penile cancer treatment will often need issues around their QoL and survivorship addressed beyond their standard cancer surveillance.

References

[1] Maddeineni S, Lau M and Sangar V. Identifying the needs of penile cancer sufferers: A systematic review of the quality of life, psychosexual and psychosocial literature in penile cancer. *BMC Urology* 2009 9:8. https://link.springer.com/article/10.1186/1471-2490-9-8.

[2] Liejte JA et al. Recurrence patterns of squamous cell carcinoma of the penis: recommendations for follow up based on a two centre analysis of 700 patients *European Urology* 54(1):161-8 August 2008.

[3] Baumgarten et al. Penile sparing surgery for penile cancer: A multicenter international retrospective cohort. *J Urol* 2018 (199):5 (1233-1237).

[4] Ornellas AA, et al. Prognostic factors in invasive squamous cell carcinoma of the penis: analysis of 196 patients treated at the Brazilian National cancer institute. *J Urol.* 2008; 180(4):1354-9.

[5] Velazquez EF, Ayala G, Liu H Chaux A, Zanotti M, Torres J et al. Histologic grade and perineural invasion are more important than tumour thickness as predictor of nodal metastasis in penile squamous cell carcinoma invading 5 to 10mm. *Am J Surg Pathol.* 2008;32(7):974-9.

[6] Tang DH, Clark PE, Giannico G, Hameed O, Chang SS, Gellert LL. Lack of P16 over expression in penile squamous cell carcinoma is associate with recurrence after lymph node dissection. *J Urol.* 2015; 193(2):519-25.

[7] Ficarra V, Zattoni F, Cunico SC, Galetti TP, Luciani L, Fandella A et al. Lymphatic and vascular embolization are independent predictive variables of inguinal lymph node involvement in patients with squamouse cell carcinoma of the penis: *Gruppo Uro-oncological* 2005;103(12):2507-16.

[8] Lopes A, Hidalgo GS, Kowalski LP, Torloni H, rossi BM, Fonsecca FP. Prognostic factors in carcinoma of the penis: multivariate analysis of 145 patients treaten with amputation and lymphadenectomy. *J Urol.*1996;156(5):1637-42.

[9] Kravvas G, Shim TN, Doiron PR et al. The diagnosis and management of male genital lichen sclerosus: a retrospective review of 301 patients. *J Eur Acad Dermatol Venereol.* 2018 Jan;32(1):91-95.

[10] Horenblas S, van Tinteren H, Delemarre JF, et al. Squamous cell carcinoma of the penis. II. Treatment of the primary tumor. *J Urol* 1992;147:1533-8; McLean M, Akl AM, Warde P, et al. The results of primary radiation therapy in the

management of squamous cell carcinoma of the penis. *Int J Radiat Oncol Biol Phys* 1993;25:623-8; Windahl T, Hellsten S. Laser treatment of localized squamous cell carcinoma of the penis. *J Urol* 1995;154:1020-3; Bandieramonte G, Santoro O, Boracchi P, et al. Total resection of glans penis surface by CO2 laser microsurgery. *Acta Oncol* 1988;27:575-8; Kroon BK, Horenblas S, Nieweg OE. Contemporary management of penile squamous cell carcinoma. *J Surg Oncol* 2005;89:43-50.

[11] McLean M et al. The results of primary radiation therapy in the management of squamous cell carcinoma of the penis. *Int J Radiat Oncol Biol Phys* 1993;25:623-8

[12] Windahl T, Hellsten S. Laser treatment of localized squamous cell carcinoma of the penis. *J Urol* 1995;154:1020-3

[13] Bandieramonte G et al. Total resection of glans penis surface by CO2 laser microsurgery. *Acta Oncol* 1988;27:575-8

[14] Kroon BK, Horenblas S, Nieweg OE. Contemporary management of penile squamous cell carcinoma. *J Surg Oncol* 2005;89:43-50

[15] Djajadiningrat RS, van WerkhovenE, Meinhardt W, van Rhijn BWG, Bex A, van der Poel HG, et al. Penile sparing surgery for penile cancer-does it affect survival? *J Urol.* 2014;192(1):120-6.

[16] Lerner SE, Jones JG, Fleischmann J. Management of recurrent penile cancer following partial or total penectomy. *Urol Clin North Am* 1994;21:729-37

[17] Djajadiningrat R, Van Werkhoven Eric, Horenblas, S. *Analysis of contemporary treatment of penile cancer at the Netherlands Cancer Institute.* Springer Science Business Media New York 2014 DOI: 10.1007/978-1-4939-0461-7_9

[18] Minhas S et al. What surgical resection margins are required to achieve oncological control in men with primary penile cancer? *BJU Int.* 2005;96(7):1040

[19] Lont AP et al. Penis conserving treatment for T1 and T2 penile carcinoma: clinical implications of a local recurrence. *J Urol*. 2006; 176(2):575-80

[20] Moses KA et al. Contemporary management of penile cancer: greater than 15-year MSKCC experience *Can J Urol* 2014;21:7201-6

[21] Pizzocaro G et al. EAU penile cancer guidelines 2009. *Eur Urol* 2010;57:1002-12

[22] Thuret R et al. A contemporary population-based assessment of the rate of lymph node dissection for penile carcinoma. *Ann Surg Oncol* 2011;18:439-46

[23] Mistry T et al. A 10-year retrospective audit of penile cancer management in the UK. *BJU Int* 2007;100:1277-81.

[24] Graafland NM et al. Repeat dynamic sentinel node biopsy in locally recurrent penile carcinoma. *BJU Int.* 2010 Apr;105(8):1121-4

[25] Djajadiningrat RS et al. Contemporary management of regional nodes in penile cancer-improvement of survival? *J Urol* 2014;191:68-73

[26] Rieken M et al. Predictors of cancer-specific mortality after disease recurrence in patients with squamous cell carcinoma of the penis. *Eur Urol* 2014;66:811-4.

[27] Zhu Y et al. New N Staging system of penile cancer provides a better reflection of prognosis. *J Urol* 2011;186(2):518-23

[28] Al Najar A et al. External validation of the proposed T and N categories of squamous cell carcinoma of the penis. *Int J Urol.* 2011; 11:312-6

[29] Marconnet L, Rigauls J, Bouchot O. Long term follow up on penile carcinoma with hgh risk for lymph node invasion treated with inguinal lymphadenectomy. *J Urol.* 2010; 183(6):2227-32.

[30] Slaton JW, Morgenstern N, Levy DA, Santos MW, Tamboli P, Ro JY, et al. Tumour stage, vascular invasion and the percentage of poorly differentiated cancer: independent prognosticators for inguinal lymph node metastasis in penile squamous cancer. *J Urol.* 2001;165(4):1138-42.

[31] Lont AP et al. Pelvic lymph node dissection for penile carcinoma: extent of inguinal lymph node involvement as an indication for pelvic lymph node involvement and survival. *J Urol.* 2007;177(3):947-52.

[32] Ravi R. Correlation between the extent of nodal involvement and survival following groin dissection for carcinoma of the penis. *Br J Urol.* 1993;72(5 pt2):817-9.

[33] Graafland NM et al. Inguinal recurrence following therapeutic lymphadeonpathy for node positive penile carcinoma: outcome and implications for management. *J Urol.* 2011;185(3):888-93.

[34] Djajadiningrat RS, van Werkhoven E, Horenblas S. Prophylactic pelvic lymoh node dissection in penile cancer patients. *J Urol.* 2015; 193(6):1976-80.

[35] Horenblas S, van Tinteren H, Delmarre JF, Moonen LM, Lustig V, van Waardenberg EW, Squamous cell carcinoma of the penis III. Treatment of regional lymph nodes. *J Urol.* 1993;149(3):492-7.

[36] Spiess PE, National Comprehensive Cancer Network New treatment guidelines for penile cancer. *J Natl Compr Canc Netw* 2013;11:659-62

[37] Thuret R, Sun M, Abdollah F, et al. Tumor grade improves the prognostic ability of American Joint Committee on Cancer stage in patients with penile carcinoma. *J Urol.* 2011 Feb;185(2):501-7.

SECTION D. PENILE RECONSTRUCTION FOLLOWING SURGICAL MANAGEMENT

In: Penile Cancer: Challenges and Controversies
Editors: F. E. Martins and M. L. Djordjevic ISBN: 978-1-53615-950-9

Chapter 11

ORGAN SPARING SURGERY AND FUNCTIONAL RESTORATION OF THE PENIS

Vladimir Kojovic* and Miroslav L. Djordjevic
School of Medicine, University of Belgrade, Belgrade, Serbia

ABSTRACT

Penile carcinoma (PC) is one of the less common tumors of the genitourinary system but it may present as a life-threatening condition with potential significant impact on the patient's sexual activity and quality of life due to possible severe psychological and functional disturbance. Malignant infiltration of the penile tissue and surgical treatment of PC can also be associated with erectile dysfunction. The ideal treatment outcome involves preservation of normal sexual and urinary functions while eradicating the disease, but this is not always possible due to the extent of the disease. Radical surgery can be an effective treatment modality, but this is often considered mutilating with a high incidence of aesthetic, functional and psychological morbidity. The development of organ preserving surgical techniques in appropriately selected patients allows for phallus preservation, reducing the negative impact on functional and cosmetic outcomes without sacrificing oncological objectives. Penile-sparing procedures have been increasingly performed and reported in recent decades, leading to minimized physical disfigurement and consequently maximizing quality of life. Therefore, goals of the surgical treatment of PC should be both eradication of the disease and preservation of as much functional penile tissue as possible. Additionally, total phallic reconstruction gives new perspectives to patients who were not candidates for organ-sparing procedures. The importance of long-term follow-up should be emphasized, especially in organ-preserving procedures. The main objective of this chapter is to highlight the treatment of PC with the possibility for preservation and restoration of erectile and sexual functions.

Keywords: penile carcinoma, erectile dysfunction, surgical treatment, sexual function

---

* Corressponding Author's E-mail: kojovic.dr@gmail.com; kojovicuromiros@gmail.com.

INTRODUCTION

In the industrialized world, particularly in developed countries of Europe and USA, penile carcinoma (PC) is an uncommon malignancy, but it is a significant health and social problem in many African, Asian, and South American countries. The incidence of PC in Europe ranges from 0.9 to 2.1 cases per 100 000 persons per year [1]. In the United States, PC accounts for only 0.4% to 0.6% of all malignant tumors of the adult male population, with an age-standardized incidence of 0.3 to 1.8 per 100 000 male inhabitants, having gradually declined over the last three decades [2, 3, 4]. The incidence of PC is higher in developing countries of Africa, South America and Asia, ranging from 1-10% of all malignancies in men [5, 6]. Brazil, Paraguay and Uganda have been recognized as the countries with the highest incidence, at a rate of 4.2-6.8 per 100 000, respectively [6, 7]. The lowest incidence of 0.1/100 000 is found among Israeli Jews [8]. An increasing incidence of PC have been reported in England and Denmark during the last decades due to changes in sexual practices, greater exposure to the sexually transmitted human papilloma viruses (HPV), and decreasing rates of childhood circumcision [9, 10]. Socioeconomic status, religious and sexual practices have a major role in the etiology of PC due to significant variation among ethnic groups, reflecting the importance of these factors [7].

The majority of PC are primary carcinomas (90%), of which 95% are squamous cell carcinoma (SCC). SCC most commonly affects men between the ages of 50 and 70, with only 19% in men under 40 and 7% in men under 30 being affected [2, 11, 12]. It occurs most commonly on the distal penis in more than 80% of men, especially the glans but also the coronal sulcus and prepuce [13, 14]. Penile SCC is a significant uro-oncological condition with approximately 640 new cases diagnosed in the UK each year and it accounts for 1% of all cancer deaths in males in the UK [15].

About one third of cases of PC are associated with HPV infection and, therefore, PC is common in regions with higher prevalence of HPV. This may account for the geographic variation in incidence [16]. The most commonly identified HPV serotypes are 16, 18, 31, 33, 45, 56, and 65 [1, 17]. Other factors positively associated with penile cancer are chronic inflammation (lichen sclerosus, phimosis), premalignant lesions, cigarette smoking, and low educational and socioeconomic status [18, 19, 20, 21]. Patients with HIV (human immunodeficiency virus) have an 8-fold increased risk for PC, but it may correspond to a higher incidence of HPV among men with HIV infection [22, 23, 24, 25]. Phimosis presents a risk factor for PC likely due to chronic inflammation which may result from inability to clean the glans and remove accumulated smegma, although smegma itself is not a carcinogen [26]. Maden et al. found that the risk of penile cancer was 3.2 times greater among men who had never been circumcised relative to men circumcised at birth and 3.0 times greater among men circumcised after the neonatal period [27, 28].

Premalignant lesions such as Bowen's disease, intraepithelial neoplasia grade III, giant condylomata (Buschke-Lowenstein tumor), erythroplasia of Queyrat and Paget's disease are associated with PC because up to one-third will transform into invasive SCC [22]. Cutaneous horn of the penis, Bowenoid papulosis and lichen sclerosus (balanitis xerotica obliterans-BXO) are sporadically associated with SCC of the penis [29, 30, 31].

The first step in the diagnosis of PC is physical examination of the penis which should include palpation of the glans and whole penile shaft. The tumor lesion is assessed with regard to size, location, fixation and involvement of the corporeal bodies. Physical examination must include palpation of the groins in search of inguinal lymph nodes (LN). The presence of LN metastases is very likely in patients with enlarged inguinal LN. However, clinically normal inguinal LN could have micrometastatic disease in approximately 25% of patients with PC [32]. Current imaging techniques are not reliable in detecting these micrometastases, so patients with clinically negative inguinal regions should undergo invasive LN staging if they have intermediate or high risk of lymphatic spread based on primary tumor characteristics [32, 33].

Ultrasound or magnetic resonance with an artificial erection can give information about tumor infiltration of the corpora [34, 35]. Biopsy may be a separate procedure from definitive surgical treatment or biopsy with frozen section confirmation can be followed by definitive local therapy. Staging of penile cancer by physical examination and imaging is critical for adequate and effective oncological treatment planning simultaneously preserving as much native tissue and function as possible.

Penile cancer is staged according to the TNM classification of malignant tumors by American Joint Committee on Cancer/Union for International Cancer Control [36]. A new TNM classification was proposed in order to distinguish invasion of the corpora cavernosa and spongiosum due to significant variation in prognosis [37]. Penile cancer is curable in early stages with the appropriate treatment, but its prognosis depends crucially on the proper management of the regional LN [1]. Five-year survival varies greatly by pathologic stage at the time of treatment: 100% survival for *in situ* tumors, 84% for pT1, 84% for pT2, and 54% for pT3-4, while 3-year survival for patients with pathologically positive LN was 65% [38]. Invasive PC is a lethal disease and without treatment most patients are dead from complications of loco-regional disease or metastasis within two years of diagnosis [39].

THE EVOLVING TREATMENT OF PENILE CANCER WITH FUNCTIONAL RESTORATION OF THE PENIS

Early diagnosis is essential in effective management and cure, and accurate staging is imperative for risk stratification and treatment planning. Treatment options depend upon tumor location, size, and clinical stage and if the tumor has changed significantly over time and continues to evolve [40]. Treatment modalities vary and may include topical chemotherapy, systemic chemotherapy, radiotherapy, laser excision/ablation, Mohs micrographic surgery, local surgical excision, circumcision, radical surgery and organ sparing surgery [41, 42].

Carcinoma *in situ* (CIS) penile lesions, such as erythroplasia of Queyrat and Bowen's disease, can be treated conservatively by local topical therapy, laser therapy, local excision or circumcision.

Topical chemotherapy agents (5-fluorouracil, imiquimod) were proven as moderately-effective first-line therapy in the treatment of penile CIS with few adverse events [43, 44].

Radiotherapy (plesiotherapy, interstitial brachytherapy, external beam radiotherapy) has been used as both primary and palliative treatments with success in the management of primary penile tumors as well as inguinal LN metastases [45]. Radiotherapy may be used in T1–2 lesions <4 cm in diameter [22, 46]. Brachytherapy achieves local control rates of 70–90% [47, 48, 49]. Local tumor recurrence rates are higher than after partial penectomy, but salvage surgery can achieve local control without jeopardizing overall survival [50, 51]. It has the benefit of leaving the penis with normal appearance and intact structures. Complications of radiation therapy are very common, such as urethral stenosis that may occur in 20–35% and glans necrosis in 10–20% of treated patients. With brachytherapy meatal stenosis occurs in >40% of patients [22, 52]. The effects of radiotherapy on sexual function are not well studied [53].

Laser therapy (CO_2, Nd:YAG, KTP) may be considered in Tis and T1 stages of disease. Laser ablation therapy showed good preservation of sexual function and satisfaction in treated patients [54, 55, 56]. Wound healing after laser therapy comprises secondary intention healing with full re-epithelialization at 8-10 weeks post-operatively. These patients need early detection of incomplete response to treatment and long-term surveillance [57, 58, 59].

Mohs micrographic surgery is a minimal invasive procedure that involves serial tissue resections with histological evaluation to ensure that a tumor-free margin is obtained. This procedure has shown favorable outcomes in patients with CIS and superficially invasive lesions of the glans and penile shaft. The advantages of the Mohs technique include tumor excision without positive margins and preservation of penile tissue with good aesthetical and functional outcomes. The disadvantage is high local tumor recurrence rate after one procedure. Therefore, patients subjected to this procedure should be carefully monitored for early signs of recurrence. However, in most cases the Mohs procedure can be repeated [60, 61, 62].

Indications for circumcision alone as a treatment of PC are preputial changes and low-grade and low-stage PC of the prepuce only. The reported tumor recurrence rate is more than 50% after two years, indicating mandatory regular and close surveillance [63,

64]. However, unfortunately, patients treated for PC have poor follow-up, especially in developing countries [65]. Most patients with penile lesions are uncircumcised in these countries.

In case of simple excision of a small tumor, negative surgical margins are essential. However, local recurrence rates may occur in up to 50% of patients [66]. This technique relies on primary closure, mobilization of local tissues, or grafting, and may not permit a cosmetically favorable result.

Despite progress in the development of the abovementioned mostly non-surgical therapies, surgery still plays a critical role in the treatment of penile cancer, especially for large tumors or tumors known or suspected to be invasive.

Traditional management of PC is partial penectomy (amputation of the glans and some extent of shaft length) with a 2 cm margin of normal tissue or total penectomy which were used even for small lesions on the glans [67]. These are mutilating procedures associated with a devastating impact on patients' physical and psychological status [68, 69, 70]. Men who had total penectomy report severely negative impact on their sexual function and quality of life [71]. Men who underwent partial penectomy reported significant decline in their erectile and orgasmic function, and sexual desire, as well as overall decreased satisfaction with sexual intercourse and a third of patients did not resume sexual activity after surgery [70]. Studies have shown that two-thirds of patients reported diminished sexual function, with psychiatric symptoms in up to 50% of them, including significant rates of impaired well-being, mental illness, avoidant behavior, post-traumatic stress, depression, and suicidal ideation [72]. Penis size is important in male perception of masculinity and virility and efforts to preserve penile length are important for psychological and functional reasons [73].

A major trend over the past few decades has been the development of less invasive surgery with the goal of providing oncologic control with minimal loss of penile tissue and preservation of function, cosmetic and psychological well-being [74, 68]. Earlier efforts to lessen the devastating impact of radical surgery included efforts to make the penile stump more prominent by mobilization and advancement of the remaining penile shaft from the suspensory ligament and even bringing the penile remnant below the scrotum with relocation of the testicles in order to maximize visibility and access to the penis and urethra [75, 76]. More recent reports have added resection of mons pubis fat and fixation of skin at base of the penis to deep structures with split-thickness skin grafting of the exposed base of the penis to allow greater visible length of the penis [77].

One of the most important developments in the treatment of PC has been the reduction of surgical margins sufficient for effective oncological control. Recent studies confirmed that patients with only 5 mm of clear margins have equal outcome as patients treated with more radical surgical interventions [78, 79, 80]. Fortunately, unnecessarily radical therapy is now discouraged, and a less morbid philosophy is well-established [22]. Patients receiving organ-sparing therapies compared to partial penectomy report better orgasmic function and fewer appearance concerns and less interference with quality of life [81].

Penile sparing surgery can provide excellent local control for superficial penile tumors as well as for appropriately selected invasive lesions with necessary strict follow-up in the early postoperative period [74]. Organ potency-sparing surgery has a positive impact on a wide spectrum of the patient's quality of life, including family, social and working relationships [68]. Organ-sparing techniques in penile cancer lead to slightly higher local tumor recurrence rates, compared with traditional partial or total penile amputation. Thus, adequate patient compliance is compulsory and an intensified follow-up for more than the usual 5 years postoperatively is required [82].

The human glans penis has a high concentration of sensory structures and nerve endings and since most cancerous lesions of the penis involve the glans, the unique anatomy of the human glans penis is particularly relevant [83]. Afferent sensory stimulation from the glans is important in the mechanisms of erection and orgasm [84]. Thus, significant loss of sensory nerve input, due to the penile tumor or its treatment, can lead to decreased erectile capability and loss of orgasmic function. Therefore, preserving the glans penis to the extent that is safely possible is a major goal of organ-preserving therapy. An innovative surgical technique for treating penile glans CIS is total glans resurfacing. This technique, first described by Bracka for treatment of lichen sclerosis, excises the glans epithelium only and replaces it with a split-thickness skin graft [85, 86]. This preserves the appearance of the natural glans tissue after healing of the graft, while the nerves to the glans remain undisturbed. Skin grafts have been shown to develop return of sensation over time [87]. The first report of this technique in penile CIS showed good functional outcomes without short-term tumor recurrence [88]. Shabbir et al. reported 25 patients with a prior biopsy-proven CIS who underwent glans resurfacing [89]. There were 10 unexpected T1-T2 tumors (40%) and a total of 12 instances of positive surgical margins (48%) with 28% undergoing further surgery, but only a 4% tumor recurrence rate.

When a tumor of the glans penis invades the glans but not the corpora cavernosa, glansectomy may provide the best compromise between tumor control and functional preservation approaches. Glansectomy uses the technique of complete penile disassembly to anatomically separate and remove the glans from the underlying corpora cavernosa [90, 91]. To recreate the appearance of a glans penis further reconstruction using split-thickness skin grafting on top of the corporeal bodies is necessary [92]. A report on the use of this technique in 15 patients found that all patients were able to have successful penetrative intercourse, orgasm and ejaculation but with decreased sensitivity of the neoglans [93]. There is no description in the literature of attempts to use the remaining dorsal nerves to try to restore erogenous sensation of the neoglans. In order to achieve sensation another technique has been described which mobilizes the penile urethra to a length of 2-3 cm longer than the tips of the corporeal bodies, and after ventral spatulation, the urethral surface is used to cover the tips of the corporeal bodies, thus recreating a more natural-appearing glans with sensation provided by urethral innervation. With a six-month follow-up after surgery, IIEF (International index of erectile function) scores for erection, ejaculation, orgasm and libido showed no significant difference compared to preoperative scores [94].

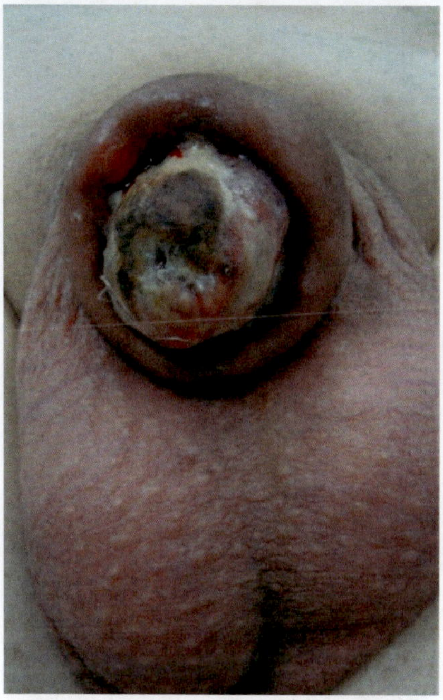

Figure 1. Penile carcinoma involved whole glans and distal urethra.

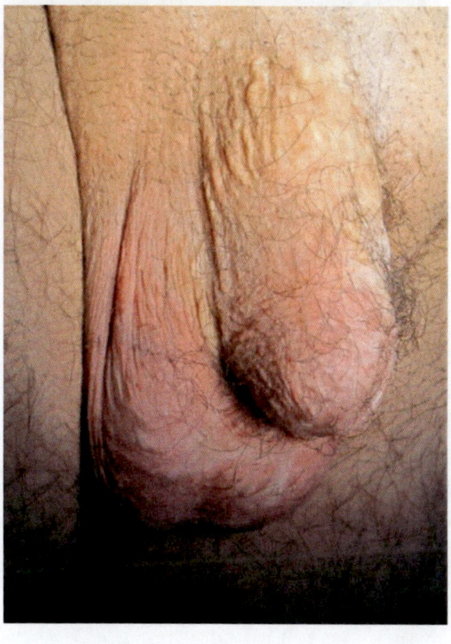

Figure 2. Penis is hidden. Glans is missing.

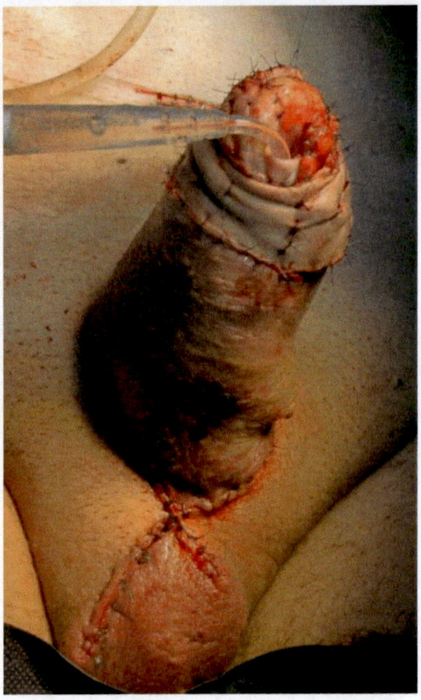

Figure 3. Penis is lengthened and covered with scrotal flaps. Glans is resurfaced using both skin and buccal mucosa grafts.

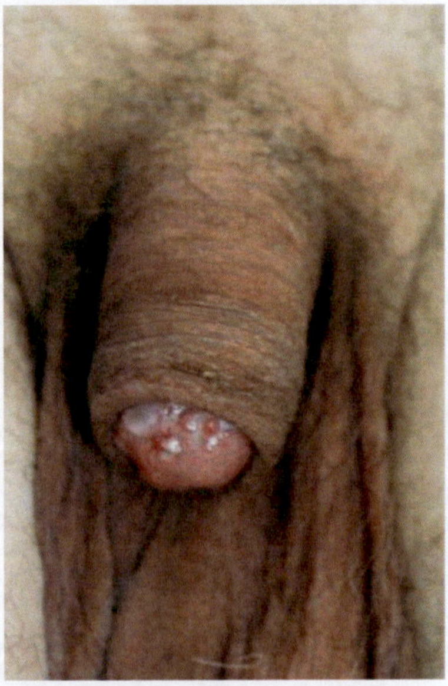

Figure 4. Appearance one year later.

After partial penectomy, lengthening and covering of the penile stump with vascularized genital flaps or free grafts derived from skin or buccal mucosa are necessary. To achieve a better outcome all these approaches can be combined (Figure 1, Figure 2, Figure 3, Figure 4).

A reconstructive option for restitution of penile skin after partial penectomy involves stage reconstruction using scrotal skin. After organ preserving surgery, the penile stump can be trapped (Figure 5), and after penile lengthening, penile skin is often insufficient to cover the whole penile body (Figure 6). The scrotal sac could be used for penile incorporation with glans fixed to the scrotal skin (Figure 7, Figure 8). The penile body with scrotal skin is divided from the scrotum several months later, achieving a satisfactory appearance of the genitalia (Figure 9, Figure 10).

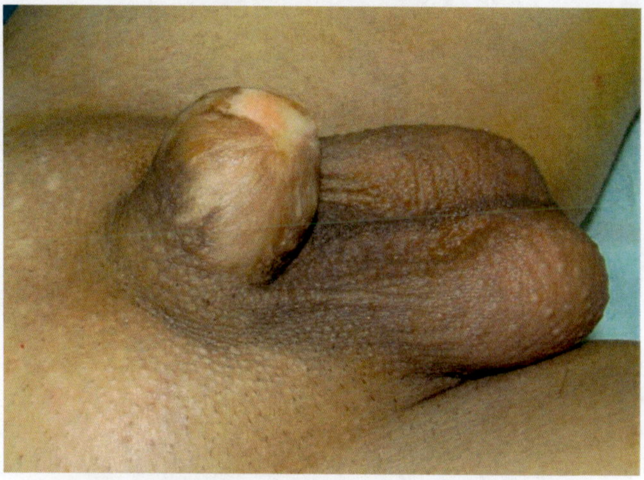

Figure 5. Penis became trapped after organ preserving surgery for penile carcinoma.

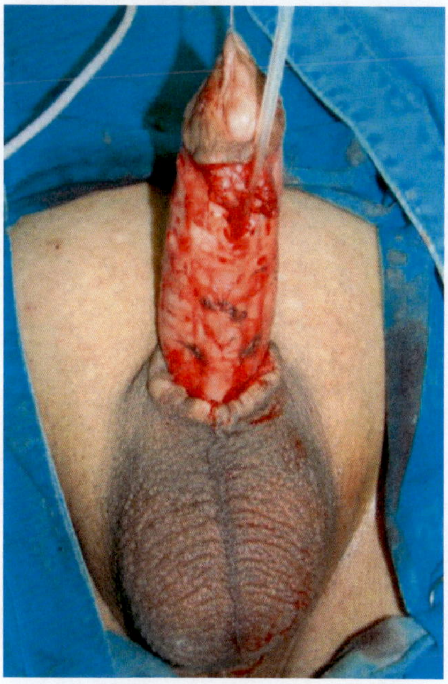

Figure 6. Penile lengthening is necessary. Penile skin is missing.

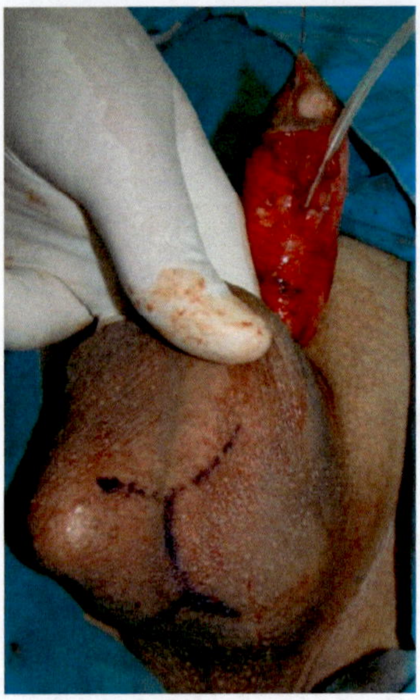

Figure 7. Design at the scrotal skin for penile transfer.

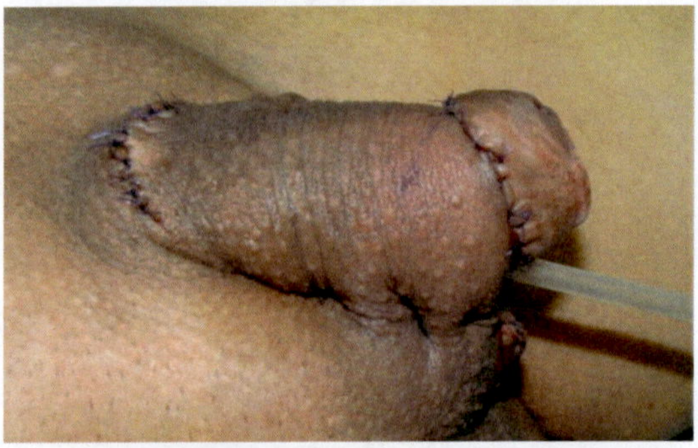

Figure 8. Penile body is incorporated into the scrotal sac. Glans is fixed to the scrotal skin to be visible.

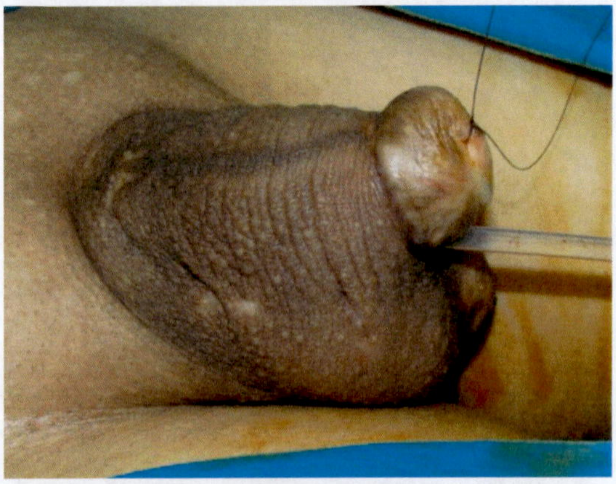

Figure 9. Appearance three months later before penile-scrotal division.

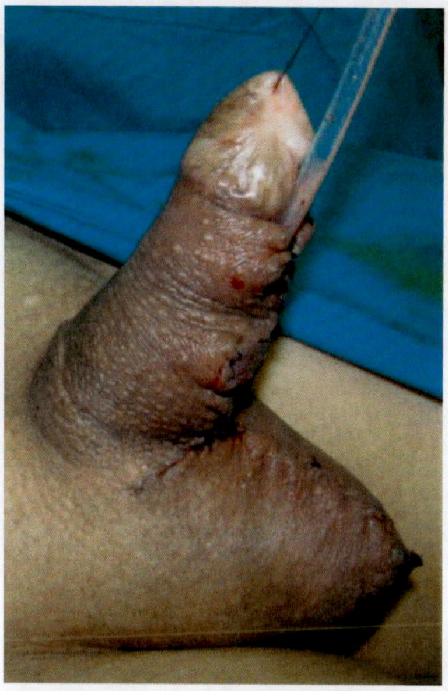

Figure 10. Penile body with scrotal skin is divided from the scrotum. Good length and appearance of the genitalia are achieved.

There are no direct, prospective comparisons of organ-preserving therapies and partial or total penectomy. Penile-preserving operations have higher rates of local tumor recurrence [40]. However, long-term survival is greater than 90% at 5 years for local-only recurrence [95]. There is no significant difference in survival rates between organ preserving and more radical therapies [96].

Total penectomy with perineal urethrostomy is a necessary procedure in patients in whom size and/or location of the penile malignant lesion does not allow complete removal with clear surgical margins. Total phallic reconstruction should be recommended to these patients. Phalloplasty may be used as a solution for different causes of penile insufficiency: congenital absence of the penis, micropenis, exstrophy-epispadias complex, accidental or iatrogenic trauma, penile cancer or transsexual population [97, 98]. The goals of phalloplasty are to create a functioning and aesthetically acceptable phallus with the ability to void standing and to achieve sexual function. Microsurgical free flap reconstruction is the method of choice for total phalloplasty. The ideal flap should be sensate and hairless, with a long pedicle, and with sufficient tissue to allow tubularization and insertion of penile prosthesis. The most commonly used flap for phalloplasty is the radial forearm flap, because it fulfills the above-mentioned requirements [99, 100]. The latissimus dorsi musculocutaneous flap has been used for phallic reconstruction in an effort to improve the donor site scar [101]. This flap has been described in Belgrade for the treatment of transsexuals and patients after severe penile trauma [102]. The final step after phalloplasty should be the implantation of penile stiffeners to enable sexual intercourse with penetration [103]. Although some patients are not satisfied with the appearance of their genitalia after total phalloplasty, eventually,

90% of them are satisfied with the final surgical result. All patients would undergo phalloplasty again if necessary, because of significantly improved sexual quality of life [104].

Significant research progress has been made in recent years in the field of bioengineering of penile tissue, although it still remains in the phase of animal studies [105, 106]. Chen et al. reported that the entire pendular penile corpora could be engineered using autologous cells. The engineered tissues are able to maintain normal intracorporeal pressures and are able to contract and relax [107]. These results are very encouraging but further studies are required. Bioengineered penile tissue opens new horizons for the treatment of patients with penile insufficiency.

Conclusion

Penile cancer and its traditional management can severely affect patient's psychosocial and psychosexual life. The ideal outcome of the treatment involves the preservation of normal sexual and urinary function while eradicating the disease. However, this is not always possible due to the extent of the disease. More recent and evolving therapies aim to preserve or reconstruct the penis both functionally and aesthetically to increase patient satisfaction. The importance of long-term follow-up should be emphasized, especially if organ-preserving procedures are employed. Finally, in patients with more aggressive disease, radical treatment is indicated, and it should be followed by some variant of complete phallic reconstruction and subsequent insertion of penile implants. These treatment modalities offer oncological control of the disease with preserved sexual function and improved quality of life to patients.

Further research is necessary to gain a greater insight into the impact of penile cancer surgery on men's psychosexual well-being and to determine the most appropriate strategies for rehabilitation of men experiencing penile cancer surgery.

Key Points

- Despite great progress in development of non-surgical treatment modalities, surgery still plays a critical role in the treatment of penile cancer, especially for large tumors or tumors known or suspected to be invasive.
- Traditional management of penile carcinoma is partial or total penectomy, which are mutilating procedures associated with a devastating impact on patients' physical and psychological status.

- Organ preserving surgical techniques, allowing phallus preservation in appropriately selected patients, reduce the negative impact on functional and cosmetic outcomes of penile amputation without sacrificing oncological goals.
- Patients with more aggressive disease are not suitable for organ-sparing procedures and radical treatment is necessary. Total penile amputation should be followed by complete phallic reconstruction and subsequent insertion of penile implants. These treatment modalities offer oncological control of the disease with preserved sexual function and improved quality of life to patients.

REFERENCES

[1] Hakenberg OW, Dräger DL, Erbersdobler A, Naumann CM, Jünemann KP, Protzel C. The Diagnosis and Treatment of Penile Cancer. *Dtsch Arztebl Int.* 2018 Sep 28; 115(39): p. 646-52.

[2] Barnholtz-Sloan JS, Maldonado JL, Pow-Sang J, Giuliano AR. Incidence trends in primary malignant penile cancer. *Urol Oncol.* 2007; 25: p. 361-7.

[3] Forman D, Bray F, Brewster DH, Gombe Mbalawa C, Kohler B, Steliarova-Foucher E, et al., editors. *Cancer Incidence in Five Continents Lyon: IARC* No. 164; 2014.

[4] Misra S, Chaturvedi A, Misra NC. Penile carcinoma: a challenge for the developing world. *Lancet Oncol.* 2004 Apr; 5(4): p. 240-7.

[5] Backes DM, Kurman RJ, Pimenta JM, Smith JS. Systematic review of human papillomavirus prevalence in invasive penile cancer. *Cancer Causes Control.* 2009 May; 20(4): p. 449-57.

[6] Bleeker MC, Heideman DA, Snijders PJ, Horenblas S, Dillner J, Meijer CJ. Penile cancer: epidemiology, pathogenesis and prevention. *World J Urol.* 2009 Apr; 27(2): p. 141-50.

[7] Christodoulidou M, Sahdev V, Houssein S, Muneer A. Epidemiology of penile cancer. *Curr Probl Cancer.* 2015 May-Jun; 39(3): p. 126-36.

[8] Pow-Sang MR, Ferreira U, Pow-Sang JM, Nardi AC, Destefano V. Epidemiology and natural history of penile cancer. *Urology.* 2010 Aug; 76(2 Suppl 1): p. S2-6.

[9] Arya M, Li R, Pegler K, Sangar V, Kelly JD, Minhas S, Muneer A, Coleman MP. Long-term trends in incidence, survival and mortality of primary penile cancer in England. *Cancer Causes Control.* 2013 Dec; 24(12): p. 2169-76.

[10] Baldur-Felskov B, Hannibal CG, Munk C, Kjaer SK. Increased incidence of penile cancer and high-grade penile intraepithelial neoplasia in Denmark 1978-2008: a nationwide population-based study. *Cancer Causes Control.* 2012 Feb; 23(2): p. 273-80.

[11] Favorito LA, Nardi AC, Ronalsa M, Zequi SC, Sampaio FJ, Glina S. Epidemiologic study on penile cancer in Brazil. *Int Braz J Urol.* 2008 Sep-Oct; 34(5): p. 587-91.

[12] Persson B, Sjödin JG, Holmberg L, Windahl T. The National Penile Cancer Register in Sweden 2000-2003. *Scand J Urol Nephrol.* 2007; 41(4): p. 278-82.

[13] Sarin R, Norman AR, Steel GG, Horwich A. Treatment results and prognostic factors in 101 men treated for squamous carcinoma of the penis. *Int J Radiat Oncol Biol Phys.* 1997 Jul 1; 38(4): p. 713-22.

[14] Pietrzak P, Corbishley C, Watkin N. Organ-sparing surgery for invasive penile cancer: early follow-up data. *BJU Int.* 2004 Dec; 94(9): p. 1253-7.

[15] *Cancer Research UK. Penile Cancer Statistics.* [Online].; 2015 [cited 2019 Jan. Available from: https:// www.cancerresearchuk.org/ health-professional/ cancer-statistics/statistics-by-cancer-type/penile-cancer.

[16] Alemany L, Cubilla A, Halec G, Kasamatsu E, Quirós B, Masferrer E et al. Role of Human Papillomavirus in Penile Carcinomas Worldwide. *Eur Urol.* 2016 May; 69(5): p. 953-61.

[17] Gao G, Smith DI. Human Papillomavirus and the Development of Different Cancers. *Cytogenet Genome Res.* 2016; 150(3-4): p. 185-93.

[18] Pompeo A, Heyns C, Abrams P, editors. *Penile Cancer. International Consultation on Penile Cancer* Santiago; November 2008.

[19] Harish K, Ravi R. The role of tobacco in penile carcinoma. *Br J Urol.* 1995 Mar; 75(3): p. 375-7.

[20] Daling JR, Madeleine MM, Johnson LG, Schwartz SM, Shera KA, Wurscher MA, Carter JJ, Porter PL, Galloway DA, McDougall JK, Krieger JN. Penile cancer: importance of circumcision, human papillomavirus and smoking in in situ and invasive disease. *Int J Cancer.* 2005 Sep 10; 116(4): p. 606-16.

[21] Koifman L, Vides AJ, Koifman N, Carvalho JP, Ornellas AA. Epidemiological aspects of penile cancer in Rio de Janeiro: evaluation of 230 cases. *Int Braz J Urol.* 2011 Mar-Apr; 37(2): p. 231-40.

[22] Hakenberg OW, Compérat EM, Minhas S, Necchi A, Protzel C, Watkin N. EAU guidelines on penile cancer: 2014 update. *Eur Urol.* 2015 Jan; 67(1): p. 142-50.

[23] Wentzel SW, Vermeulen LP, Beukes CA, Thiart J, Joubert G, Goedhals J. Human immunodeficiency virus (HIV) infection in men with penile carcinoma is associated with increased prevalence of human papilloma virus infection and younger age at presentation. *S Afr J Surg.* 2018 Sep; 56(3): p. 47-50.

[24] Stankiewicz E, Kudahetti SC, Prowse DM, Ktori E, Cuzick J, Ambroisine L et al. HPV infection and immunochemical detection of cell-cycle markers in verrucous carcinoma of the penis. *Mod Pathol.* 2009 Sep; 22(9): p. 1160-8.

[25] Engels EA, Pfeiffer RM, Goedert JJ, Virgo P, McNeel TS, Scoppa SM et al. Trends in cancer risk among people with AIDS in the United States 1980-2002. *AIDS.* 2006 Aug 1; 20(12): p. 1645-54.

[26] Van Howe RS, Hodges FM. The carcinogenicity of smegma: debunking a myth. *J Eur Acad Dermatol Venereol.* 2006 Oct; 20(9): p. 1046-54.

[27] Maden C, Sherman KJ, Beckmann AM, Hislop TG, Teh CZ, Ashley RL et al. History of circumcision, medical conditions, and sexual activity and risk of penile cancer. *J Natl Cancer Inst.* 1993 Jan 6; 85(1): p. 19-24.

[28] Letendre J, Saad F, Lattouf JB. Penile cancer: what's new? *Curr Opin Support Palliat Care.* 2011 Sep; 5(3): p. 185-91.

[29] Barbagli G, Palminteri E, Mirri F, Guazzoni G, Turini D, Lazzeri M. Penile carcinoma in patients with genital lichen sclerosus: a multicenter survey. *J Urol.* 2006 Apr; 175(4): p. 1359-63.

[30] Philippou P, Shabbir M, Ralph DJ, Malone P, Nigam R, Freeman A, et al. Genital lichen sclerosus/balanitis xerotica obliterans in men with penile carcinoma: a critical analysis. *BJU Int.* 2013 May; 111(6): p. 970-6.

[31] Pietrzak P, Hadway P, Corbishley CM, Watkin NA. Is the association between balanitis xerotica obliterans and penile carcinoma underestimated? *BJU Int.* 2006 Jul; 98(1): p. 74-6.

[32] Graafland NM, Lam W, Leijte JA, Yap T, Gallee MP, Corbishley C, et al. Prognostic factors for occult inguinal lymph node involvement in penile carcinoma and assessment of the high-risk EAU subgroup: a two-institution analysis of 342 clinically node-negative patients. *Eur Urol.* 2010 Nov; 58(5): p. 742-7.

[33] Alkatout I, Naumann CM, Hedderich J, Hegele A, Bolenz C, Jünemann KP, et al. Squamous cell carcinoma of the penis: predicting nodal metastases by histologic grade, pattern of invasion and clinical examination. *Urol Oncol.* 2011 Nov-Dec; 29(6): p. 774-81.

[34] Lont AP, Besnard AP, Gallee MP, van Tinteren H, Horenblas S. A comparison of physical examination and imaging in determining the extent of primary penile carcinoma. *BJU Int.* 2003 Apr; 91(6): p. 493-5.

[35] Kayes O, Minhas S, Allen C, Hare C, Freeman A, Ralph D. The role of magnetic resonance imaging in the local staging of penile cancer. *Eur Urol.* 2007 May; 51(5): p. 1313-8.

[36] Sobin L, Gospodarowicz M, Wittekind C, editors. *TNM Classification of Malignant Tumours. International Union against Cancer.* 7th ed. West Sussex; 2009.

[37] Leijte JA, Gallee M, Antonini N, Horenblas S. Evaluation of current TNM classification of penile carcinoma. *J Urol.* 2008 Sep; 180(3): p. 933-8.

[38] Moses KA, Winer A, Sfakianos JP, Poon SA, Kent M, Bernstein M, et al. Contemporary management of penile cancer: greater than 15 year MSKCC experience. *Can J Urol.* 2014 Apr; 21(2): p. 7201-6.

[39] Kroon BK, Horenblas S, Nieweg OE. Contemporary management of penile squamous cell carcinoma. *J Surg Oncol.* 2005 Jan 1; 89(1): p. 43-50.

[40] Hegarty PK, Eardley I, Heidenreich A, McDougal WS, Minhas S, Spiess PE, et al. Penile cancer: organ-sparing techniques. *BJU Int*. 2014 Dec; 114(6): p. 799-805.

[41] Brady KL, Mercurio MG, Brown MD. Malignant tumors of the penis. *Dermatol Surg*. 2013 Apr; 39(4): p. 527-47.

[42] Sharma P, Zargar-Shoshtari K, Spiess PE. Current surgical management of penile cancer. *Curr Probl Cancer*. 2015 May-Jun; 39(3): p. 147-57.

[43] Alnajjar HM, Lam W, Bolgeri M, Rees RW, Perry MJ, Watkin NA. Treatment of carcinoma in situ of the glans penis with topical chemotherapy agents. *Eur Urol*. 2012 Nov; 62(5): p. 923-8.

[44] Torelli T, Catanzaro MA, Nicolai N, Giannatempo P, Necchi A, Raggi D, et al. Treatment of Carcinoma In Situ of the Glans Penis With Topical Imiquimod Followed by Carbon Dioxide Laser Excision. *Clin Genitourin Cancer*. 2017 Jun; 15(3): p. e483-e487.

[45] Crook J. Contemporary Role of Radiotherapy in the Management of Primary Penile Tumors and Metastatic Disease. *Urol Clin North Am*. 2016 Nov; 43(4): p. 435-48..

[46] Azrif M, Logue JP, Swindell R, Cowan RA, Wylie JP, Livsey JE. External-beam radiotherapy in T1-2 N0 penile carcinoma. *Clin Oncol (R Coll Radiol)*. 2006 May; 18(4): p. 320-5.

[47] Hasan S, Francis A, Hagenauer A, Hirsh A, Kaminsky D, Traughber B, et al. The role of brachytherapy in organ preservation for penile cancer: A meta-analysis and review of the literature. *Brachytherapy*. 2015 Jul-Aug; 14(4): p. 517-24.

[48] Crook J, Jezioranski J, Cygler JE. Penile brachytherapy: technical aspects and postimplant issues. *Brachytherapy*. 2010 Apr-Jun; 9(2): p. 151-8.

[49] Crook JM, Haie-Meder C, Demanes DJ, Mazeron JJ, Martinez AA, Rivard MJ. American Brachytherapy Society-Groupe Européen de Curiethérapie-European Society of Therapeutic Radiation Oncology (ABS-GEC-ESTRO) consensus statement for penile brachytherapy. *Brachytherapy*. 2013 May-Jun; 12(3): p. 191-8.

[50] de Crevoisier R, Slimane K, Sanfilippo N, Bossi A, Albano M, Dumas I, et al. Long-term results of brachytherapy for carcinoma of the penis confined to the glans (N- or NX). *Int J Radiat Oncol Biol Phys*. 2009 Jul 15; 74(4): p. 1150-6.

[51] Escande A, Haie-Meder C, Mazeron R, Maroun P, Cavalcanti A, de Crevoisier R, et al. Brachytherapy for Conservative Treatment of Invasive Penile Carcinoma: Prognostic Factors and Long-Term Analysis of Outcome. *Int J Radiat Oncol Biol Phys*. 2017 Nov 1; 99(3): p. 563-70.

[52] Seibold J, Strnad V, Fietkau R. Organ-sparing treatment of penile cancer with interstitial pulsed-dose-rate brachytherapy. *Strahlenther Onkol*. 2016 Jul; 192(7): p. 467-72.

[53] Crook JM, Jezioranski J, Grimard L, Esche B, Pond G. Penile brachytherapy: results for 49 patients. *Int J Radiat Oncol Biol Phys*. 2005 Jun 1; 62(2): p. 460-7.

[54] Tang DH, Yan S, Ottenhof SR, Draeger D, Baumgarten AS, Chipollini J, et al. Laser ablation as monotherapy for penile squamous cell carcinoma: A multi-center cohort analysis. *Urol Oncol.* 2018 Apr; 36(4): p. 147-52.

[55] Zreik A, Rewhorn M, Vint R, Khan R, Hendry D. Carbon dioxide laser treatment of penile intraepithelial neoplasia. *Surgeon.* 2017 Dec; 15(6): p. 321-4.

[56] Skeppner E, Windahl T, Andersson SO, Fugl-Meyer KS. Treatment-seeking, aspects of sexual activity and life satisfaction in men with laser-treated penile carcinoma. *Eur Urol.* 2008 Sep; 54(3): p. 631-9.

[57] Pereira N, Cabral AR, Vieira R, Figueiredo A. Conservative treatment of penile carcinoma - a retrospective study of 10 years. *An Bras Dermatol.* 2013 Sep-Oct; 88(5): p. 844-6.

[58] Meijer RP, Boon TA, van Venrooij GE, Wijburg CJ. Long-term follow-up after laser therapy for penile carcinoma. *Urology.* 2007 Apr; 69(4): p. 759-62.

[59] van Bezooijen BP, Horenblas S, Meinhardt W, Newling DW. Laser therapy for carcinoma in situ of the penis. *J Urol.* 2001 Nov; 166(5): p. 1670-1.

[60] Machan M, Brodland D, Zitelli J. Penile Squamous Cell Carcinoma: Penis-Preserving Treatment With Mohs Micrographic Surgery. *Dermatol Surg.* 2016 Aug; 42(8): p. 936-44.

[61] Shindel AW, Mann MW, Lev RY, Sengelmann R, Petersen J, Hruza GJ, et al. Mohs micrographic surgery for penile cancer: management and long-term followup. *J Urol.* 2007 Nov; 178(5): p. 1980-5.

[62] Wells MJ, Taylor RS. Mohs micrographic surgery for penoscrotal malignancy. *Urol Clin North Am.* 2010 Aug; 37(3): p. 403-9.

[63] Martins FE, Rodrigues RN, Lopes TM. Organ-preserving surgery for penile carcinoma. *Adv Urol.* 2008. 2008; 2008: p. 634216.

[64] Li J, Zhu Y, Zhang SL, Wang CF, Yao XD, Dai B, et al. Organ-sparing surgery for penile cancer: complications and outcomes. *Urology.* 2011 Nov; 78(5): p. 1121-4.

[65] Chalya PL, Rambau PF, Masalu N, Simbila S. Ten-year surgical experiences with penile cancer at a tertiary care hospital in northwestern Tanzania: a retrospective study of 236 patients. *World J Surg Oncol.* 2015 Feb 22; 13: p. 71.

[66] Horenblas S, van Tinteren H. Squamous cell carcinoma of the penis. IV. Prognostic factors of survival: analysis of tumor, nodes and metastasis classification system. *J Urol.* 1994 Maz; 151(5): p. 1239-43.

[67] Das S. Penile amputations for the management of primary carcinoma of the penis. *Urol Clin North Am.* 1992 May; 19(2): p. 277-82.

[68] Gulino G, Sasso F, Palermo G, D'Onofrio A, Racioppi M, Sacco E, et al. Sexual outcomes after organ potency-sparing surgery and glans reconstruction in patients with penile carcinoma. *Indian J Urol.* 2013 Apr; 29(2): p. 119-23.

[69] Hegarty PK, Rees RW, Borley NC, Ralph DJ, Minhas S. Contemporary management of penile cancer. *BJU Int.* 2008 Sep; 102(8): p. 928-32.

[70] Romero FR, Romero KR, Mattos MA, Garcia CR, Fernandes Rde C, Perez MD. Sexual function after partial penectomy for penile cancer. *Urology*. 2005 Dec; 66(6): p. 1292-5.

[71] Opjordsmoen S, Waehre H, Aass N, Fossa SD. Sexuality in patients treated for penile cancer: patients' experience and doctors' judgement. *Br J Urol.* 1994 May; 73(5): p. 554-60.

[72] Maddineni SB, Lau MM, Sangar VK. Identifying the needs of penile cancer sufferers: a systematic review of the quality of life, psychosexual and psychosocial literature in penile cancer. *BMC Urol.* 2009 Aug 8; 9: p. 8.

[73] Tiggemann M, Martins Y, Churchett L. Beyond muscles: unexplored parts of men's body image. *J Health Psychol.* 2008 Nov; 13(8): p. 1163-72.

[74] Baumgarten A, Chipollini J, Yan S, Ottenhof SR, Tang DH, Draeger D, et al. Penile Sparing Surgery for Penile Cancer: A Multicenter International Retrospective Cohort. *J Urol.* 2018 May; 199(5): p. 1233-7.

[75] Greenberger ML, Lowe BA. Penile stump advancement as an alternative to perineal urethrostomy after penile amputation. *J Urol.* 1999 Mar; 161(3): p. 893-4.

[76] de Souza LJ. Subtotal amputation for carcinoma of the penis with reconstruction of penile stump. *Ann R Coll Surg Engl.* 1976 Sep; 58(5): p. 398-400.

[77] Hage JJ. Simple, safe, and satisfactory secondary penile enhancement after near-total oncologic amputation. *Ann Plast Surg*. 2009 Jun; 62(6): p. 685-9.

[78] Minhas S, Kayes O, Hegarty P, Kumar P, Freeman A, Ralph D. What surgical resection margins are required to achieve oncological control in men with primary penile cancer? *BJU Int*. 2005 Nov; 96(7): p. 1040-3.

[79] Philippou P, Shabbir M, Malone P, Nigam R, Muneer A, Ralph DJ, et al. Conservative surgery for squamous cell carcinoma of the penis: resection margins and long-term oncological control. *J Urol.* 2012 Sep; 188(3): p. 803-8.

[80] Gunia S, Koch S, Jain A, May M. Does the width of the surgical margin of safety or premalignant dermatoses at the negative surgical margin affect outcome in surgically treated penile cancer? *J Clin Pathol*. 2014 Mar; 67(3): p. 268-71.

[81] Kieffer JM, Djajadiningrat RS, van Muilekom EA, Graafland NM, Horenblas S, Aaronson NK. Quality of life for patients treated for penile cancer. *J Urol.* 2014 Oct; 192(4): p. 1105-10.

[82] Sohn M, Dietrich M, Wirthmann A, Rieger UM. Reconstructive surgery in penile cancer. *Urologe A.* 2018 Apr; 57(4): p. 428-34.

[83] Halata Z, Munger BL. The neuroanatomical basis for the protopathic sensibility of the human glans penis. *Brain Res.* 1986 Apr 23; 371(2): p. 205-30.

[84] Tajkarimi K, Burnett AL. The role of genital nerve afferents in the physiology of the sexual response and pelvic floor function. *J Sex Med.* 2011 May; 8(5): p. 1299-312..

[85] Depasquale I, Park AJ, Bracka A. The treatment of balanitis xerotica obliterans. *BJU Int*. 2000 Sep; 86(4): p. 459-65.

[86] Håkansson U, Kirrander P, Uvelius B, Baseckas G, Torbrand C. Organ-sparing reconstructive surgery in penile cancer: initial experiences at two Swedish referral centres. *Scand J Urol*. 2015 Apr; 49(2): p. 149-54.

[87] Waris T, Astrand K, Hämäläinen H, Piironen J, Valtimo J, Järvilehto T. Regeneration of cold, warmth and heat-pain sensibility in human skin grafts. *Br J Plast Surg.* 1989 Sep; 42(5): p. 576-80.

[88] Hadway P, Corbishley CM, Watkin NA. Total glans resurfacing for premalignant lesions of the penis: initial outcome data. *BJU Int.* 2006 Sep; 98(3): p. 532-6.

[89] Shabbir M, Muneer A, Kalsi J, Shukla CJ, Zacharakis E, Garaffa G, et al. Glans resurfacing for the treatment of carcinoma in situ of the penis: surgical technique and outcomes. *Eur Urol*. 2011 Jan; 59(1): p. 142-7.

[90] Mitchell ME, Bägli DJ. Complete penile disassembly for epispadias repair: the Mitchell technique. *J Urol.* 1996 Jan; 155(1): p. 300-4.

[91] Djordjevic ML, Perovic S, Korac G. Penile carcinoma: organ-sparing surgery. *Urology.* 2006; 68(Suppl 1): p. 216–7.

[92] Bracka A. Glans resection and plastic repair. *BJU Int*. 2010 Jan; 105(1): p. 136-44.

[93] Morelli G, Pagni R, Mariani C, Campo G, Menchini-Fabris F, Minervini R, et al. Glansectomy with split-thickness skin graft for the treatment of penile carcinoma. *Int J Impot Res.* 2009 Sep-Oct; 21(5): p. 311-4.

[94] Gulino G, Sasso F, Falabella R, Bassi PF. Distal urethral reconstruction of the glans for penile carcinoma: results of a novel technique at 1-year of followup. *J Urol.* 2007 Sep; 178(3): p. 941-4.

[95] Leijte JA, Kirrander P, Antonini N, Windahl T, Horenblas S. Recurrence patterns of squamous cell carcinoma of the penis: recommendations for follow-up based on a two-centre analysis of 700 patients. *Eur Urol.* 2008 Jul; 54(1): p. 161-8.

[96] Djajadiningrat RS, van Werkhoven E, Meinhardt W, van Rhijn BW, Bex A, van der Poel HG, et al. Penile sparing surgery for penile cancer-does it affect survival*? J Urol*. 2014 Jul; 192(1): p. 120-5.

[97] Lumen N, Monstrey S, Selvaggi G, Ceulemans P, De Cuypere G, Van Laecke E, et al. Phalloplasty: a valuable treatment for males with penile insufficiency. *Urology.* 2008 Feb; 71(2): p. 272-6.

[98] Djordjevic ML, Bumbasirevic MZ, Vukovic PM, Sansalone S, Perovic SV. Musculocutaneous latissimus dorsi free transfer flap for total phalloplasty in children. *J Pediatr Urol.* 2006 Aug; 2(4): p. 333-9.

[99] Chang TS, Hwang WY. Forearm flap in one-stage reconstruction of the penis. *Plast Reconstr Surg.* 1984 Aug; 74(2): p. 251-8.

[100] Garaffa G, Spilotros M, Christopher NA, Ralph DJ. Total phallic reconstruction using radial artery based forearm free flap phalloplasty in patients with epispadias-exstrophy complex. *J Urol.* 2014 Sep; 192(3): p. 814-20.
[101] Perovic SV, Djinovic R, Bumbasirevic M, Djordjevic M, Vukovic P. Total phalloplasty using a musculocutaneous latissimus dorsi flap. *BJU Int.* 2007 Oct; 100(4): p. 899-905.
[102] Djordjevic ML, Bumbasirevic MZ, Krstic Z, Bizic MR, Stojanovic BZ, Miocinovic R, et al. Severe penile injuries in children and adolescents: reconstruction modalities and outcomes. *Urology.* 2014 Feb; 83(2): p. 465-70.
[103] Hoebeke P, de Cuypere G, Ceulemans P, Monstrey S. Obtaining rigidity in total phalloplasty: experience with 35 patients. *J Urol.* 2003 Jan; 169(1): p. 221-3.
[104] Callens N, De Cuypere G, T'Sjoen G, Monstrey S, Lumen N, Van Laecke E, et al. Sexual quality of life after total phalloplasty in men with penile deficiency: an exploratory study. *World J Urol.* 2015 Jan; 33(1): p. 137-43.
[105] An G, Ji C, Wei Z, Chen H, Zhang J. Engineering of corpus cavernosum using vascular endothelial growth factor-expressing muscle-derived stem cells seeded on acellular corporal collagen matrices. *Urology.* 2013 Feb; 81(2): p. 424-31.
[106] Orabi H, Lin G, Ferretti L, Lin CS, Lue TF. Scaffoldless tissue engineering of stem cell derived cavernous tissue for treatment of erectile function. *J Sex Med.* 2012 Jun; 9(6): p. 1522-34.
[107] Chen KL, Eberli D, Yoo JJ, Atala A. Bioengineered corporal tissue for structural and functional restoration of the penis. *Proc Natl Acad Sci U S A.* 2010 Feb 23; 107(8): p. 3346-50.

Biographical Sketch

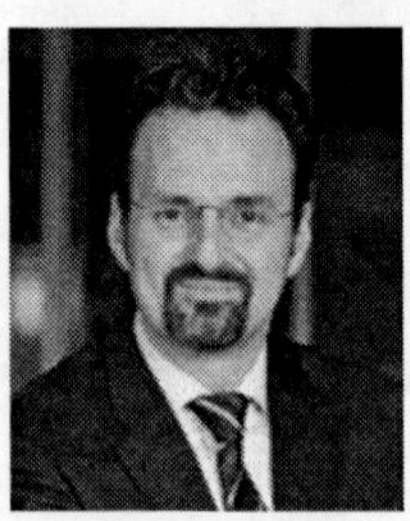

Vladimir Kojovic, MD, PhD
Urologist and Pediatric Surgeon
Assistant Professor

Vladimir Kojovic, MD, PhD, is a Serbian consultant urologist, pediatric surgeon and microsurgeon. Dr. Kojovic completed both his pediatric surgical and urologic residency training at the Medical School, University of Belgrade. He was trained in Belgrade school for genital surgery and gender confirming surgery. Dr. Kojovic is the author and co-author of many papers and book chapters in field of genital reconstructive surgery. He received awards and recognitions for his work at prestigious international scientific meetings.

Dr. Kojovic's areas of expertise include genital reconstructive surgery, gender confirming surgery and congenital anomalies of genitals. Dr. Vladimir Kojovic is currently an assistant professor at the Faculty of Medicine, University of Belgrade and he is a full-time surgeon at Institute for Mother and Child Health Care of Serbia.

In: Penile Cancer: Challenges and Controversies
Editors: F. E. Martins and M. L. Djordjevic
ISBN: 978-1-53615-950-9

Chapter 12

THE ROLE OF PENILE TRANSPLANTATION AFTER PENILE CANCER SURGERY

Andre van der Merwe*
Division of Urology, Department of Surgical Sciences,
Stellenbosch University and Tygerberg Hospital,
Cape Town, South Africa

ABSTRACT

Penile transplantation would only be safe in penile cancer cases if long term remission is achieved. The risk of early metastases or local recurrence under the influence of immunosuppression is significant. Recurrence of penile cancer is grade and stage dependent.

Having this assured during surveillance, patients could be considered for penile transplantation from around four to five years of remission. Informed consent is vital and should include all the toxic side effects of immunosuppression and the stringent follow-up schedule.

The consequences of non-adherence should be clear. A psychological evaluation should be done by a psychologist and social worker experienced in dealing with transplant patients.

Batteries of blood tests are performed over time which gives each time a good opportunity to remind about the risks and informed consent. The ideal case for penile transplantation would be a total penectomy or proximal sub-total penectomy as a radical penectomy may be too difficult, and a partial penectomy does not justify the risks of joining a penile transplant program. Return of erectile function can be expected. The psychological integration of the new penis does not seem to be problematic in the few cases done so far worldwide.

Penile transplantation is an option for qualifying men in long term remission not wanting a phalloplasty after oncological surgery.

* Corresponding Author's E-mail: arvdm@sun.ac.za.

Keywords: penile transplantation, penile cancer, quality of life, sexual function, ethical concerns, reconstructive surgical procedures, penile defects, vascularized complex allotransplant

Introduction

Penile allotransplantation was met with great caution initially, but it appears to be acceptable treatment in the correct circumstances.[1, 2] Penile transplantation creates hope for normal sexual function, urinary function and appearance after the devastating loss accompanied by total-, sub-total- or radical penectomy. Current reconstructive methods do not create a phallus with similar appearance and function. [3, 4] The psychological impact after the loss of a penis is devastating to the patient as well as his partner. In penile cancer, the patient already received the diagnosis of a dreaded disease. While trying to come to terms with this, he loses his penis with an impact on body image and sexual function.

In patients with early penile cancer sexual function would still be possible and a sudden loss of sexual function would have a major impact on the patient and his partner. Immunosuppression in previous penile cancer patients could risk recurrence due to the compromised immune system. Therefore, an extended time of remission would be mandatory before considering penile transplantation as a substitute for traditional phalloplasty. Anatomical challenges will be significant in particular radical penectomy where the corpora cavernosa is removed from the pubic bone.

Is Penile Transplantation Possible after Penile Cancer?

The first United States of America (USA) penile transplantation was done in Boston in 2016 [5]. This was worldwide the second successful penile transplantation after the first successful transplantation in South Africa in 2014 [6]. The patient was a 64-year-old male who had a sub-total penectomy and left inguinal groin dissection four years earlier. He was in total remission since penectomy. After penile transplantation he declares marked improvement in body image; he has improving erectile function and sensation is progressing past the base of the penis [7].

Risk of Recurrence of Penile Cancer

More than 90% of local and distant recurrence would have occurred at four years post penectomy [8]. It is therefore imperative to wait at least four years before performing the transplantation. As the skin over the recipient penis stump is removed during penile transplantation, the risk for local recurrence would be even less. At informed consent, the risk of later recurrence should be communicated to potential transplant recipients.

Anatomical Considerations

At harvesting, the penis is removed with the urethra as proximal as possible similar to the technique of radical penectomy. After removal of the penis, it is flushed with ice-cold transplant solution at around 3 degrees Celcius. Flushing is done via the dorsal arteries of the penis, cavernosal arteries if possible, and with direct injection into the corpora cavernosa – much like the approach treating priapism. The fluid draining from the penis should be clear. The penis is cooled to three to four degrees Celcius. Bench work for preparation of the penis for transplantation is commenced immediately after the penis is cooled sufficiently. This bench should be prepared in advance and have an operating microscope, good theatre light, vascular- and microsurgical instruments and seated chairs for the surgeon and two assistants. The bench should be outside of the main theatre in an area where very few staff members will transit. The exposed graft is at risk to be colonised by micro-organisms that will flourish once implanted in the recipient.

1. The corpora cavernosa controls the length of the transplanted penis. It is possible to adjust this length by transecting the corpora more proximal or more distal. The length of corpora should be in balance with the amount of skin needed. The skin should be generous; in every successful transplanted case worldwide, so far, a small area of skin at the base of the penis had to be debrided as it was necrotic. The corpora should only be transected after the dorsal neurovascular bundle had been elevated for about two or three centimetres distal to the transection line. The tunica of the corpora should be transected on its own, and after this, the spongy tissue inside stretched before transected. The transection of this tissue should be conical pointing towards the proximal part of the graft allowing for more erectile tissue to be incorporated and longer length of the cavernosal arteries. Anastomosing cavernosal arteries is extremely difficult due to size and the fact that they retract into the spongiosal tissue making it difficult to find.

2. Corpus spongiosum and urethra should be preserved as long as possible to allow wide spatulation and anastomosis later.
3. Skin retained should be more than what one consider will be needed. Excess skin can be trimmed later. Bloodvessels in the skin should be evaluated and preserved for anastomosis – in particular veins that will enhance venous drainage.
4. Cavernosal arteries should be left as long as possible using the conical dissection technique described above. The arteries should be marked with small clips to make identification easier and prevent retraction.
5. Dorsal nerves of the penis should be identified dorso-laterally and dissected free so that the nerves are about three to four centimetres longer than the proximal corpora. Care should be taken not to damage the dorsal arteries or branches of those vessels. These branches can have a similar appearance to the dorsal nerves in the bench preparation of the penis.
6. Dorsal veins of the penis can be single or multiple. Each one should be preserved as venous drainage is critically important. These veins should be dissected free from the rest of the neurovascular bundle to make anastomoses easier with draining veins in the recipient.
7. Dorsal arteries of the penis should be dissected free form the neurovascular bundle. They have multiple small branches that should be secured properly to prevent penile haematoma post-operatively. It is pivotal to realise that dorsal vessels increase rapidly in size proximally. They should be harvested as proximal as possible under the pubic bone to make anastomosis with for example the deep inferior epigastric vessels.

The penis is preserved and sealed after preparation during the cold ischaemic time in three plastic bags, the inner one containing 500ml of transplant solution to prevent freezing of the penis.

The elements to consider in the recipient are:

1. Arterial blood supply. An excellent inflow into the graft is needed to prevent vessel thrombosis and supply nourishment to the penis. Inflow should be maximal to allow for normal spontaneous- and nocturnal erections. Normal nocturnal erections are essential in the maintenance of the penis. Potential sources of arterial blood supply to the graft are from the deep inferior epigastric arteries and superficial pudendal arteries. A saphenous vein graft may also be used from the femoral artery to the deep dorsal arteries of the penis if this has been saved by groin lymph node dissections in the cases of positive nodal disease. It is important to avoid the dorsal arteries of the recipient penis as a source of blood supply to the graft as these will be damaged and obliterated after

the penectomy similar to the circumcision-related penile cases the South Africa group performed transplantation for.

2. Venous drainage takes place via a number of routes. All need to be maximised to reduce postoperative swelling from venous congestion that will increase infection and skin necrosis. The dorsal veins of the penis drain the glans penis and possibly also skin and corpora cavernosa. In during the two penile transplantations at South Africa, it was observed that flushing transplant solution via the dorsal arteries caused a return of fluid via the dorsal veins, corpora cavernosa and corpus spongiosum. One can conclude that interconnections between different parts of the penis are probably more pronounced than previously believed [9]. Options for drainage is the deep inferior epigastric veins and long saphenous veins, if still present. The dorsal veins to the recipient penis should be avoided as above.
3. Dorsal nerves of the penis should be dissected free from the remaining penile tissue in the recipient. The orgasmic function is via the dorsal nerves. Therefore all efforts should be made to find them using microscope dissection if needed. Planning during the donor harvesting should be such that the donor dorsal nerves are about three to four centimetre longer than the graft as part of the neurovascular bundle. This allows for nerve anastomoses without the need of a nerve graft. A nerve graft in the first USA case that received penile transplantation for penile cancer might have caused the delay in sensation recovery. Anastomosed nerves grow at about 5 mm per week. In the South Africa cases, this growth was about half the normal rate. Retarded nerve ingrowth is presumably caused by immunosuppression. In both South African cases, full sensation returned within eight months of surgery. In penile cancer cases without nerve grafts, the same rate could be expected.
4. Corpora cavernosa should be fixed with a few dissolvable polyglycolic acid sutures ventrally to allow movement free anastomosis of the corporeal arteries.

The surgery would be greatly affected by the recipient genital remainder after penectomy.

In the case of sub-total penectomy, such as the first USA case, anatomy would lend it to surgery similar to penile transplantation after penile loss from ritual circumcision such as the two cases done in South Africa.

Pre-Transplant Investigations

Investigations have the goal to help select cases, exclude cases where the risks are unacceptably high such as unfavourable psychological profile or anatomy, plan surgery, plan immunosuppression and build a team to work towards successful penile transplantation. Active infections such as tuberculosis and HIV should be excluded. A transplant immunologist manages amongst other blood groups, previous exposure to cytomegalovirus (CMV) and donor-specific antibodies (DSA). In simple cases where there are only a pendulous penis defect, pre-operative angiograms and computed tomography (CT) or magnetic resonance imaging (MRI) scans might be an unnecessary cost.

However, after radical penectomy, it would be very helpful to know the extent of the remaining corpora, if any. Also, to know the presence of bulbar arteries in the recipient who had a radical penectomy before would be critical to establish normal blood flow to the spongiosum, glans and urethra.

Proposed Approaches after Different Levels of Penectomy

Subtotal Penectomy

One such case has been successfully performed in the USA. Arterial blood supply was from the femoral vessels with a vein graft to the dorsal arteries of the penis. Venous drainage was to the dorsal recipient vein of the penis — the recipient dorsal arteries were obliterated as expected. Another technique could be to make incisions on the lateral sides of the lower rectus muscle for about 20 centimetres and then using the deep inferior epigastric vessels under a skin bridge to be anastomosed in the skin wound to the dorsal vessels of the penis. The corpora cavernosa is sutured in a watertight fashion with 2/0 polyglycolic acid. The urethras are spatulated wide, and the mucosa sutured separately from the adventitia to allow blood to flow in the spongial tissue for venous drainage as well as erections. A urethral catheter should not be used as this might create movement on the penis that might affect the new vascular supply or create infection at the urethral anastomosis site. An adequate size (F16 – F18) suprapubic catheter should be inserted before the vascular anastomoses are started.

Total Penectomy

A very similar approach to the above may be proposed. Expected differences would include that the recipient penile stump will have to be dissected and mobilised as much as possible. The anastomosis may have to be performed in a more proximal manner that will increase the complexity of the procedure. The recipient urethral stump might be very deep and will have to be mobilised as much as possible to allow for a tension-free and spatulated anastomosis as above.

See Figure 1 of an example of a penile transplantation where the recipient had a defect similar to total penectomy.

Radical Penectomy

After a radical penectomy, the challenges to perform successful penile transplantation will be near insurmountable and has not been attempted yet. Fortunately, momentum to perform penile transplantation in trans men is gaining ground. A very similar approach can be followed after radical penectomy.

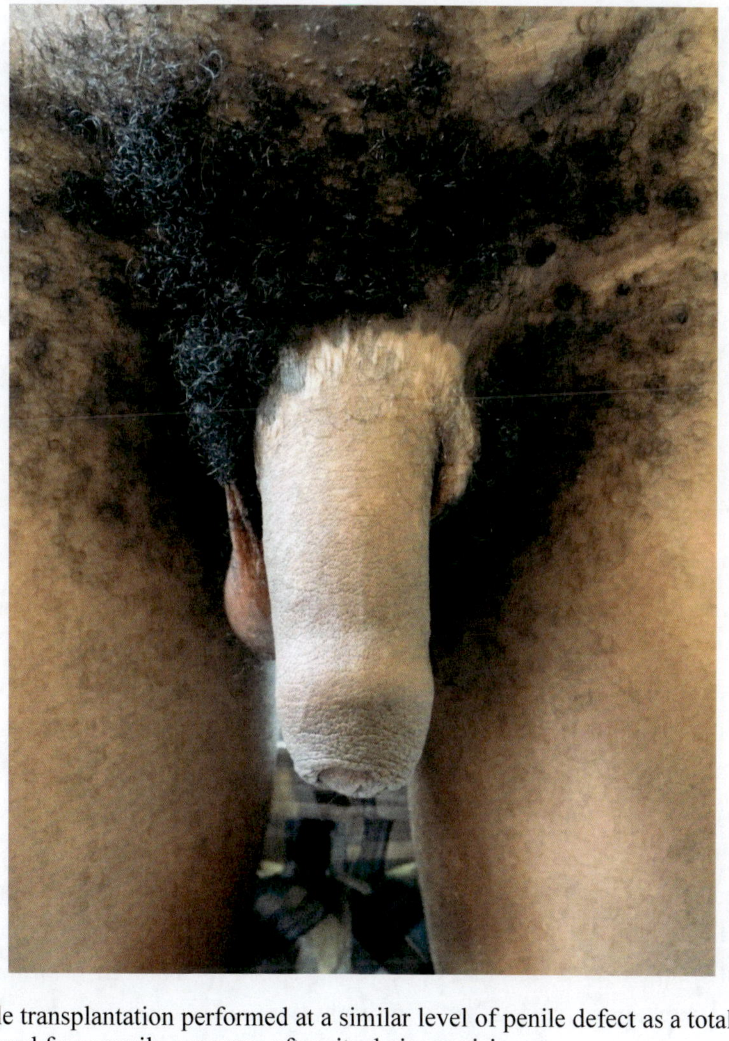

Figure 1. Penile transplantation performed at a similar level of penile defect as a total penectomy. This case suffered from penile gangrene after ritual circumcision.

Principles from a Gothenburg group doing cadaver dissections towards penile transplantation in transmen discovered that the best approach towards securing blood supply to the graft would be by doing a block dissection of blood vessels and nerves from a combined pelvic and perineal approach [10]. This will allow for the bulbo-urethral arteries to be preserved. These arteries play an important role in the perfusion of the corpus spongiosum during erections. The graft's dorsal arteries and veins could with this dissection be more proximally anastomosed. The anastomosis might be in the pelvis increasing the complexity of the surgery. The bulk of donor tissue will be more than any other approach and much time will tell have to be spent on identifying the different vessels and structures. On-bench, angiograms might be useful. The disfigurement of the donor would also be significantly more than any other approach. This will have to be conveyed in the informed consent process to the grieving family. All efforts should be made to cover the defect with skin flaps and produce a simple skin flap to resemble a phallus to preserve the dignity of the donor.

IMMUNOSUPPRESSION

While a detailed description is out of the scope of this chapter, it is vitally important that immunosuppression should be as little as possible. The second USA case might have received the perfect regime with a bone marrow infusion of donor bone marrow to induce immunological tolerance. This worked very well as the recipient, a young war veteran, is maintained on a single dose of tacrolimus [5].

ETHICAL CONSIDERATIONS

Patients are at increased risk for cancer recurrence when immunosuppression starts. In addition, the cumulative risk of the side effects on immunosuppression such as renal failure and haematological cancers makes for careful consideration. The recipients are a vulnerable population that would easily engage in an *innovative alliance* where the patient encourages his doctor to do risky surgery as it is perceived as safe enough. *Therapeutic misconception* is very difficult to manage as patients will focus on the perfect outcome where their manhood is recovered. The severe risks and side effects in balance with a good outcome should be repeatedly communicated to patients. As the work-up for these cases is lengthy with psychological evaluations as well as a battery of blood tests at frequent intervals, the opportunity exists to share all information with the patient over an extended period with multiple contact sessions, and he can make an informed decision.

The value of *informed consent* cannot be overestimated. The first case done at South Africa University had a period of non-compliance at around 30 weeks post-operative and lost a large portion of this graft despite returning his immunosuppression levels to high normal and boosting with steroids. Even hyperbaric oxygen for the maximum duration did not save most of the penis. The patient was accepting the complication as he had understood the risks before surgery well and was told on many occasions to be adherent to medication otherwise the graft will reject. As in many young non-adherent recipients of solid organ transplantation, it was the skin rash from the medication that made him stop his medication. As informed consent was in place, a major psychological disaster was avoided. *Patient autonomy* is an ethical principle that allows the patient to decide on his fate.

To prevent a penile transplant program as the risks are perceived too much is *paternalistic* and therefore ethically wrong. In those that qualify for the transplantation informed consent remains the pivotal ethical principle. The cost of penile transplantation should not be more than the cost of renal transplantation. In the case of penile transplantation, no dialysis is needed which negate the cost of vascular access procedures.

Conclusion

Penile transplantation is safe if the careful selection of cases is made. After surgery for penile cancer, more difficulties might be encountered than in simple cases such as traumatic loss of the pendulous penis.

Key Points

- Penile transplantation is feasible and has great improvement in quality of life for the recipient.
- In penile cancer patients, extra caution should be applied to reduce the risk of inducing recurrence of penile cancer. Recipients must be carefully selected to avoid psychological deterioration after transplantation such as depression (induced by steroid immunosuppression) or psychosis.
- Anatomical considerations for transplantation will be influenced by the level of penile amputation at curative surgery. This will influence the level of corporeal and urethral harvesting in the donor. The more radical the penectomy in the recipient, the more proximal the donor penis needs to be harvested.
- Ethical matters revolve around not wanting to harm the recipient, patient autonomy, avoiding well-meant paternalism (to decide for the recipient to avoid

surgery due to implied risks) and avoiding an innovative alliance between an eager surgeon and a desperate patient.

REFERENCES

[1] Dubernard, J. M. Penile transplantation? *Eur. Urol.,* 2006; 50:664 - 665.

[2] Sopko, N. A., Burnett, A. L. Penile transplantation is here. *Lancet,* 2017; 390:1008 - 1010.

[3] Andreasson, M., Georgas, K., Elander, A., Selvaggi, G. Patient-Reported Outcome Measures Used in Gender Confirmation Surgery: A Systematic Review. *Plast. Reconstr. Surg.,* 2018; 141:1026 - 1039.

[4] Jacobsson, J., Andreasson, M., Kolby, L., Elander, A., Selvaggi, G. Patients' Priorities Regarding Female-to-Male Gender Affirmation Surgery of the Genitalia-A Pilot Study of 47 Patients in Sweden. *J. Sex. Med.,* 2017; 14:857 - 864.

[5] Cetrulo, C. L., Jr., Li, K., Salinas, H. M., Treiser, M. D., Schol, I., Barrisford, G. W., McGovern, F. J., Feldman, A. S., Grant, M. T., Tanrikut, C., Lee, J. H., Ehrlichman, R. J., Holzer, P. W., Choy, G. M., Liu, R. W., Ng, Z. Y., Lellouch, A. G., Kurtz, J. M., Austen, W. G., Jr., Winograd, J. M., Bojovic, B., Eberlin, K. R., Rosales, I. A., Colvin, R. B., Ko, D. S. C. Penis Transplantation: First US Experience. *Ann. Surg.,* 2018; 267:983 - 988.

[6] van der Merwe, A., Graewe, F., Zuhlke, A., Barsdorf, N. W., Zarrabi, A. D., Viljoen, J. T., Ackermann, H., Spies, P. V., Opondo, D., Al-Qaoud, T., Bezuidenhout, K., Nel, J. D., Bailey, B., Moosa, M. R. Penile allotransplantation for penis amputation following ritual circumcision: a case report with 24 months of follow-up. *Lancet,* 2017; 390:1038 - 1047.

[7] Szafran, A. A., Redett, R., Burnett, A. L. Penile transplantation: the US experience and institutional program set-up. *Transl. Androl. Urol*., 2018; 7:639 - 645.

[8] Leijte, J. A., Kirrander, P., Antonini, N., Windahl, T., Horenblas, S. Recurrence patterns of squamous cell carcinoma of the penis: recommendations for follow-up based on a two-centre analysis of 700 patients. *Eur. Urol.,* 2008; 54:161 - 168.

[9] Tuffaha, S. H., Sacks, J. M., Shores, J. T., Brandacher, G., Lee, W. P., Cooney, D. S., Redett, R. J. Using the dorsal, cavernosal, and external pudendal arteries for penile transplantation: technical considerations and perfusion territories. *Plast. Reconstr. Surg.,* 2014; 134:111e-119e.

[10] Selvaggi, G., Wesslen, E., Elander, A., Wroblewski, P., Thorarinsson, A., Olausson, M. En Bloc Surgical Dissection for Penile Transplantation for Trans-Men: A Cadaveric Study. *Biomed. Res. Int.,* 2018; 2018:6754030.

In: Penile Cancer: Challenges and Controversies
Editors: F. E. Martins and M. L. Djordjevic
ISBN: 978-1-53615-950-9

Chapter 13

PSYCHO-SEXUAL AND SOCIAL EFFECTS OF PENILE CANCER THERAPIES AND IMPACT ON QUALITY OF LIFE

Jorge Daza and John P. Sfakianos*
Department of Urology, Icahn School of Medicine at Mount Sinai, New York, New York, US

ABSTRACT

Penile carcinoma has a wide range of treatments ranging from organ sparing surgery, partial or radical penectomy, systemic chemotherapy and/or radiotherapy depending on the stage of the disease. As expected, the more radical treatments generate more adverse consequences including lower urinary tract conditions such as urethral strictures and sexual function impairment, which bring severe psychological and social effects. The negative effects of treatments for penile carcinoma demand a multidisciplinary approach of each case and the inclusion of instruments that allow the assessment of the quality of life of the patients after the therapy during their follow up. Patients should be directly involved in the decision-making process when choosing the most appropriate treatment and he must understand the nature of every therapy and potential consequences. Organ sparing techniques should be encouraged if they do not compromise the oncological outcome of the patients.

Keywords: psychosexual, social, quality of life, penile cancer, treatment impact, penectomy, sexual function

* Corresponding Author's E-mail: john.sfakianos@mountsinai.org.

Introduction

Penile cancer has a strong association with human papillary virus (HPV). The incidence of the disease has been found to be more prevalent in African and South American countries where the incidence of HPV has been reported to be remarkably higher [1, 2]. The choice of the surgical treatment for each patient whether it is an organ sparing approach or more radical treatment such as partial penectomy can impact severely the quality of life of the patient, not only for its functional implications but also sexually, socially and psychologically [3]. Furthermore, some of these patients will require systemic therapy and other subsets, in the most advanced stages of the disease, will be only candidates for palliative treatment [4]. Thus, a multidisciplinary approach to address all the impacted areas derived from the oncological treatment seems to be very helpful for these patients.

Impact of CO_2 and Laser Therapies on Psycho-Sexual Function

The sexual and psychological function after penile cancer treatment has been poorly studied. As expected, the psychological impairment is strongly related with the type of treatment in each case (Table 1). Not surprisingly, the more conservative surgical treatments have less severe adverse effects on the psycho-sexual component of the patient.

Glans resurfacing, along with other conservative therapies, has a role in the treatment for superficial non-invasive disease. A study on the sexual function of seven patients with penile carcinoma who had glans resurfacing showed that all patients were sexually active three to five months after surgery. The sexual function of the patients was assessed through the International Index of Erectile Function (IIEF-5) and a non-validated 9-item questionnaire six months after the treatment. All patients reported that the sensation on their glans was either the same or better after surgery. Furthermore, all of them had erections within two to three weeks of surgery and six patients reported sexual intercourse 3 months after the procedure. Interestingly, overall satisfaction rate with glans resurfacing was reported as high. Indeed, five patients considered that their sexual life had improved [5].

A study on the outcomes of sexual function, after laser treatment for penile carcinoma, of 40 patients showed that 75% of those who were sexually active prior to the procedure resumed the sexual activity afterwards. Moreover, the authors evaluated the satisfaction of the patients regarding their sexual life after therapy by using the Fugl-Meyer Life Satisfaction Check List Score (LiSat-11) and found that 50% of cases were satisfied. Dyspareunia was found in only 10% of the patients [6]. On the other hand, a retrospective Swedish study after laser therapy for *carcinoma in situ* (CIS) including 67 patients with a mean age of 63 years, reported that overall general satisfaction with life including their sexual component, was similar to the overall Swedish population. However they found a decrease in manual or oral sexual stimulation [7]. Likewise, no sexual dysfunction was reported in a cohort of 19 patients after laser therapy [8]. The impact on sexual function after CO_2 laser therapy for penile cancer was evaluated in a study that included 224 patients and alterations in potency or sexual activity were not identified [9].

In summary, glands resurfacing, CO_2 and laser therapies have a low impact on sexual life of patients with penile carcinoma. The overall satisfaction with conservative therapies, specifically with glans resurfacing has been reported as high. Dyspareunia seems to be one of the most prevalent sexual impairment of patients who undergo laser treatment. However, these observations were found in retrospective studies with small samples, hence they have to be validated in more representative studies

Psycho-Sexual Function after Radical Treatment

Despite the benefits of conservative therapies in patients with penile carcinoma, many cases may need more radical treatments to provide better oncological outcomes. Amputation of the glans penis 2 cm proximal to the tumor was for long time a widely used therapy in penile carcinoma cases. Remarkably, an analysis of 68 cases who underwent glansectomy reported that 79% of patients did not report a decline in spontaneous erection, rigidity and penetrative capacity and 75% had full recovery of orgasm [10]. In another study, all twelve patients returned to "normal" sexual activity one month after surgery [11].

Sexual function after partial penectomy has been poorly studied. A series of 14 patients who underwent partial penectomy reported that 26% of patients had decreased or no sexual function after the surgery using the Overall Sexual Functioning Questionnaire (OSFQ). Surprisingly, no significant levels of anxiety or depression were reported [12]. In contrast, an analysis on 18 patients who had a partial penectomy showed that 55.6% of patients described erectile function suitable for intercourse using the IIEF-15 survey. However, only a third kept their preoperative frequency of intercourse. In the patients with no sexual activity, 50% reported that the main reason for the lack of activity was feeling of shame as a consequence of smaller penis size and absence of glans [13].

Table 1. Summary of the main articles published in the literature evaluating sexual function and quality of life after treatment for penile carcinoma [24]

Study	Number of patients	Treatment	Evaluation	Mean FU (months)	Results
Windhal et al. J Urol 2004 [5]	36	Laser	Face-to-face interview	36	75% had resumed sexual activity; 72% reported unaltered erectile function; 50% were satisfied with their sexual life; 10% had dyspareunia; 78% considered satisfying cosmetic results
Skeppner et al. Eur Urol 2008 [6]	46	Laser	Face-to-face interview	54	65% had resumed sexual activity; 75% were satisfied with life as a whole; 54% were satisfied with their sexual life; 76% were satisfied with their sexual health
Hadway et al. BJU Int 2006 [9]	7	Total glans resurfacing	IIEF-5	Median: 30	All patients who were previously sexually active were sexually active within 3-5 months of surgery
Li et al. Urology 2011	29	Radical circumcision and/or wide local excision	IIEF-5	Median: 26.5	In the group of patients with no to mild erectile dysfunction prior to surgery, 21/22 had the same rating of sexual function as before
Opjordsmoen et al. Br J Urol 1994 [20]	30	Local excision/laser beam treatment [5] Radiotherapy [12] Partial penectomy [9] Total penectomy [4]	IES, GHQ-12, EORTC QLQ C-30	80	Patients treated with partial or total penectomy had a worse outcome with regard to sexual function than patients treated conservatively; 50% had mental symptoms at follow-up
D'Ancona et al. Urology 1997 [13]	14	Partial penectomy	OSFQ, SPQ, GHQ-12, HAD	11.5	In 64% the overall sexual function was normal or slightly decreased; Sexual interest and satisfaction remained normal or slightly reduced in 9 and 12 patients, respectively
Ficarra et al. Prog Urol 1999 [14]	17	Partial penectomy [11] Total penectomy [4] Radiotherapy [2]	GHQ-12, HADS, SPQ, OSFQ,	69	The global sexual function was compromised in 76.5%; 29.5% presented with anxiety and 6% with depression
Ficarra et al. Urol Int 2000 [21]	16	Partial penectomy	GHQ-12, HADS	69	6% were depressed; 31% were found to have anxiety
Romero et al. Urology 2005 [12]	18	Partial penectomy	Personal interview + IIEF-15	23.5	55.6% reported erectile function that allowed sexual intercourse; 33.3% maintained their preoperative sexual intercourse frequency and were satisfied with their sexual relationship and their overall sex life
Gulino et al. J Urol 2007 [16]	14	Partial penectomy	IIEF	13	71% had spontaneous and/or induced erections; IIEF scores in the ejaculation and orgasm domains did not significantly change
Alei et al. Ann Ital Chir 2012 [15]	10	Partial penectomy	IIEF-5	40	The average IIEF score in the preoperative period was 21.6 points, one month postoperatively it was 13 points, 40 months postoperatively it was 19.7 points (mild erectile dysfunction)

In another study of 17 patients of which 15 were treated with partial or total penectomy and two with radiotherapy, compromise in the sexual function was reported in 76.5% of the patients by using the OSFQ scale. Patients with wider area of resection reported worse sexual function and 35% reported limitations in their perception of health and social problems [14]. Nonetheless, Alei et al. showed an improvement in erectile function over time in a series of ten patients [15].

Gulino et al. have reported their experience on distal reconstruction of the glans using distal urethra in a series of 14 cases. All patient reported subjective and objective thermal and tactile epicritic sensibility in the area of the neoglans and 71% noticed spontaneous and/or induced rigid erections. Remarkably, IIEF scores in ejaculation and orgasm components did not change significantly after surgery [16]. Total phallic reconstruction is fairly limited after total or near-total penile amputation [17-19]. Currently, cosmetically acceptable results are obtainable, but reports of function recovery have not been achieved.

Quality of Life

Multiples instruments have been used to evaluate the impact on quality of life derived from health care. The Impact of events scale, General Health Questionnaire (GHQ) and the EORTC QLQ C-30 questionnaire were used to evaluate comprehensively the quality of life of 30 patients who had undergone local excision/laser beam treatment (n = 5), radiotherapy (n = 12), partial penectomy (n = 9) or total penectomy (n = 4). Patients treated with partial or total penectomy had worse sexual function than patients treated conservatively, however, no other differences were found in the rest of the components of quality of life. Therefore, we can presume that patients who had more aggressive treatments usually adapt adequately. Nonetheless, 50% of the patients developed psychological symptoms at follow up. This subset of patients showed less satisfaction rates and less social interaction. Seven men reported that, if they could choose again, they would have preferred a less aggressive treatment regardless of the impact on long-term oncological outcomes in order to increase sexual function. Remarkably, the majority of the patients included in the study prioritized a better long-term survival [20].

D'Anconna et al. studied the social activity, sexual function, depression, and anxiety levels among other domains of the quality of life of patients who had undergone partial penectomy for penile carcinoma. Instruments such as GHQ-12 and Hospital Anxiety and Depression (HAD) scale questionnaires were utilized. No significant changes were found in living conditions, family life and social interactions. However, they found that negative impact on sexual activity and the discomfort with the need to sit when urinating were the most important challenges that the patients were facing. Furthermore, loss of sexual pleasure, fear of dying and the dramatic impact of the latter on their relatives' life were fairly concerning aspects for the patients. When asked about mechanisms that help them to overcome their fears, certainly encouragement of their wives and families appeared in the first place [12].

Ficarra and colleagues also used the GHQ along with HAD scale to compare the effects of surgical treatments for genitourinary (GU) malignancies on the quality of life of the patients versus those who underwent treatments for benign prostatic hyperplasia. They could not find significant differences in the levels of depression but the impact on anxiety was significantly increased in patients who had undergone treatments for GU carcinoma. Among the analyzed group, 16 patients had squamous cell carcinoma (SCC) of the penis. They found that one patient (6%) suffered from depression after the therapy. Moreover, 31% of patients who had a partial penectomy reported some level of anxiety. Compare to other GU malignancies such as prostate cancer, urothelial carcinoma and renal cell carcinoma, the depression levels were similar, but the anxiety levels increased by more than 2-fold in patients treated for penile carcinoma. After all the aforementioned findings, the authors concluded that patients who underwent partial penectomy for SCC of the penis showed significant impairment in the overall state of health, especially in anxiety levels in contrast to those who were treated for benign conditions [21].

Witty et al. found that a prevalent concern for several patients was the potential inability to provide pleasure to their partner and this seems to be more troublesome than the inability to pleasure themselves [22].

In order to find potential elements to predict better adaptive capacity in the patients who are being treated for penile carcinoma, Drager and colleagues identified that younger patients, those who were under chemotherapy or diagnosed with a recurrence were more integrated to psychosocial care networks in a cohort of 40 patients who received either surgical treatment (n = 29) or chemotherapy (n = 11). Remarkably, all the patients regardless of treatment, age or tumor stage reported an increase need for psychosocial support. This finding was more pronounced in patients diagnosed with cancer recurrence [23]. However, only 67% of the cases had received inpatient psychosocial support. Among those who received surgical treatment, 96.5% underwent an organ-sparing surgery.

CONCLUSION

Penile carcinoma is a life-threatening condition that in some cases requires aggressive and mutilating treatments for oncological control. As expected, the more radical approaches can dramatically impact the functional capacity of the genitourinary tract. Moreover, sexual activity and quality of life will face significant challenges after treatment. Therefore, a multimodal therapy seems to be the most indicated for these cases, which include psychological input. Patients should be provided all the necessary information during the decision-making process and if the case is suitable for conservative treatments, such approaches should be strongly considered as it has been shown that they provide less impact on the life of patients. Furthermore, a comprehensive follow up needs to be performed by a multidisciplinary group that can provide psychological support besides the required attention to the oncological condition. Certainly, instruments used to evaluate different domains of the quality of the life of the patients help in the postoperative evaluation, therefore all the professionals involved in the health care of these cases need to be familiar and use them as metrics to report potential changes in sexual, psychological and social condition. Efforts need to be maximized in order to find new and better ways to reestablish the functional and cosmetic characteristic of genitourinary tract. Better design studies are needed in order to be able to do accurate recommendations to health care professionals in order to approach psycho-sexual and social dysfunction in an effective way.

KEY POINTS

- Penile carcinoma treatments can impact severely the quality of life of the patients.
- Besides functional implications, patients may suffer of sexual, social and psychological consequences.
- More conservative treatments (CO2, laser and glans resurfacing) have less severe adverse effects on the psycho-sexual component of the patient.
- Wider area of resection reported worse sexual function and limitations in their perception of health and social problems than patients with more organ preservation (glansectomy).
- Multiples instruments have been used to evaluate the impact on quality of life derived from health care. These tools should be applied to every case during the follow up.
- Multidisciplinary follow up needs to be done in order to provide psychological support besides the required attention to the oncological condition.

REFERENCES

[1] Hakenberg OW, Comperat EM, Minhas S, Necchi A, Protzel C, Watkin N. EAU guidelines on penile cancer: 2014 update. *European Urology.* 2015;67(1):142-50.

[2] Misra S, Chaturvedi A, Misra NC. Penile carcinoma: a challenge for the developing world. *The Lancet Oncology.* 2004;5(4):240-7.

[3] Maddineni SB, Lau MM, Sangar VK. Identifying the needs of penile cancer sufferers: a systematic review of the quality of life, psychosexual and psychosocial literature in penile cancer. *BMC urology.* 2009;9:8.

[4] Network. NCC. NCCN Clinical Practice Guidelines in Oncology - *Penile Cancer* 2.2017 Available from: https://www.nccn.org/professionals/physician_gls/pdf/penile.pdf.

[5] Hadway P, Corbishley CM, Watkin NA. Total glans resurfacing for premalignant lesions of the penis: initial outcome data. *BJU International.* 2006;98(3):532-6.

[6] Windahl T, Skeppner E, Andersson SO, Fugl-Meyer KS. Sexual function and satisfaction in men after laser treatment for penile carcinoma. *The Journal of urology.* 2004;172(2):648-51.

[7] Skeppner E, Windahl T, Andersson SO, Fugl-Meyer KS. Treatment-seeking, aspects of sexual activity and life satisfaction in men with laser-treated penile carcinoma. *European urology.* 2008;54(3):631-9.

[8] van Bezooijen BP, Horenblas S, Meinhardt W, Newling DW. Laser therapy for carcinoma in situ of the penis. *The Journal of urology.* 2001;166(5):1670-1.

[9] Bandieramonte G, Colecchia M, Mariani L, Lo Vullo S, Pizzocaro G, Piva L, et al. Peniscopically controlled CO2 laser excision for conservative treatment of in situ and T1 penile carcinoma: report on 224 patients. *European urology.* 2008;54(4):875-82.

[10] Austoni E GA, Colombo F, Cazzaniga A, Ceresoli A, Grasso Macola G, et al. Reconstructive Surgery for Penile Cancer with Preservation of Sexual Function (Abstract 183). *European Urology Supplements.* 2008 Mar 1;7(3):116.

[11] Li J, Zhu Y, Zhang SL, Wang CF, Yao XD, Dai B, et al. Organ-sparing surgery for penile cancer: complications and outcomes. *Urology.* 2011;78(5):1121-4.

[12] D'Ancona CA, Botega NJ, De Moraes C, Lavoura NS, Jr., Santos JK, Rodrigues Netto N, Jr. Quality of life after partial penectomy for penile carcinoma. *Urology.* 1997;50(4):593-6.

[13] Romero FR, Romero KR, Mattos MA, Garcia CR, Fernandes Rde C, Perez MD. Sexual function after partial penectomy for penile cancer. *Urology.* 2005;66(6):1292-5.

[14] Ficarra V, Mofferdin A, D'Amico A, Zanon G, Schiavone D, Malossini G, et al. Comparison of the quality of life of patients treated by surgery or radiotherapy in epidermoid cancer of the penis. *Progres en urologie: Journal de l'Association francaise d'urologie et de la Societe francaise d'urologie.* 1999;9(4):715-20.

[15] Alei G, Letizia P, Sorvillo V, Alei L, Ricottilli F, Scuderi N. Lichen sclerosus in patients with squamous cell carcinoma. Our experience with partial penectomy and reconstruction with ventral fenestrated flap. *Annali italiani di chirurgia.* 2012;83(4):363-7.

[16] Gulino G, Sasso F, Falabella R, Bassi PF. Distal urethral reconstruction of the glans for penile carcinoma: results of a novel technique at 1-year of followup. *The Journal of urology.* 2007;178(3 Pt 1):941-4.

[17] Garaffa G, Raheem AA, Christopher NA, Ralph DJ. Total phallic reconstruction after penile amputation for carcinoma. *BJU international.* 2009;104(6):852-6.

[18] Gerullis H, Georgas E, Bagner JW, Eimer C, Otto T. Construction of a penoid after penectomy using a transpositioned testicle. *Urologia internationalis.* 2013;90(2): 240-2.

[19] Hage JJ. Simple, safe, and satisfactory secondary penile enhancement after near-total oncologic amputation. *Annals of plastic surgery.* 2009;62(6):685-9.

[20] Opjordsmoen S, Fossa SD. Quality of life in patients treated for penile cancer. A follow-up study. *British journal of urology.* 1994;74(5):652-7.

[21] Ficarra V, Righetti R, D'Amico A, Pilloni S, Balzarro M, Schiavone D, et al. General state of health and psychological well-being in patients after surgery for urological malignant neoplasms. *Urologia internationalis.* 2000;65(3):130-4.

[22] Witty K, Branney P, Evans J, Bullen K, White A, Eardley I. The impact of surgical treatment for penile cancer – patients' perspectives. European journal of oncology nursing: *The official journal of European Oncology Nursing Society.* 2013;17(5):661-7.

[23] Drager DL, Protzel C, Hakenberg OW. Identifying Psychosocial Distress and Stressors Using Distress-screening Instruments in Patients With Localized and Advanced Penile Cancer. *Clinical genitourinary cancer.* 2017;15(5):605-9.

[24] Audenet F, Sfakianos JP. Psychosocial impact of penile carcinoma. *Andrology and Urology.Translational* 2017;6(5):874-8.

In: Penile Cancer: Challenges and Controversies
Editors: F. E. Martins and M. L. Djordjevic
ISBN: 978-1-53615-950-9

Chapter 14

PENILE PROSTHESIS IMPLANTATION FOLLOWING PHALLOPLASTY

Ervin Kocjancic*[1,*]*, MD and Jorge H. Jaunarena*[2,†]*, MD

[1]Department of Urology, University of Illinois at Chicago, Chicago, Illinois, US
[2]Department of Urology, Instituto Alexander Fleming and Centro de Urologia CDU, Buenos Aires, Argentina

ABSTRACT

The ideal neophallus should have good appearance and functionality. The final step of a successful phalloplasty, after achieving sensitivity and standing urination, is gaining erectile function. Nowadays, the most accepted approach is implanting a penile prosthesis.

Radial forearm free flap seems to be the best neophallus for prosthesis implantation, and this should be done between 6 to 12 months after phalloplasty. Key surgical steps include preservation of the neurovascular pedicle, careful dilation of the neophallus, covering the prosthesis with a synthetic or biologic sheath and adequately fixing the prosthesis to the symphysis pubis. Different prostheses have been tried in multiple series, and there doesn't seem to be a specific model of choice. There is consensus, though, in the use of inflatable penile prostheses (IPP) over malleable prostheses, because of a lower risk of erosion.

Several reports in the literature have shown that complications and revision surgeries are very frequent after penile prosthesis implantation. It is very important to discuss these obstacles with the patient and to be ready to deal with them. Despite this, patient satisfaction is very high. Psychological and psychosexual support are crucial before and after the procedure and should be part of standard care.

* Corresponding Author's E-mail: ervkoc@gmail.com.
† Corresponding Author's E-mail: jorgejaunarena@gmail.com.

Successfully implanting a penile prosthesis in a neophallus is a challenging procedure. Nevertheless, it is definitely worthy since it is like bringing to life a neophallus, something that will comfort both the patient and the surgeon. Further investigations are needed, with focus in surgical outcomes, prevention of complications and patient and partner quality of life and satisfaction.

Keywords: phalloplasty, penile prosthesis, neophallus, erectile function, patient satisfaction, surgical complications

Introduction

The penis is a symbol of manhood not only for its conspicuous morphology but also its functionality: it allows standing urination and penetrative intercourse [1]. Thus, penile reconstructive surgery bears a double challenge, since the goals are not simply esthetic, but also functional. Several authors have described the ideal neophallus, which should be built in the least possible number of stages with a reproducible technique, should have a good aspect and should grant standing urination, sensitivity and stiffness [1–3]. The objective of achieving rigidity in the neophallus is directed not only to patient, but also to partner satisfaction, which is not easily achieved [4]. In spite of all these difficulties, a functional neophallus may restore dignity and self-esteem to the patient, making it a high-reaching goal [5, 6].

The first report of a phalloplasty with cartilage implant was done by the Soviet surgeon Nikolaj Bogoraz in 1936 [7]. In this case the neophallus was formed with a pedicled graft from abdominal skin, and was stiffened using rib cartilage. Interestingly, the author reported that the patient was able to have satisfactory intercourse and that the wife was very satisfied. Different approaches for phalloplasty have been used ever since, as well as different techniques for stiffening a neophallus. These have included osteocutaneous grafts, implantable splints and external prosthetic epithesis [8]. The first inflatable penile prosthesis (IPP) was introduced by Scott and colleagues in 1973 [9] and Puckett and Montie replicated the procedure in a transgender patient four years later [9–12]. With the advent of AMS700 and Mentor 3-piece IPP in 1983 [13], these models became the most frequently used.

Is There a Better Neophallus to Implant a Prosthesis on?

There are some phalloplasty techniques that do not require a prosthesis to allow penetrative intercourse. The latissimus dorsi myocutaneous free flap stiffens by contraction of the latissimus muscle, but this also shortens the neophallus [12, 14]. The osteocutaneous fibula or osteocutaneous radial forearm flaps use bone as a stiffener [12].

Despite the alternative of creating a neophallus with an autologous stiffener sounds appealing, most reconstructive surgeons have moved away from this approach. Nowadays, the most accepted technique is the insertion of a penile prosthesis [12].

There is no consensus regarding which is the best type of neophallus, but most authors will agree that the Radial forearm free flap (RFFF) is the best alternative [12, 15]. Falcone et al. analyzed 247 transgender patients who had a phalloplasty and posteriorly an IPP implantation in a single center [4]. Cox regression analysis showed that patients with a RFFF were significantly less likely to require revision surgery than those with an infra-umbilical pubic flap (PFP) (HR 0.74, $p = 0.013$). On the contrary, age, surgeon and number of cylinders did not show statistical significance. There weren't significant predictors of infection and mechanical failure. The authors hypothesize that the PFP results in a larger neophallus that has less tactile sensitivity and often requires two cylinders to achieve an adequate erection, thus increasing the risk of erosion.

A large metaanalysis published by Remington et al. analyzed patient satisfaction and sexual function as secondary outcomes in cis and trans men who had a phalloplasty [16]. They found that patients from the RFFF group, both cis and trans, had significantly higher satisfaction rates than those receiving other types of neophalli (86% versus 76% respectively, $p < 0.01$). Also, RFFF patients had better sexual function, despite the difference wasn't statistically significant (57% versus 39% in transmen, $p = 0.56$ and 79% versus 69% in cismen, $p = 0.06$). These differences are probably explained by the fact that RFFF is more frequently used than other techniques and therefore surgeons have greater expertise.

TIMING FOR PROCEDURE

Most authors agree that patients should wait between 6 to 12 months after phalloplasty before undergoing a penile prosthesis (PP). Levine et al. reported in 1993 that after 4 to 6 months, tactile and erogenous sensation could be achieved, granting protective sensation during penetrative intercourse [17]. Schechter and Safa refer that though testicular implants may be placed 3 months after phalloplasty, the PP should be implanted between 9 to 12 months, since protective sensation is crucial for retaining the erectile device [15]. Falcone et al. also add that this time should be enough to detect and solve any urethral complications that could endanger the neophallus and increase infection rates after PP implantation [4]. In their series, they report a range of 12 to 37 months before PP.

Finally, another group described a staged approach for IPP, in which they placed the reservoir when performing the glansplasty, but waited 3 additional months for placing the cylinders and pump [4, 18]. The rationale is that an inguinal incision has to be performed to harvest the full-thickness skin graft for the glansplasty, and it is therefore simple to deepen the incision to the preperitoneal space to place the reservoir. It is important to leave the reservoir inflated, and a deactivation plug is placed in the tip of the tubbing, which is left in the scrotum or labia majora [19].

SURGICAL PROCEDURE

Initial Considerations

According to the International Consultation on Sexual Medicine, preoperative antibiotics with gram-positive and gram-negative coverage should be given, with therapeutic antibiotic levels attained before making the surgical incision (Level of evidence (LE) 2, grade of recommendation (GR) B) [13]. Shaving versus clipping to remove pubic hair is left to the surgeon's discretion (LE 4, GR C) [13]. Surgeons should use alcohol-based skin preparations in the operating room as the operative site scrub (LE 1, GR A), since clorhexidine-alcohol scrub reduces deep and superficial wound infections [13].

The patient is placed in a supine position. Lithotomy position may be used in case a perineal dissection is required to access the proximal neocrura [20]. After a 10-minute scrub and usual draping, a Foley catheter is placed over a cystoscopically-inserted guidewire [12]. A 4 cm transverse incision is made just below the level of the pubic bone. Other authors prefer ischial [21], parascrotal [4, 11, 19, 22] or penoscrotal incisions [20]. During initial dissection, it is critical to identify and avoid the neurovascular pedicle of the neophallus, as well as the neourethra [20]. Table 1 summarizes the surgical approaches of different authors. A video of the author's technique [23] can be accessed at AUA University (https://auau.auanet.org/).

Neophallus Dilation

Using initial sharp dissection with Metzembaum scissors, two pockets are created within the proximal end of the neophallus. Again, care is taken not to injure the neurovascular pedicle nor the urethra [23]. The surgeon may palpate the Foley catheter in order to avoid urethral injury. Should this happen, the procedure should be cancelled, and the Foley catheter left in place for two weeks [4, 11, 19, 22]. Another PP attempt can be done after 6 months [4, 11, 19, 22].

Table 1. Surgical technique. Aspects of the surgical approach and types of prosthesis used in the different series

Series	Incision	Penile Prosthesis Model	Number of cylinders	Envelope	Reservoir	Dilation	Pubic fixation
Hoebecke 2009	Parascrotal	6.9% Dynaflex, 38.7% AMS700 CX/CXM, 13.3% AMS700 CX Inhibizone, 36.5% Ambicor, 4.6% Coloplast Titan	63% Single, 37% Dual	Initially Polyethilene terephthalate (Dacron®), after 2006 only tip extenders without Dacron®	Paravesical, single incision	Hegar	Non-reabsorbable suture to the sock or tip extender
Segal 2015	Penoscrotal	AMS700 CX/CXR	89% Single, 11% Dual	Pericardium allograft, acellular dermal matrix, None	Secondary incision, site depends on previous scars	When present, proximal cavernous bodies are opened anterolaterally and dilated	Rear tip extenders or allograft sheath are fixed to the pubic symphysis
Zuckerman 2015	Bilateral ischial	68% Malleable (Duraphase or Spectra), 32% Inflatable (AMS700 CX/CXR or Coloplast Titan)	6% Single, 94% Dual	Polytetrafluoroethylene (Gore-tex®) neotunica	Retropubic, secondary incision	Hegar or Brooks	Non-reabsorbable suture to the neotunica
Neuville 2016	Parascrotal	95% Ambicor, 5% AMS700 CXR/CX / AMS600	94% Single, 6% Dual	Polyester graft at the base of the IPP	NA (most had an Ambicor IPP)	Hegar	Non-reabsorbable suture to the graft
Falcone 2017	Parascrotal	69% AMS700 CX, 9.4% AMS700 CXM/R, 17.7% Coloplast Titan, 3.9% Ambicor	63% Single, 37% Dual	Polyethilene terephthalate (Dacron®) sock on the tip and rear of the IPP	3 months before, inguinal incision	18 Hegar	Non-reabsorbable suture to the sock
Kocjancic 2018	Transverse prepubic	100% AMS700	20% Single, 80% Dual	Acellular dermal matrix	Retropubic, single incision	10 Hegar	Non-reabsorbable suture to the rear tip extenders

Progressive dilation with Hegar dilators creates the space for the neocorpora. Patients with previous prosthesis explants or urethral fistulae may present with more fibrosis, therefore requiring especially delicate maneuvers. It is also recommendable to begin with large dilators, because they are associated with less risk of perforation than smaller ones [23]. In cases where 2 cylinders are planned, dilators should be directed dorsolaterally, toward the 2 O'clock and 10 O'clock positions, to prevent cylinder crossover [12].

Prosthesis Fixation

Adequate prosthesis fixation is a key principle of this surgery, since a mobile prosthesis can generate discomfort, erosion and malfunction. In cases where the proximal corpora are present, the scar is incised and the proximal cavernosal body is dilated [20]. If the plan is to insert only one cylinder, the surgeon may choose the most appropriate side to dilate [20]. Some authors consider that even in the presence of proximal cavernosal bodies, pubic anchoring is better since the corpora are usually atrophic and weak after trauma or radical surgery [21].

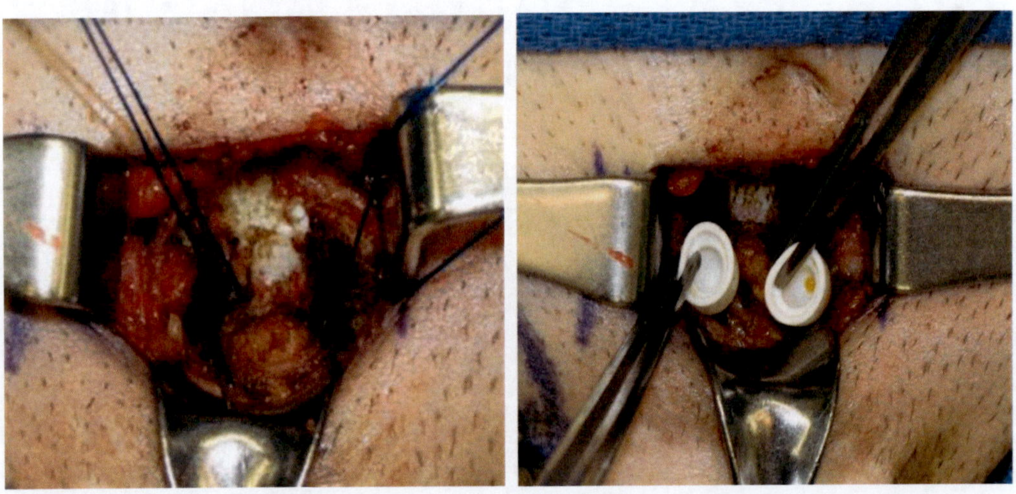

A B

Figure 1. (A) Pubis symphysis dissection and placement of stay sutures. (B) Rear tip extender positioning.

When cavernosal bodies are not present or accessible, fixation to the pubic bone or ischiopubic rami should be performed (Figure 1). For this, the surgeon can carve a periosteal flap to create a cortical indentation where to anchor stay sutures that will fix the rear of the prosthesis, the rear tip extender or the sheath to the bone [8, 12]. An alternative is to fix the non-reabsorbable sutures to the pubic periosteum [22]. Also, the surgeon can drill a corticotomy in the pubic symphysis and generate a cavity where to insert the rear tip extenders [24].

Neocorpora Cavernosa

Different authors have described the use of a sheath to cover the PP like a "pseudo corpora cavernosa" [12]. This aids in fixing the PP proximally and cushions the tip of the prosthesis distally [8]. Biologic materials include acellular dermal matrix [12] and pericardium allograft [20], whereas synthetic materials comprise vascular grafts made of polyester [22] (Hemashield Gold, Maquet Getinge Group, Rastatt, Germany), Gore-Tex® [21] (Polytetrafluoroethylene, Gore Medical, Flagstaff, USA) or Dacron® [4, 11, 19, 22] (Polyethilene terephthalate, Invista, Kansas, USA). Hoebecke et al. found that the Dacron socks were associated with IPP malfunction due to erosion, and ceased using these grafts late in their series [4, 11, 19, 22]. On the opposite side, Segal et al. moved from not using a sheath towards placing a pericardium allograft and found a decrease in erosion rate [20].

We prefer biologic grafts because of their softer nature and better interaction with neophallus tissue. The acellular dermal matrix is sewn in a tubular fashion over a 10.5 Hegar dilator. Afterwards, the neocorpora are placed over the IPP in the backbench (Figure 2). Finally, the IPP with the neocorpora are placed in the neophallus using the Furlow instrument and the Keith needle [23]. The stay sutures fixed to the pubis are threaded through the rear tip extenders, thus giving stability and support to the PP.

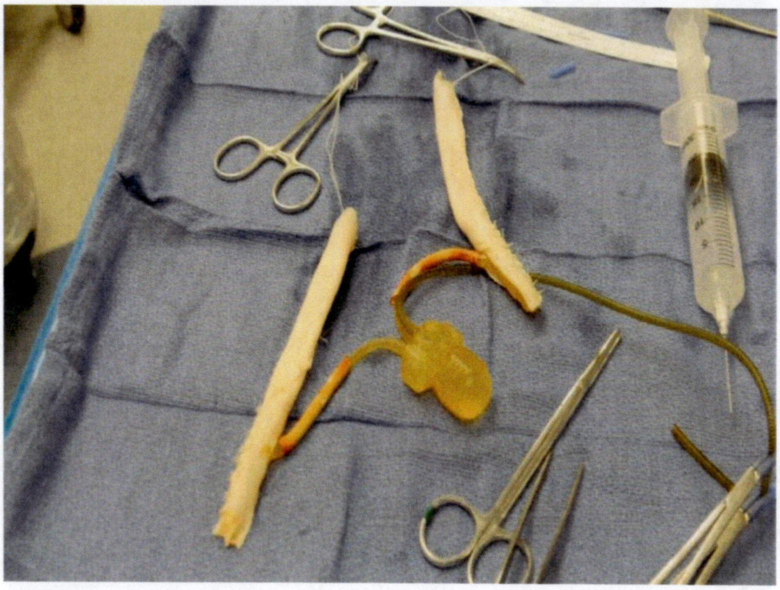

Figure 2. Acellular dermal matrix neocorpora wrapping the IPP.

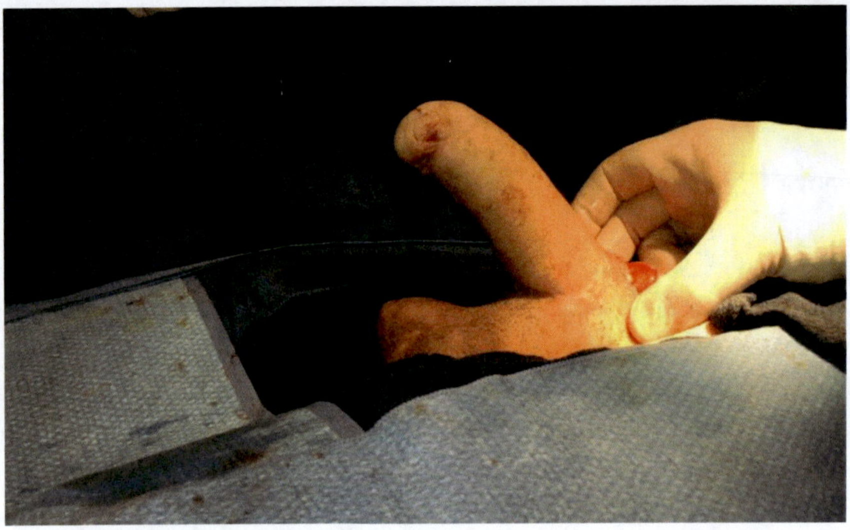

Figure 3. Final aspect of the neophallus with the IPP in place.

Selection of the Appropriate Prosthesis

Although multiple devices are available, inflatable devices are preferred nowadays, as shown on Table 1. Despite the malleable PP is cheaper, less complicated in design and easier to implant, the permanent rigidity may increase the risk of erosion through the skin or urethra [8, 12]. Another advantage of the IPP is that the possibility to cycle from flaccid to erect state optimizes concealment [13]. In a retrospective analysis, Zuckerman et al. found a non-significant trend towards a higher complication rate in patients with malleable prosthesis (28% versus 10%, $p = 0.10$) [21].

IPP model selection is currently up to surgeon's preference. Using Kaplan Meier's method and log rank test, Falcone et al. compared AMS 700CX, AMS700 CXM/R, Ambicor and Coloplast Titan [4]. Overall 5-year survival rate was 78%, and there weren't significant differences in survival among the mentioned models. Ambicor may show an advantage in patients with large scars in the lower abdomen, because an additional reservoir isn't necessary, but the drawbacks include less rigidity during erection and a harder pump [12].

There is a tendency towards the use of a single cylinder, although there is significant variability among the different series (see Table 1). The decision depends on the surgeon's preference and is usually based on the girth of the neophallus [8]. Some surgeons have recommended against dual implantation because of worse esthetic results secondary to misplacement of one of the cylinders [11].

Table 2. Outcomes and complications. Detail of the outcomes in different series including complications and satisfaction rate

Series	Patients (n)	Reason for surgery	Phalloplasty	Prosthesis (n)	Follow-up (months)	5-year survival (%)	Infection rate (%)	Revision rate (%)	Mechanical failure rate (%)	Penetrative intercourse (%)	Satisfaction (%)
Garaffa 2008	15	100% Penile cancer	100% RFFF	7	18.2	NA	14	14	NA	71	NA
Leriche 2008	38	100% Gender confirmation	100% RFFF	NA	110	NA	NA	29	NA	51	90
Hoebecke 2009	129	100% Gender confirmation	100% RFFF	185	30	AMS 3 piece 50%, Dynaflex 42%	12	41	18.4	NA	NA
Segal 2015	9	55% Bladder extrophy, 22.5% trauma, 22.5% ambiguous genitalia	100% RFFF	NA	9.6	NA	33.33	55.55	0	16.7	NA
Zuckerman 2015	31	48% gender confirmation, 23% trauma, 7% penile cancer, 19% others	96% RFFF, 4% groin flap	NA	59.7	70	10	23	NA	81	NA
Neuville 2016	69	89.9% Gender confirmation, 5.8% malformation, 4.3% trauma	71% RFFF, 29% suprapubic	95	48	Median survival 4.2 years	4.2	37.7	4.2	NA	NA
Falcone 2017	247	100% Gender confirmation	64% RFFF, 36% suprapubic	328	20	78	8.5	43	15.4	77	88

RFFF Radial Forearm Free Flap; NA Not Available.

Final Details

The prosthesis pump is usually placed at the contralateral side of the vascular pedicle of the neophallus in the scrotum. The prosthesis is partially activated during the first week, and is deactivated on day 7. The patient is taught how to cycle the prosthesis between weeks 3 and 6 and is encouraged to engage in penetrative intercourse after week 6 [4, 11, 19, 22].

Postoperative Outcomes and Complications

Good quality evidence is lacking in these matters. All the reports of PP after phalloplasty are retrospective, most of them have less than 50 patients and most phalloplasties are in trans men. Table 2 shows the outcomes and complications of the most significant series.

Opposite from IPP implantation in the native penis, which has a 5-year overall survival from 77% to 91% [13], IPP in the neophallus has a lower survival rate and much higher revision, complication and mechanical failure rates (see Table 2). Interestingly, satisfaction rates seem to be similar between native penis and neophallus patients (81% to 97% and 88% to 90% respectively).

A summary of frequent complications is shown in Table 3 [8, 12]. There are several hypotheses to explain the higher complication rate in patients with neophallus. Firstly, the absence of corpora cavernosa may be associated with a higher risk of malposition [11]. Apart from that, the lack of native tunica albuginea and its replacement with ectopic materials may be a reason for the high extrusion rate. Mechanical failure is also related to this, since friction between vascular grafts and the IPP can damage the tubings [4, 11, 19, 22].

Also, the neophallus tissue has less vascularization than the native penis, secondary to scar formation and single arterial supply, thus explaining the higher infection rate. Finally, patients who undergo neophallus and IPP are much younger than patients who undergo IPP for erectile dysfunction, which may explain the higher mechanical failure rates secondary to a more frequent and vigorous sexual intercourse [11].

Table 3. Summary of frequent complications

Complication	%
Infection	8 - 50
Extrusion or erosion	4 - 8
Device migration	15 - 30
Early mechanical failure	11 - 15
Patient disatisfaction	19

Quality of Life

It must be noted that out of all the revised publications, only 2 assessed quality of life (QOL) and satisfaction after IPP in neophallus, and this was done using non-validated questionnaires [4, 25]. Even though all the other authors refer excellent patient satisfaction, this wasn't assessed objectively.

One study evaluated sexual QOL in 10 men who had a phalloplasty and IPP for different reasons including penile cancer, trauma and bladder exstrophy [6]. All the patients had a high level of satisfaction with their neophallus, but when asked specifically about sexual and psychological issues, answers were less consistent. Patients referred inhibition and fear of sexual rejection, and in one case the subject didn't dare to attempt a sexual encounter. Regarding genital appraisal, patients reported dissatisfaction with the size (20%), artificial appearance (50%) and difficulties for undressing publicly. On the other hand, an important finding was that all patients were able to achieve orgasm with ejaculation, 80% through penetrative intercourse and 20% through masturbation. Patients who had a higher penile remnant at the base of the neophallus referred better erogenous sensitivity than those who didn't. The authors conclude that it is crucial to establish realistic expectations with patients and that psychosexual support must be offered before and after the surgery.

Another group compared sexual QOL after phalloplasty in cis-men with (9) and without (4) an IPP [5]. Using the International Index of Erectile Function (IIEF), the authors found that IPP patients did significantly better than non-IPP patients in all domains except sexual desire. Paradoxically, there were no significant differences in the Pediatric Penile Perception Score (PPPS) and the Sexual Quality of Life for Men (SQOL-M). These findings were attributed to the small sample size.

Even though both publications had a low number of patients, there are some elements to take into account. Patients seem to be very satisfied with having a neophallus and an IPP, but that doesn't make their lives any easier. These patients definitively need constant support from a multidisciplinary team, in order to assimilate their condition and relate socially and sexually with other people. It is necessary to include sexual QOL and psychological assessment as part of future research, especially in larger, multicentric projects.

Conclusion

Successfully implanting a penile prosthesis in a neophallus is a challenging procedure. Nevertheless, it is definitely worthy since it is like bringing to life a neophallus, something that will comfort both the patient and the surgeon. After surgery, several complications are to be expected, which is why the surgical team and the patient need to be warned and prepared. Psychological and psychosexual support are key issues before and after the procedure and should be part of standard care. Further investigations are needed, with focus in surgical outcomes, prevention of complications and patient and partner QOL and satisfaction.

Key Points

- Implantation of a penile prosthesis is the ultimate step after phalloplasty. Inflatable penile prosthesis is nowadays preferred over malleables because of better concealment and less risk or erosion.
- It is recommended to wait between 6 to 12 months after phalloplasty to implant a penile prosthesis. This allows for early complication troubleshooting and development of neophallus protective sensitivity.
- Key surgical steps include careful dilatation of the neophallus, adequate anchoring of the prosthesis using the native crura or pubic symphysis and constructing a neotunica albuginea with synthetic materials or allografts.
- Depending on surgeon's preference and neophallus characteristics, one or two cylinders may be used.
- Complication rate is high, and includes infection, erosion or extrusion, device migration, mechanical failure and patient dissatisfaction. Patient and surgeon should be prepared and motivated to deal with these issues.
- Psychosexual support before and after surgery is crucial and should be offered to all patients.

References

[1] Rashid M, Tamimy MS. Phalloplasty: The dream and the reality. *Indian J Plast Surg* 2013;46:283–93.

[2] Gilbert DA, Horton CE, Terzis JK, Devine CJ Jr, Winslow BH, Devine PC. New concepts in phallic reconstruction. *Ann Plast Surg* 1987;18:128–36.

[3] Monstrey S, Ceulemans P, Hoebeke P. Sex Reassignment Surgery in the Female-to-Male Transsexual. *Semin Plast Surg* 2011;25:229–44.

[4] Falcone M, Garaffa G, Gillo A, Dente D, Christopher AN, Ralph DJ. Outcomes of inflatable penile prosthesis insertion in 247 patients completing female to male gender reassignment surgery. *BJU Int* 2018;121:139–44.

[5] Young EE, Friedlander D, Lue K, Anele UA, Khurgin JL, Bivalacqua TJ, et al. Sexual Function and Quality of Life Before and After Penile Prosthesis Implantation Following Radial Forearm Flap Phalloplasty. *Urology* 2017;104:204–8.

[6] Callens N, De Cuypere G, T'Sjoen G, Monstrey S, Lumen N, Van Laecke E, et al. Sexual quality of life after total phalloplasty in men with penile deficiency: an exploratory study. *World J Urol* 2015;33:137–43.

[7] Schultheiss D, Gabouev AI, Jonas U. Nikolaj A. Bogoraz (1874-1952): pioneer of phalloplasty and penile implant surgery. *J Sex Med* 2005;2:139–46.

[8] Dy GW, Sun J, Granieri MA, Zhao LC. Reconstructive Management Pearls for the Transgender Patient. *Curr Urol Rep* 2018;19:36.

[9] Scott FB, Bradley WE, Timm GW. Management of erectile impotence. Use of implantable inflatable prosthesis. *Urology* 1973;2:80–2.

[10] Puckett CL, Montie JE. Construction of male genitalia in the transsexual, using a tubed groin flap for the penis and a hydraulic inflation device. *Plast Reconstr Surg* 1978;61:523–30.

[11] Hoebeke PB, Decaestecker K, Beysens M, Opdenakker Y, Lumen N, Monstrey SM. Erectile implants in female-to-male transsexuals: our experience in 129 patients. *Eur Urol* 2010;57:334–40.

[12] Kocjancic E, Iacovelli V. Penile Prostheses. *Clin Plast Surg* 2018;45:407–14.

[13] Levine LA, Becher EF, Bella AJ, Brant WO, Kohler TS, Martinez-Salamanca JI, et al. Penile Prosthesis Surgery: Current Recommendations From the International Consultation on Sexual Medicine. *J Sex Med* 2016;13:489–518.

[14] Vesely J, Hyza P, Ranno R, Cigna E, Monni N, Stupka I, et al. New technique of total phalloplasty with reinnervated latissimus dorsi myocutaneous free flap in female-to-male transsexuals. *Ann Plast Surg* 2007;58:544–50.

[15] Schechter LS, Safa B. Introduction to Phalloplasty. Clin Plast Surg 2018;45:387–9.

[16] Remington AC, Morrison SD, Massie JP, Crowe CS, Shakir A, Wilson SC, et al. Outcomes after Phalloplasty: Do Transgender Patients and Multiple Urethral Procedures Carry a Higher Rate of Complication? *Plast Reconstr Surg* 2018;141:220e – 229e.

[17] Levine LA, Zachary LS, Gottlieb LJ. Prosthesis placement after total phallic reconstruction. *J Urol* 1993;149:593–8.

[18] Garaffa G, Christopher NA, Ralph DJ. Total phallic reconstruction in female-to-male transsexuals. *Eur Urol* 2010;57:715–22.

[19] Garaffa G, Ralph DJ. Penile Prosthesis Implantation in Phalloplasty in Female-to-Male Transsexuals. *Management of Gender Dysphoria*, 2015, p. 311–6.

[20] Segal RL, Massanyi EZ, Gupta AD, Gearhart JP, Redett RJ, Bivalacqua TJ, et al. Inflatable penile prosthesis technique and outcomes after radial forearm free flap neophalloplasty. *Int J Impot Res* 2015;27:49–53.

[21] Zuckerman JM, Smentkowski K, Gilbert D, Storme O, Jordan G, Virasoro R, et al. Penile Prosthesis Implantation in Patients with a History of Total Phallic Construction. *J Sex Med* 2015;12:2485–91.

[22] Neuville P, Morel-Journel N, Maucourt-Boulch D, Ruffion A, Paparel P, Terrier J-E. Surgical Outcomes of Erectile Implants After Phalloplasty: Retrospective Analysis of 95 Procedures. *J Sex Med* 2016;13:1758–64.

[23] Kocjancic E, Jaunarena J, Sofer L, Morgantini L, Schechter L. V11-04 Inflatable Penile Prosthesis Implantation Post Phalloplasty. *J Urol* 2018;199:e1162–3.

[24] Cohen AJ, Bhanvadia RR, Pariser JJ, Hatcher DM, Gottlieb LJ, Bales GT. Novel Technique for Proximal Bone Anchoring of Penile Prosthesis After Radial Forearm Free Flap Neophallus. *Urology* 2017;105:2–5.

[25] Leriche A, Timsit MO, Morel-Journel N, Bouillot A, Dembele D, Ruffion A. Long-term outcome of forearm flee-flap phalloplasty in the treatment of transsexualism. *BJU Int* 2008;101:1297–300.

SECTION E. CHALLENGES AND CONTROVERSIES

In: Penile Cancer: Challenges and Controversies
Editors: F. E. Martins and M. L. Djordjevic
ISBN: 978-1-53615-950-9

Chapter 15

IS PREVENTION AND EARLY DIAGNOSIS OF PENILE CANCER POSSIBLE?

C. Dunford, L. Vyas, T. Tharu and S. Minhas*
Imperial College Healthcare NHS Trust, London, England

ABSTRACT

Penile cancer is a rare and debilitating disease with a prevalence of approximately 1% worldwide. There are three main aspects to the etiology: phimosis together with chronic inflammation, and association with the Human Papilloma virus (HPV). The differences in prevalence of these risk factors may account for variations in incidence. High risk HPV 16 and 18 are those thought to cause almost all cases of penile intra-epithelial neoplasia (PeIN) and up to half the cases of invasive squamous cell carcinoma (SCC) of the penis. Although HPV is treatable, prevention of HPV with vaccination may reduce the risk of penile cancer. Vaccination programs have been proven in cervical cancer for both efficacy and cost effectiveness. Subsequently its use has expanded to men in order to prevent all HPV related disease. Whilst, HPV vaccination in men is effective, the prophylactic benefit in the prevention of penile cancer is yet to be reported in large randomised control trials. Cost effective modelling predicts it should be economically viable to expand the vaccination program to include females and males and as such this is now increasingly used in practice in many countries worldwide. Other modifiable risk factors that contribute to over half of invasive penile cancer cases include smoking, obesity, sex education and good penile hygiene. In this chapter we discuss the complexities of penile cancer prevention and early detection of this rare disease.

Keywords: penile cancer, early detection, causes, risk factors, prevention, staging

---

* Corresponding Author's E-mail: sminhas@btinternet.com.

Learning Objectives

- To understand pathogenesis and prevention of penile cancer
- To understand the challenges faced in penile cancer prevention and early detection including the multi-factoral etiology
- To understand the complexities of HPV prevention in males including vaccination, its efficacy and cost effectiveness

Evidence-Based Medicine (EBM)

Defined as the conscientious, explicit and judicious use of current best evidence, EBM practice in medicine has really taken hold in the last two decades. It challenges the clinician to use clinical experience, patient values and best evidence in their decision making [1]. But more than that, it focuses the mind on the important questions, delivering research and pushing the boundaries of traditional medicine. That's not to say that traditional medicine wasn't based on evidence, far from it as the concept of EBM was first discussed in the mid-19Th century. But today it would be defined as lower level evidence from a consensus panel of experts, and whilst it has served clinicians well in the past, it has led to the demand for higher level evidence with which to base clinical decisions on. Expert panel guidelines from the European and American Associations of Urology for example, summarise the current evidence base and where it may be lacking, continue to make expert panel recommendations [2, 3]. However, as the clinician grows ever more literate in critical appraisal and research, they demand higher level evidence including systematic reviews, meta-analyses and long-term data with which to base decisions on.

The statisticians would suggest good quality evidence requires data, and lots of it. The first issue is that penile cancer is rare so, by definition, the evidence is based on small numbers which can skew the data when analysed and mislead its interpretation. There is long term data pertaining to treatment of established penile cancer, but prevention and early diagnosis is a relative 'new kid on the block', so the long-term data isn't there yet. Other cancer research helps us draw parallels, for example cervical cancer prevention, but to the purist, these are suppositions and a starting point for the research question rather than the answer.

Introduction

Penile cancer is rare in western countries with just over 2000 new cases diagnosed in the US[1]. Proven risk factors include geographical location, hygiene, social and cultural factors together with circumcision and HPV (Human Papilloma Virus). HPV and penile cancer have a strong relationship with over half of men with penile cancer harbouring HPV. However, interestingly penile cancer is rare in circumcised men especially when this occurs in newborns.

Epidemiology

Penile cancer is uncommon in Western countries causing only 0.1% of all cancer deaths and an incidence of < 1 in 100, 000. However, it occurs more frequently in South America, South East Asia and parts of Africa where it reaches 1 - 2% prevalence [2, 4, 5]. It commonly affects men aged 50 - 70 years, usually occurs on the glans penis, with 95% of cases being squamous cell carcinoma [2-4, 6, 7]. The incidence varies with race, ethnicity and geographical areas. In North America Hispanics, Alaskans, Native Americans and African Americans have higher respective incidences of penile cancer, than non-Hispanics [2, 7, 8]. More interesting is the increasing rates of penile cancer recently reported in the USA, UK and parts of Scandinavia [2, 9, 10]. This is potentially a consequence of improved data collection and the increased reporting of cases in these industrialised countries as well as expanding population diversity from global migration.

Although small numbers of men are affected by penile cancer the disease is also noted to cause considerable physical and psychological impact. The majority of penile cancers are curable when detected early, therefore it is essential to focus on defining parameters for early detection and better still prevention of this disease [6, 7].

Prevention

Risk Factors for Penile Cancer

In order to prevent penile cancer, it is crucial to gain a detailed understanding of the pathogenesis of risk factors (see Figure 1). Risk factors which are well documented are include the presence of a prepuce, penile hygiene, chronic inflammation, smoking, low socio-economic status, age and human papilloma (HPV) virus infection [2, 4, 9]. Age at

[1] https://www.cancer.org/cancer/penile-cancer/about/key-statistics.html

diagnosis and socio-economic status are not easily modifiable. Conversely, Smoking status certainly is modifiable and 'stop smoking' campaigns have contributed to all cancer prevention[2].

Modifiable Risk Factors

Obesity

Similar to smoking, obesity is linked to all malignancies, but there is robust evidence pertaining the strong association between obesity and penile cancer [11]. A population-based study using matched controls showed a significant association between obesity and developing invasive penile cancer, it reported 53% increase in risk of developing the disease for every 5-point BMI increase over 25 (i.e., overweight) [12]. Whilst it is impressive this study group went on to validate the link with obesity in a controlled population study, it must be interpreted with caution in view of the wide confidence intervals. BMI also appears to have no impact on the stage of disease at diagnosis [13], therefore more robust research is required to define the effect of obesity at the cellular level. On a more practical note weight loss programs are already part of the public health message globally, for prevention of all disease pathologies, and therefore will largely contribute to penile cancer prevention.

The Prepuce

The majority of modifiable risk factors in penile cancer include preputial pathology. There is a wealth of evidence describing the association between the presence of the prepuce and its link with chronic inflammation, lichen sclerosis as well as poor penile hygiene depicted by phimosis. HPV infection similarly affects the foreskin and is potentially modifiable, therefore it is important to understand the prevention of penile cancer development.

Risk factors for penile cancer
Phimosis
HPV infection
Obesity
Smoking
Low socio-economic status
PUVA (phototherapy UVA treatment for psoriasis)

* modifiable risk factors

Figure 1. Risk factors for penile cancer.

[2] https://www.ncbi.nlm.nih.gov/pmc/articles/PMC4248563/

Factors associated with penile cancer (not causal)
Chronic inflammation- lichen sclerosis, recurrent balanitis, posthitis
Precursors penile lesions- erythroplasia de Queyrat, Bowen's disease (both PeIN)
Poor penile hygiene
Multiple sexual partners/ lack of barrier contraception(increasing HPV infection)

Figure 2. Factors associated with penile cancer (not causal).

The evidence around the prepuce itself is mixed. Whilst the presence of a prepuce that is retractile is unlikely to be pathological [2, 10], the presence of phimosis is associated with a significantly increased risk of invasive penile cancer [2, 10, 14, 15]. The exact pathogenesis in invasive penile cancer development is unknown, as smegma is not carcinogenic and chronic inflammation e.g., lichen sclerosis has only been identified as an associative rather than causal effect [2, 6, 16] (see Figure 2). However, one Swedish study in 2014 analysed 771 adult patients with Lichen Sclerosis. Whilst a third were reported to have a phimosis, overall only 1% were found to have invasive penile cancer compared with premalignant conditions. Thus, the authors concluded follow up was advisable in patients with penile lichen sclerosis [17].

Circumcision is not always the answer as a study in 2011 showed. A systematic review by Larke et al. demonstrated that circumcision does not reduce the risk of penile intra-epithelial neoplasia, which might seem a likely target in an early detection and prevention in a health model. Furthermore, whilst childhood circumcision could reduce the rates of invasive penile cancer initially, after 17 years, no benefit was seen. Similarly, no benefit was seen in invasive cancer rates following circumcision in adult men [18]. However, in pre-malignant conditions circumcision may prevent further progression.

It is important to contextualise PeIN in the penile cancer pathway. Currently only a third of PeIN cases will develop invasive squamous cell carcinoma (SCC). Circumcision involves removing half of the tissue, which can develop penile cancer, but as a rare disease, the number needed to treat to prevent one case is 300,000 circumcisions[3]. A huge number of neonates would have an unnecessary procedure, which is clearly not a cost-effective strategy. There are also cost implications to consider as well.

A less invasive option was reported in a recent systematic review. Circumcision along with reduction in the number of sexual partners and the use of barrier contraception appeared to improve penile cancer prevention. However, the odds ratio commented in the meta-analysis had wide ranging confidence intervals and as such should be interpreted with caution [19]. Nevertheless, barrier contraception is a simple and cost-effective method for men who find this acceptable.

On review of the dermatological literature on genital lichen sclerosis, there is evidence on the presence of HPV infection in 35% of penile lichen sclerosis cases. However, no causality in pathogenesis of lichen sclerosis has been identified, but rather it

[3] https://www.aafp.org/about/policies/all/neonatal-circumcision.html

is considered that 'passenger HPV' incidentally was found [20]. Both factors support the view that sex education, reducing the number of sexual partners and advocating barrier contraception would promote disease prevention by reducing HPV infection, to impact both penile cancer and other cancer prevention (e.g., cervical cancer) [21].

Human Papilloma Virus (HPV)

The human papilloma virus is the more captivating and the biggest breakthrough in the last 10 years for penile cancer treatment and prevention Current literature suggests 50% of all penile cancer cases are causally associated with HPV [22, 23, 24]. HPV is a non-enveloped circular strand of genomic material (DNA) which is the most common form of sexually transmitted infection in both males and females. There are over 150 different types of HPV, but the relevant ones to the genitalia can be subdivided into high and low risk mucosal types. HPV 6 and 11 for example are low risk and responsible for genital warts. HPV 16, 18, 31, 45, 56, 65 are high risk subtypes found in 30 - 40% of invasive penile cancer specimens, and 70 - 100% of PeIN specimens [9, 11]. HPV infection in men is usually self-limiting and clearance occurs at a median time of 7.5 months, but can take longer, up to 12.2 months in high risk subtypes [25, 26, 27]. Most infections are asymptomatic, but those that do not clear usually go on to manifest as genital warts or subsequently a primary diagnosis of penile cancer. There is no treatment available to eradicate HPV and therefore prevention could be used to reduce tumour burden instead.

The exact mechanism of carcinogenesis is poorly understood. Theoretical intracellular pathways include possible tumour suppressor gene modification as the viral genome is incorporated into the host cell's genome. p16, p53, SCC antigen, Ki-67, cyclin D1 and proliferating cell nuclear antigen are examples of intracellular signalling pathways and tumour suppressor genes that have been most extensively studied [5, 22,28, 29]. Interestingly, HPV status has been identified as a good prognostic indicator when treating head and neck cancer with chemoradiation [9, 27]. There is some evidence that the presence of tumour suppressor gene p16 for example is a better prognostic indicator in patients with established penile cancer [11, 13]. It is thought that p16 for example, has oncogenic effects via the viral proteins E6 and E7 which act on the p53 and retinoblastoma tumour suppressor gene pathways respectively [30, 31]. This has been particularly demonstrated in cervical cancer and further studies are required to assess whether this would translate to men. HPV infection results in both genomic alterations and epigenetic alterations that can be predictive of survival [27] but not all the evidence in penile cancer agrees and in one review, only two out of eight studies concluded the presence of HPV had prognostic value in penile cancer [9].

In contrast to this HPV has been found more prevalent in two particular penile cancer histological subtypes, warty and basaloid [9, 27], both of which traditionally have been associated with worse prognosis when compared with other subtypes [2], however the exact nature and impact of this association is yet to be determined.

Is HPV a suitable target for prevention and early detection? It is important to keep this discussion in context. 30 - 40% of invasive penile cancer is HPV positive, versus 70-100% of pre-malignant conditions, although only 30% will progress to invasive penile cancer [2] unlike conversion rates in cervical or head and neck cancer, which are higher. The likely difference is the result of the nature of the epithelium in which it infects. In the case of the penis; it is keratinised, unlike when it infects the cervix, which has been postulated as the reason for the marked immune response seen in women infected with HPV compared with men [9]. It is this lower immune response which is thought to impact the conversion rates to invasive carcinoma.

The prevalence of penile cancer has increased recently in the USA [9], despite the controlling for other risk factors like phimosis and smoking cessation. It may be that the benefits of these are too early to report, and certainly as mentioned before, up to date epidemiological data is pending.

Perhaps we will start to see a rise in HPV positive tumour cells in invasive penile cancer [9]. Currently though, HPV 16 or 18 infection of the penis will not necessarily develop into SCC. Evidence suggests a 2% conversion rate to PeIN with HPV 16 in 24 months, and following that, only 30% will develop invasive SCC. This disease progression is markedly slower than low risk subtypes like HPV 11 where 20% will develop benign condylomata within 8 months [25, 26].

It is not clear whether barrier methods are completely protective against HPV infections. In a small study of 3 men who had previous neonatal circumcisions and later developed penile cancer; all of them had a history of penile condyloma and one oncogenic HPV present [32]. However, in an adult setting barrier method is highly effective [33] with 35% reduced risk compared to controls [34]. There was also a reduced time to clear the disease in circumcised men [34].

Despite this the presence of HPV as a driver for pathogenesis in penile cancer created the case for targeting HPV in penile cancer prevention. Vaccination against HPV is now standard practice worldwide and successful in reducing cervical cancer rates [9, 19, 35, 36]. This has prompted the concept of male HPV vaccination.

The HPV Vaccine

HPV infection is found in almost all cases of invasive cervical carcinoma [6, 9, 27, 37, 38], therefore the HPV vaccine was originally developed as for women against cervical cancer. In contrast HPV infection is only present in half of men with invasive penile carcinoma [5, 11, 30]. The nonvalent HPV vaccine was initially developed and was soon overtaken by the bivalent (HPV 16 and 18) and quadrivalent (HPV 6,11,16 and 18) vaccines [6]. The quadrivalent vaccine has proven the more active protecting against the common strains of HPV 6 and 11 (low risk- but causing genital warts) and HPV 16 and 18 (high risk- associated with PeIN and SCC development).

This vaccine showed such tremendous success in cervical cancer prevention that it was trialled in a multi-centre, double blind, placebo controlled, randomised controlled trial in males aged 16-23 years of age, with favourable results demonstrating a significant reduction in HPV infection and genital lesions with the vaccine, regardless of sexual history or circumcision status [37]. No cases of PeIN developed in the vaccine arm insinuating that vaccine use may reduce both cancerous and precancerous lesions. Despite these recommendations for routine vaccination in the US did not occur until 2011 and is still not recommended in some parts of Western Europe. A recent systematic review has looked at the evidence base for HPV vaccination in males [36]. This review has reported that whilst studies have shown favourable outcomes for vaccinating young men and dismissed prior concerns immunogenicity, all their primary outcomes have been the presence of HPV infection post vaccination. No studies have looked at either SCC or PeIN prevention as secondary outcomes [36]. While HPV may be implemented in almost all cases of PeIN, only one third progress to invasive carcinoma and overall, HPV appears causative in half of invasive SCC cases.

On further scrutiny of Guiliano's study the reported 3 cases of HPV infection in the vaccination arm of the trial on per protocol analysis [40] may not have been true vaccine failures. In their discussion they reported the possibility of laboratory limitations in the PCR technique used to identify the HPV DNA. In the HIM study, a large multi-national, longitudinal cohort study looking at the natural history of HPV infection, 2 cases of PeIN where identified to have single infections with low risk HPV subtypes 6 and 11. However the authors did postulate that there could be low viral load of high risk subtype present that their laboratory techniques were not sensitive enough to identify [25]. Whilst one would accept vaccine failures in any population, it does demonstrate the limitations in PCR DNA detection and thus the need for further advances in diagnostic laboratory investigations.

Originally it was thought that herd immunity would be transferred when vaccinating girls on the overwhelming evidence of cervical cancer prevention. However significant populations, namely men who have sex with men (MSM) and the transgender community were not protected in this scenario. The advisory committee on Immunization Practices (ACIP) have recently made recommendations for the use of vaccine and the male groups it would benefit the most. This poses further cost implications.

As of July 2018, NICE recommended the quadrivalent vaccine be offered to all boys aged 12-13 in the UK. The planned implementation date for this is the academic year 2019/2020. Prior to this the UK had only vaccinated girls since 2008 and men who have sex with men more recently [19]. The authors are therefore are eager to see the long-term data on outcomes including cost effective analyses and impact this may have on the prevention of penile cancer in the future. Currently no urological guidelines discuss HPV vaccination or its role in penile cancer prevention. It is important these new advances are incorporated into guidelines in the future.

Health Economics

The health economics of HPV vaccination are complex. Studies of health economics often use Markov models to predict the likelihood of events happening in a population exposed to a disease like HPV, and measure the number of disease cases prevented, quality adjusted life years (QALYs) and incremental cost effectiveness ratios (ICERs). Governments make public health decisions on best evidence of a vaccination program and take into account information including: the natural history of the disease, the size disease population affected (incidence and prevalence), the economic burden of treating this disease, and whether the vaccine itself is effective in disease prevention. Wilson and Jungner principles for screening should also be taken into consideration. All of this has to be balanced with potential side effects and long-term complications of the vaccine, as well as the uptake of vaccination for herd immunity to take effect.

Firstly, the case for HPV vaccination to prevent penile cancer has limited cost effectiveness as it is such a rare disease. HPV is not the sole etiological factor, and whilst we can describe considerable physical and psychological impact to the individual affected patient, this does not translate to economic burden in this single disease, which is mainly prevalent in the 50-70-year age group. It is difficult to analyse the effects of vaccination in men as there are no studies looking at the cost effectiveness of vaccinating boys and its impact on penile cancer specifically. Rather the evidence in the literature argues for vaccination of boys in the context of overall HPV disease prevention and its sequelae. Originally it was thought that herd immunity would deliver this through girls being vaccinated. Using the principle that 100% of cervical cancer is caused by HPV and eradicating HPV in women would lead to herd immunity in men. However, this did not translate into clinical practice likely to be owing to differing disease etiology in non-cervical HPV disease, differing immunogenicity in male populations, discussed previously, and men who have sex with men. As such the promised reduction in other HPV cancers and benign diseases were not so dramatic with vaccination in girls only [6, 36, 37].

The prevalence of HPV related disease is variable geographically and therefore public health funding and vaccination programs should be made locally. Unfortunately, most literature for cost effectiveness is for girls and cervical cancer which then extends to a wider context. A recent systematic review looked at cost effectiveness of a universal HPV vaccination program and commented that all models tend not to take into account the ecological bias, described as sexual behaviour, which varies in different populations over time. They concluded that the evidence they reviewed for universal expansion perhaps over estimated cost effectiveness in terms of QALYs and ICERs added [39]. Individual countries who have published analysis on cost effectiveness, for example

Belgium [41], the Netherlands [42] and Venezuela [43] have all proven a positive impact on cost for girls vaccinated to prevent cervical cancer. However, they often conclude further information should be sought about non-cervical HPV disease prevention benefit and consideration of extending vaccination to boys.

An interesting point made in the study from Belgium was that the program was economically viable and prevented significant cases of cervical cancer in girls vaccinated before and after their sexual debut [41]. This is something reflected in the UK vaccination program, girls can receive the vaccine any time before 18. However, boys are only vaccinated between the ages of 12 and 13. This is because the vaccine is not cost effective later and boys should subsequently benefit from herd immunity [44].

To improve ICERs the drive is always to lower vaccination costs [39-42]. Using the UK model, originally bivalent vaccine (against HPV 16 and 18) were offered from 2008 [6,45]. However, the Venezuelan study did not demonstrate any cost effective difference however between using the bivalent and quadrivalent vaccine in their population model [43] and therefore the UK, like many other countries, now offer the quadrivalent vaccine (against HPV 6,11, 16 and 18) that delivers a wider range of public health effects [6, 43, 44]. These include prevention of other HPV related cancers and benign genital disease. Again, the authors look tentatively to the literature to see if the cost effectiveness predictive modelling holds true in the future.

Self-Examination and Early Diagnosis

Penile cancer is visible on the skin surface and as such its early detection is reliant on being able to correctly identify the lesion early, ideally in a pre-malignant phase. This requires patient and clinician education. It cannot be augmented by the latest biomarker, therefore clinical acumen is key. Penile cancer is diagnosed on biopsy and imaging is used for staging rather than identification. The rarity of penile cancer means it simply does not meet Jung and Wilson's criteria for screening. However, it can be extremely debilitating with psychological repercussions. Patient education to regularly carry out self-examination, particularly in those non-circumcised individuals, and stressing the importance of addressing any phimosis early, would likely improve outcomes [6]. This is one of the most cost-effective preventative methods, although, not often followed. Clinician education and clear efficient referral pathways to specialist centres who deal with penile cancer regularly improve early detection rates [6, 43].

Conclusion

Primary prevention of penile cancer is crucial in order to reduce the morbidity occurring from treatment. Patient education for modifiable risk factors such as weight loss, sexual health, barrier contraception, cessation of smoking, improved hygiene and self-examination are simple preventative methods. Although neonatal circumcision reduces the risk for penile cancer the number needed to treat together with the possibility of complication negates routine practice.

Increasing evidence associating HPV to penile cancer renders a vaccine programme appealing. Although, current evidence reports a benefit to girls to reduce cervical cancer risk; for boys, vaccination for the sole purpose to prevent penile cancer lacks clear evidence and cost-effective analyses. Despite this, if male vaccination is considered in a wider context such as prevention of both malignant and non-malignant conditions there would an increase and improved cost effectiveness. The use of quadrivalent vaccine prior to first sexual contact has the highest proven efficacy and is therefore the most frequently used regimen.

A holistic approach of education, vaccination and keeping abreast of new advances is imperative to any clinician encountering adolescents and pre-malignant penile conditions. With increasing countries using vaccine programs the future epidemiological effect is thrilling. It will be interesting to see the overall effect of these globally and whether this changes the sequelae of this disease.

Key Points

- Penile cancer is rare, but the prevalence is increasing worldwide
- Pathogenesis of penile cancer has two main driving forces: phimosis and chronic inflammation; HPV infection
- HPV appears etiological in half of invasive penile cancer cases (high risk HPV 16 and 18)
- HPV vaccine is the newest strategy in penile cancer prevention with proven efficacy in males
- Cost effective modelling is in all HPV related disease and suggests vaccination of boys is economically viable
- Modification of other risk factors in penile cancer should not be forgotten in penile cancer prevention: smoking cessation, weight loss programs, sex education, good penile hygiene
- Early detection remains reliant on patient and clinician education

REFERENCES

[1] David, L Sackett. Evidence Based Medicine. *Seminars in Gerantology*, 21(1), 3-5, 1997.

[2] European Association of Urology: *Penile cancer guidelines* www.uroweb.org/guidelines/penile-cancer.

[3] American Association of Urology *Penile Cancer guidelines* www.auanet.org/carcinomas/squuamouscellcarcinomas.

[4] Bleeker, MC; Heideman, DA; Snijders, PJ; et al. Penile cancer: epidemiology, pathogenesis and prevention. *World J Urol*, 2009, 27, 141-50. 10.1007/s00345-008-0302-z.

[5] Alemany, L; Cubilla, A; Halec, G; Kasamatsu, E; Quirós, B; Masferrer, E; Tous, S; Lloveras, B; Hernández-Suarez, G; Lonsdale, R; Tinoco, L; Alejo, M; Alvarado-Cabrero, I; Laco, J; Guimerà, N; Poblet, E; Lombardi, LE; Bergeron, C; Clavero, O; Shin, HR; Ferrera, A; Felix, A; Germar, J; Mandys, V; Clavel, C; Tzardi, M; Pons, LE; Wain, V; Cruz, E; Molina, C; Mota, JD; Jach, R; Velasco, J; Carrilho, C; López-Revilla, R; Goodman, MT; Quint, WG; Castellsagué, X; Bravo, I; Pawlita, M; Muñoz, N; Bosch, FX; de Sanjosé, S. HPV VVAP study group. Role of Human Papillomavirus in Penile Carcinomas Worldwide. *Eur Urol.*, 2016 May, 69(5), 953-61.

[6] Shabbir, M; Barod, R; Hegarty, P; Minhas, S. Primary prevention and vaccination for penile cancer. *Ther Adv Urol.*, 2013 Jun, 5(3), 161–169.

[7] Douglawi, A; Masterson, T. Updates on the epidemiology and risk factors for penile cancer *Transl Androl Urol.*, 2017 Oct, 6(5), 785–790.

[8] Hernandez, BY; Barnholtz-Sloan, J; German, RR; et al. Burden of invasive squamous cell carcinoma of the penis in the United States, 1998-2003. *Cancer*, 2008, 113, 2883-91.

[9] Kidd, L; Chaing, S; Chipollini, J; Guiliano, AR; Spiess, PE; Sharma, P. Relationship between human papillomavirus and penile cancer—implications for prevention and treatment. *Translational Andrology and Urology.*, 2017 Oct, 6(5), 791–802.

[10] Tsen, HF; et al. Risk factors for penile cancer: results of a population-based case-control study in Los Angeles County (United States). *Cancer Causes Control*, 2001, 12, 267; Larke, NL; Thomas, SL; dos Santos Silva, I; Weiss, HA. Male circumcision and penile cancer: a systematic review and meta-analysis. *Cancer Causes Control.*, 2011, Aug, 22(8), 1097-110.

[11] Barnes, KT; Smith, BJ; Lynch, CF; et al. Obesity and invasive penile cancer. *Eur Urol*, 2013, 63, 588-9. Barnes, KT; McDowell, BD; Button, A; et al. Obesity is associated with increased risk of invasive penile cancer. *BMC Urol*, 2016, 16, 42.

[12] Barnes, KT; McDowell, BD; Button, A; et al. Obesity is associated with increased risk of invasive penile cancer. *BMC Urol*, 2016, 16, 42.

[13] Djajadiningrat, RS; van Werkhoven, E; Horenblas, S. Penile cancer stage, survival and body mass index. *Urol Int*, 2015, 94, 220-4.

[14] Maden, C; et al. History of circumcision, medical conditions, and sexual activity and risk of penile cancer. *J Natl Cancer Inst*, 1993, 85, 19.

[15] Afonso, LA; et al. High-risk human papillomavirus infection of the foreskin in asymptomatic men and patients with phimosis. *J Urol*, 2016, 195, 1784.Ingles, DJ; Pierce Campbell, CM; Messina, JA; Stoler, MH; Lin, HU; Fulp, WJ; Abrahamsen, M; Sirak, BA; O'Keefe, MT; Papenfuss, M; Gage, C; Carvalho da Silva, R; Gonzalez Sosa, R; Rojas Juarez, O; Villa, LL; Lazcano Ponce, E; Giuliano, AR. Human papillomavirus virus (HPV) genotype- and age-specific analyses of external genital lesions among men in the HPV Infection in Men (HIM) Study. *J Infect Dis*, 2015, 211, 1060-7.

[16] Archier, E; et al. Carcinogenic risks of psoralen UV-A therapy and narrowband UV-B therapy in chronic plaque psoriasis: a systematic literature review. *J Eur Acad Dermatol Venereol*, 2012, 26, Suppl 3, 22.

[17] Kantere, D; Lowhagen, GB; Alvengren, G; et al. The clinical spectrum of lichen sclerosus in male patients - a retrospective study. *Acta Derm Venereol*, 2014, 94, 542-6.

[18] Larke, NL; Thomas, SL; dos Santos Silva, I; Weiss, HA. Male circumcision and penile cancer: a systematic review and meta-analysis. *Cancer Causes Control.*, 2011, Aug, 22(8), 1097-110.

[19] Zhu, YP; Jia, ZW; Dai, B; et al. Relationship between circumcision and human papillomavirus infection: a systematic review and meta-analysis. *Asian J Androl*, 2017, 19, 125-31.

[20] Bunker, CB; Shim, TN. Male genital lichen sclerosus. *Indian J Dermatol*, 2015, 60, 111-7.

[21] UK National Health Service patient advice website: HPV vaccination www.nhs.uk/ conditions/ vaccinations/ hpv-human-papillomavirus-vaccine/ #hpv-vaccination-for-men-and-boys.

[22] Shabbir, M; Barod, R; Hegarty, P; Minhas, S. Primary prevention and vaccination for penile cancer. *Ther Adv Urol.*, 2013 Jun, 5(3), 161–169.

[23] Boda, D; Docea, AO; Calina, D; Ilie, MA; Caruntu, C; Zurac, S; Neagu, M; Constantin, C; Branisteanu, DE; Voiculescu, V; Mamoulakis, C; Tzanakakis, G; Spandidos, DA; Drakoulis, N; Tsatsakis, AM. Human papilloma virus: Apprehending the link with carcinogenesis and unveiling new research avenues. *Int J Oncol.*, 2018 Mar, 52(3), 637–655.

[24] Backes, DM; Kurman, RJ; Pimenta, JM; et al. Systematic review of human papillomavirus prevalence in invasive penile cancer. *Cancer Causes Control.*, 2009, 20, 449-57.

[25] Miralles-Guri, C; Bruni, L; Cubilla, AL; et al. Human papillomavirus prevalence and type distribution in penile carcinoma. *J Clin Pathol.*, 2009, 62, 870-8.

[26] Ingles, DJ; Pierce Campbell, CM; Messina, JA; Stoler, MH; Lin, HU; Fulp, WJ; Abrahamsen, M; Sirak, BA; O'Keefe, MT; Papenfuss, M; Gage, C; Carvalho da Silva, R; Gonzalez Sosa, R; Rojas Juarez, O; Villa, LL; Lazcano Ponce, E; Giuliano, AR. Human papillomavirus virus (HPV) genotype- and age-specific analyses of external genital lesions among men in the HPV Infection in Men (HIM) Study. *J Infect Dis*, 2015, 211, 1060-7.

[27] Sudenga, SL; Ingles, DJ; Pierce Campbell, CM; Lin, HU; Fulp, WJ; Messina, JA; Stoler, MH; Abrahamsen, M; Villa, LL; Lazcano Ponce, E; Giuliano, AR. Genital Human Papillomavirus Infection Progression to External Genital Lesions: The HIM Study. *Eur Urol*, 2016, 69, 166-73.

[28] Zargar-Shoshtari, K; Sharma, P; Spiess, PE. Insight into novel biomarkers in penile cancer: Redefining the present and future treatment paradigm? *Urol Oncol.*, 2018 Oct, 36(10), 433-439.

[29] Stratton, KL; Culkin, DJ. A Contemporary Review of HPV and Penile Cancer. *Oncology (Williston Park)*, 2016, 30, 245-9.

[30] Ferreux, E; Lont, AP; Horenblas, S; et al. Evidence for at least three alternative mechanisms targeting the p16INK4A/cyclin D/Rb pathway in penile carcinoma, one of which is mediated by high-risk human papillomavirus. *J Pathol.*, 2003, 201, 109-18.

[31] Sand, FL; Rasmussen, CL; Frederiksen, MH; Andersen, KK; Kjaer, SK. Prognostic Significance of HPV and p16 Status in Men Diagnosed with Penile Cancer: A Systematic Review and Meta-analysis. *Cancer Epidemiol Biomarkers Prev.*, 2018 Oct, 27(10), 1123-1132.

[32] Saibishkumar EP, Crook J, Sweet J. Neonatal circumcision and invasive squamous cell carcinoma of the penis: a report of 3 cases and a review of the literature. *Can Urol Assoc J.* 2008;2:39-42

[33] Auvert B, Sobngwi-Tambekou J, Cutler E, et al. Effect of male circumcision on the prevalence of high-risk human papillomavirus in young men: results of a randomized controlled trial conducted in Orange Farm, South Africa. *J Infect Dis.* 2009;199:14-9

[34] Tobian AAR, Serwadda D, Quinn TC, et al. Male circumcision for the prevention of HSV-2 and HPV infections and syphilis. *N Engl J Med.* 2009;360:1298-309

[35] Gray RH, Serwadda D, Kong X, et al. Male circumcision decreases acquisition and increases clearance of high-risk human papillomavirus in HIV-negative men: a randomized trial in Rakai, Uganda. *J Infect Dis.* 2010;201:1455-62

[36] Walboomers, JM; Jacobs, MV; Manos, MM; et al. Human papillomavirus is a necessary cause of invasive cervical cancer worldwide. *J Pathol.*, 1999, 189, 12-9.

[37] Heidegger, I; Borena, W; Pichler, R. The role of human papilloma virus in urological malignancies. *Anticancer Res.*, 2015, 35, 2513-9.

[38] Favato, G; Easton, T; Vecchiato, R; Noikokyris, E. Ecological validity of cost-effectiveness models of universal HPV vaccination: A systematic literature review. *Vaccine.*, 2017 May, 9, 35(20), 2622-2632.

[39] Harder, T; Wichmann, O; Klug, SJ; van der Sande, MAB; Wiese-Posselt, M. Efficacy, effectiveness and safety of vaccination against human papillomavirus in males: a systematic review. *BMC Med.*, 2018, 16, 110.

[40] Giuliano, AR; Palefsky, JM; Goldstone, S; Moreira, ED; Jr. Penny, ME; Aranda, C; Vardas, E; Moi, H; Jessen, H; Hillman, R; Chang, YH; Ferris, D; Rouleau, D; Bryan, J; Marshall, JB; Vuocolo, S; Barr, E; Radley, D; Haupt, RM; Guris, D. Efficacy of quadrivalent HPV vaccine against HPV Infection and disease in males. *N Engl J Med*, 2011, 364, 401-11.

[41] Demarteau, N; Van Kriekinge, G; Simon, P. Incremental cost-effectiveness evaluation of vaccinating girls against cervical cancer pre- and post-sexual debut in Belgium. *Vaccine.*, 2013, Aug 20, 31(37), 3962-71.

[42] Setiawan, D; Luttjeboer, J; Westra, TA; Wilschut, JC; Suwantika, AA; Daemen, T; Atthobari, J; Wilffert, B; Postma, MJ. The cost-effectiveness of HPV vaccination in addition to screening: a Dutch perspective. *Expert Rev Vaccines.*, 2015 Apr, 14(4), 589-604.

[43] Bardach, AE; Garay, OU; Calderón, M; Pichón-Riviére, A; Augustovski, F; Martí, SG; Cortiñas, P; Gonzalez, M; Naranjo, LT; Gomez, JA; Caporale, JE. Health economic evaluation of Human Papillomavirus vaccines in women from Venezuela by a lifetime Markov cohort model. *BMC Public Health.*, 2017, Feb 2, 17(1), 152.

[44] National Institute for Health and Care Excellence (NICE) *Suspected Cancer: recognition and referral* (NG12) 2017. www.nice.org.uk.

[45] Jit, M; Chapman, R; Hughes, O; Choi, YH. Comparing bivalent and quadrivalent human papillomavirus vaccines: economic evaluation based on transmission model. *BMJ.*, 2011, Sep 27, 343, d5775.

In: Penile Cancer: Challenges and Controversies
Editors: F. E. Martins and M. L. Djordjevic
ISBN: 978-1-53615-950-9

Chapter 16

Penile Cancer Management and Decision-Making by Stage: A Changing Field?

Joren Vanthoor, MD, Hein Van Poppel, MD, PhD and Maarten Albersen*, MD, PhD
Department of Urology, University Hospitals Leuven, Leuven, Belgium

Abstract

Penile cancer is a rare disease in Western-Europe and the United States. Therefore, the disease remains a diagnostic and therapeutic challenge for physicians. Current management of the disease is mainly based on retrospective data, as there is a lack of controlled trial or large series. The rare encounter of penile cancer combined with limited evidence regularly results in a suboptimal guideline adherence. When it is diagnosed, the disease is psychologically devastating to the patient. Since narrower surgical margins do not seem to affect overall survival rates in local disease, there has been a paradigm shift over the years towards the adoption of organ-sparing surgery (OSS) for low-stage penile cancer. Surgical organ-sparing techniques allow better quality of life and sexual function. As lymphatic spread is associated with poor outcome, the management of inguinal lymph nodes is crucial for prognosis. Consequently, it is very important to perform adequate surgical lymph node staging in selected cases with impalpable lymph nodes. This should be done depending on the risk factors of the primary tumor. Lymph node metastases should be treated with radical lymphadenectomy. Guidelines currently recommend the use of adjuvant chemotherapy in patients with pN2/N3 disease, the role of adjuvant radiotherapy is still unclear. Novel second-line treatment modalities, for example EGFR targeted therapies or immunotherapy, have been proposed. This chapter aims to provide

* Corresponding Author's E-mail: maarten.albersen@uzleuven.be.

an overview of the diagnosis and the management options for the different stages of penile cancer, based on evidenced-based recommendations and current literature.

Keywords: penile cancer, decision-making, staging, organ sparing surgery, outcomes, overall survival, risk factors, recurrence rates

INTRODUCTION

In the Western world, penile cancer is diagnosed in only 1/100.000-1.000.000 men, which makes it a rare cancer [1]. The rarity of the disease, especially in countries where routine circumcision has been adopted, makes it a diagnostic and therapeutic challenge for physicians treating these patients.

Current management of the disease is nearly exclusively based on small retrospective series, and in all aspects of management of penile cancer, high quality evidence is lacking. The rare encounter of penile cancer in daily clinical practice combined with limited evidence based recommendations unfortunately frequently results in suboptimal management [2]. Especially in surgical staging of the groin areas, it has been shown that this procedure is largely underused in the community and under-staging and delayed treatment of lymphatic groin metastasis unfortunately directly impact disease related morbidity and mortality [3]. In countries where centralized healthcare is offered, under-staging rates have dropped dramatically resulting in improved survival, while at the same time the adoption of organ-sparing surgical approaches is higher [4]. Centralization however, is not evident everywhere and only few countries and governments have effectively supported and adopted such an approach. In Europe, the European Commission has taken the initiative to develop reference networks for rare diseases, with penile cancer being a topical focus in eUROGEN, the reference network for rare diseases supported and driven by the European Association of Urology (EAU) ©. These networks aim to provide the best care to patients with rare diseases even when reference centers are not in the immediate vicinity.

For localized disease, we have observed over the past two decades a paradigm shift toward the universal adoption of organ-sparing surgery as it has become apparent - although based on retrospective analyses- that excessive wide resection margins in penile cancer are often not needed but rather complete tumor eradication with often only a few millimeters of surgical margins offering excellent oncological outcomes while preserving maximal normal penile tissue [5]. Although patients treated with organ-sparing approaches have higher risks of local recurrence, these do not seem to impact cancer specific survival rates but do preserve the capacity to have sexual intercourse, to void standing upright and when combined with sophisticated reconstructive techniques, the aspect of the penis can be near-normal after surgical amputation of the distal portion of the penis [6–8]. Alternatives such as topical therapies, laser surgery, brachytherapy and external beam radiotherapy have all been explored with encouraging results when carefully selected as potential organ-preserving approaches to the local tumor [9].

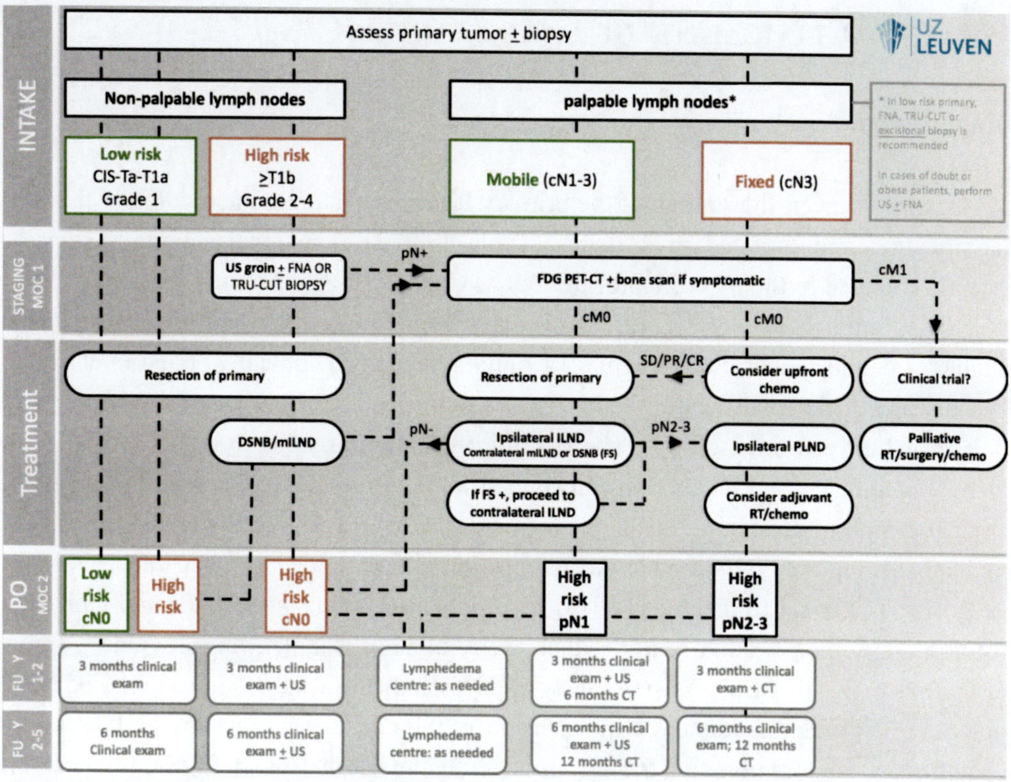

Figure 1. Standardized clinical care pathway for penile cancer at the University Hospitals Leuven, based on the EAU, NCCN and ESMO guidelines [1, 10, 11]. DSNB = dynamic sentinel node biopsy; mILND = modified inguinal lymphadenectomy; PLND = pelvic lymphadenectomy; SD = stable disease; PR = partial response; CR = complete response.

For advanced disease, we have very limited evidence-based options and the responses to chemotherapy and radiotherapy have for the most part been disappointing, and have been characterized by unacceptably high rates of locoregional recurrence and systemic toxicity. The use of adjuvant chemoradiotherapy following inguinal and pelvic lymph node dissection is under heavy debate although there seems to be a subgroup of patients benefitting from this approach but responders today remain difficult to identify upfront.

In our own institute, we have developed a patient pathway for penile cancer patients which can be used to guide decision when encountering a patient presents with a new diagnosis of penile cancer (Figure 1). The care pathway is based on the NCCN (National Comprehensive Cancer Network), EAU (European Association of Urology) and ESMO (European Society of Medical Oncology) guidelines [1, 10, 11]. This chapter aims to provide an overview of the management options of penile cancer per stage, whilst other chapters in this textbook will explore all the options mentioned here in more detail.

Clinical Stage 1 and Stage 2 (CIS-T1-2-3)

Diagnosis and Staging

In penile cancer, the staging of the primary lesion is performed according to the TNM classification and grouped in 4 stages (Table 1 & 2). The local staging system has recently changed in the 8th edition of the AJCC Cancer Staging Manuel for penile cancer, which was published in 2017 [12]. There have been some important adaptations in the staging of penile cancer. For example, T1 tumors have been sub-categorized into T1a and T1b disease. This modification refers to the significant different risk on lymph node metastasis between the 2 groups. The risk for T1a tumors ranges from 10% to 18%, and from 33% to 50% for T1b tumors. This is particularly important in whether to perform a surgical lymph node staging of the groins or not. Perineural invasion (PNI) is a reliable predictor for regional lymph node metastasis, and is been added as a separate criterion to categorize T1a and T1b disease [12, 13]. Lymphovascular invasion (LVI) and high-grade histology are the 2 other criteria that were already adapted in previous editions. Furthermore, T3 disease was previously used to indicate urethral invasion. Today, T2 tumors are classified as tumors with invasion in the corpus spongiosum, and T3 tumors are defined as tumors invading the corpus cavernosum. Both T2 and T3 disease can either or not include involvement of the urethra. These changes signify the prognostically more important level of corporal invasion rather than the urethral invasion.

In staging the primary tumor, it is important to perform an extensive clinical examination which should describe anatomical morphologically extend and invasion of the penile structures. Clinical examination in most cases, especially in experienced hands, can readily identify whether a tumor has invaded in the distal corpora cavernosa or tunica albuginea. When there is a strong clinical suspicion of penile cancer, it is not necessary to perform a biopsy. However, when a non-surgical treatment is planned (i.e., topical therapy, radiotherapy and laser surgery) or there is doubt about the nature of the lesion, it is recommended to take a biopsy of the tumor [1, 9]. It should be noted that there may be intratumoral heterogeneity, which can lead to under-staging of the primary tumor after performing an incisional biopsy.

Magnetic resonance imaging (MRI) with an artificially induced erection after intracavernous injection of prostaglandin E1 or another vasodilatory agent is advised in cases where there is doubt on whether there is corporal or tunical invasion at clinical examination [1, 14]. In those cases, an MRI or alternatively a Doppler ultrasound, can assist in planning the type of local surgery. For example, this can make an important difference in the decision to perform either a glansectomy or a distal partial penectomy.

Table 1. The American Joint Committee on Cancer (AJCC) TNM staging system of penile cancer [12]

TUMOR (T) – Primary tumor	
Tx	The primary tumor cannot be evaluated.
T0	No evidence of primary tumor.
Tis	Carcinoma in situ, which is an early, noninvasive precancerous growth.
T1	The tumor has invaded 1 or more outer layers of the penis. These layers may include the dermis, the lamina propria, the dartos fascia or the subepithelial connective tissue depending on the localization of the tumor. Based on the grade of differentiation of the tumor and whether there is lymphovascular invasion, T1 tumors are divided into 2 substages. T1a: The tumor has not grown into blood vessels, lymph vessels or nerves, and is not poorly differentiated (<G3, see below). T1b: The tumor has grown into blood vessels, lymph vessels or nerves, and/or is poorly differentiated (G3-G4).
T2	The tumor has invaded the corpus spongiosum with or without invasion of the urethra. The corpus spongiosum is an internal chamber of the penis that runs along the bottom and into the head of the penis.
T3	The tumor has invaded the corpus cavernosum with or without invasion of the urethra. Either 1 of 2 internal chambers that run along the top of the shaft of the penis.
T4	The tumor has invaded other adjacent structures such as the pubic bone, the scrotum or the prostate.
NODE (N) – Regional lymph nodes	
Clinical classification	
cNx	The regional lymph nodes cannot be assessed.
cN0	There are no palpable or visibly enlarged inguinal lymph nodes.
cN1	There is a palpable mobile unilateral inguinal lymph node.
cN2	There are palpable mobile multiple or bilateral lymph nodes.
cN3	Fixed inguinal nodal mass or pelvic lymphadenopathy, unilateral or bilateral
Pathological classification	
pNX	The cancer has not spread to the regional lymph nodes.
pN0	The cancer has not spread to the regional lymph nodes.
pN1	The cancer has spread to 1 or 2 unilateral inguinal lymph nodes.
pN2	The cancer has spread to 3 or more inguinal lymph nodes bilateral inguinal lymph node(s) metastasis.
pN3	Extension of the inguinal lymph node metastasis, the cancer has grown into the surrounding tissue and/or the cancer has spread to pelvic lymph node(s).
METASTASIS (M)	
M0	There is no distant metastasis.
M1	Metastasis to parts of the body that not include the penis and the regional lymph nodes.

Table 2. Stage grouping of penile cancer based on AJCC TNM staging system

Cancer stage grouping	
Stage I (T1a, N0, M0)	A low-grade cancer that has grown just below the surface layer of the skin. There is no lymphovascular of perineural invasion, and the tumor is not poorly differentiated. The cancer has not spread to lymph nodes (N0) or to distant parts of the body (M0).
Stage IIA (T1b, T2, N0, M0)	The cancer is high grade or has grown into blood vessels, lymph vessels, or nerves (T1b). Or it has grown into the corpus spongiosum with or without urethral invasion (T2). The cancer has not spread to lymph nodes (N0) or to distant parts of the body (M0).
Stage IIB (T3, N0, M0)	The cancer has grown into the corpus cavernosum with or without urethral invasion. It has not spread to lymph nodes (N0) or distant parts of the body (M0).
Stage IIIA (T1-T3, N1, M0)	The tumor has not grown beyond the penis and urethra. It has spread to 1 to 2 groin lymph nodes on the same side of the body (N1), but not too distant parts of the body (M0).
Stage IIIB (T1-T3, N2, M0)	The tumor has not grown beyond the penis and urethra. It has spread to 3 or more groin lymph nodes (N2). It has not spread outside the groin lymph nodes, to the pelvic lymph nodes, or to distant parts of the body (N3, M0).
Stage IV (T4, any N, M0; any T, N3, M0; any T, any N, M1):	Any of the following: The cancer has grown into nearby tissues such as the pubic bone, the scrotum, or the prostate (T4, any N, M0). The cancer has grown outside of a lymph node and into surrounding tissue, or it has spread to 1 or more pelvic lymph nodes (any T, N3, M0).

Regional Staging

In stage 1 disease, there are no palpable inguinal lymph nodes. However, it is possible that micrometastatic spread has already occurred. It has been shown that nomograms and conventional imaging are unreliable in predicting and detecting lymph node involvement. Therefore, it is very important to perform adequate surgical lymph node staging in selected cases [15, 16]. The NCCN and EAU guidelines discern 3 risk groups, based on the risk of micrometastatic disease. The risk groups are listed below:

- Low risk tumors (Tis, Ta G1-2 or T1 G1), in which there is a very low risk of harboring micrometastatic disease.
- Intermediate risk tumors (T1 G2) in which the risk of harboring micrometastatic disease is 7 to 9% in series with centralized pathological review [17, 18].
- High risk tumors (>T1b or high-grade tumor) in which the risk of harboring micrometastatic disease goes up to 33%. When subdivided by T-stage, T1 high-risk disease harbors a risk of 13%, T2 of 21% and T3 of 33%. The odds ratio of

harboring micrometastatic disease for grade 3 tumors is 4.9 and 2.2 for tumors with LVI [19].

For this reason, both the NCCN and EAU guidelines advocate to carry out surgical lymph node staging in cases of intermediate and high-risk localized penile cancer with non-palpable lymph nodes. If surgical staging doesn't reveal (micro)metastatic disease, it is not necessary to perform further staging using imaging such as PET-CT scan or CT scan [1, 10].

Treatment Options

When encountering a penile cancer patient with a clinical stage T1 of T2 disease, which is localized to the penis, the various treatment options for the localized tumor should be discussed with the patient. According to the EAU guidelines, the aim of treatment of the primary tumor is complete tumor removal with as much organ preservation as possible without compromising oncological control [1]. Practically, this means that tumors eligible for organ-sparing surgery (OSS) would be clinical CIS, cT1, cT2 and cT3.

The principles on which the concept of organ-sparing surgery are based (each detailed further below):

1. The tumor is most commonly diagnosed at the distal aspect of the penis. Most common localization of penile cancer is on the glans, followed by the prepuce. Only about 1/10 tumors are located at least partially on the penile shaft. This makes a large proportion of these local tumors eligible for OSS by amputating only a very distal or very small portion of the distal penis.
2. The margins can be minimal.
3. Local recurrence is more prevalent OS but is does not impact survival.
4. The patient must be compliant to strict follow-up.

Margins

Classical teaching dictated that the surgical margins in penile carcinoma should be at least 20mm or more. However, Hoffman and colleagues showed in 1999 that a tumor free margin of less than 10mm harbored no increased chance for local recurrence [20]. In 2000, Agrawal showed that most lesions have spread less than 5 mm beyond a microscopic margin, and Minhas and colleagues showed in 2005 showed that lesions that were removed with a section margin of less than 10mm resulted in low local recurrence rates [21, 22].

More recently, Philippou and colleagues demonstrated in 2012 that a margin of less than 5mm did not predict for higher rate of local recurrence, and that no patient with involved margins had undergone intraoperative frozen section margins [23]. Therefore, it is important that in OSS, intraoperative frozen section margins are employed to ensure resection of the tumor with minimal but negative surgical margins. In 2018, Sri and colleagues demonstrated that a clear margin of less than 1mm showed an increased risk of local recurrence compared to more than 1mm, with a 5.9 relative risk ratio [5]. These authors also showed that most recurrences had lymphovascular invasion or cavernosal spread, suggesting an embolic mechanism rather than continuous spread is a worthy predictor of local recurrence for penile cancer. These results illustrate that a minimal margin between 1 and 5 mm can be respected, and that this margin should be save in terms of local recurrence risk.

Local Recurrence Does Not Impact Disease Specific Survival

In 2008, Leijte and colleagues demonstrated a disease specific survival of 92% in a group of 109 out of 700 patients in who OSS was performed and experienced local recurrence [24]. Philippou and colleagues showed in 2012 that the cases of local recurrence are amenable to further surgery with no significant impact on the 5-year disease specific survival (91.7%) [23]. Djajadiningrat and colleagues in 2014, and Albersen and colleagues in 2018 both performed a multivariate cox regression analysis for disease specific survival and showed that the local occurrence did not impact disease specific survival in penile cancer patients treated with organ-sparing surgery [7, 25].

Meticulous Follow-Up

Local recurrence is common following OSS. These rates range from 4 to 10% for cold-knife surgical series, and 20 to 30% for series with high percentages of laser surgery (26). Most recurrences (92%) are observed in the first 5 years after OSS [24]. For this reason the EAU and NCCN guidelines recommend visits 3 monthly after OSS in the first 2 years, semi-annually during years 3 to 5 and then yearly till 10 years after surgery [1, 10]. These data signify that patients should be willing to comply with meticulous follow-up following OSS, as the risk of local recurrence might be a little bit higher than with conventional partial penectomy or total penectomy. However, follow-up schedules are rather based on lymphatic status rather than the risk of local recurrence.

Techniques for Organ-Sparing Surgery

Various techniques have been described to treat penile cancers with OSS. For lesions confined to the prepuce, or small lesions located on the base of the glans and/or the corona, *circumcision* either or not in combination with *wide local excision* (WLE) of the tumor can be performed. In case of perimeatal lesions, this may involve distal urethrectomy and meatal reconstruction, with buccal mucosa for example. For circumferential coronal lesions, small lesions on the glans and/or corona which are unsuitable for wide local excision, a *hemi-glansectomy* can be performed [27]. A *glansectomy* can be employed if there are large lesions on the glans and corona in which local excision would leave a non-reconstructible glans, in perimeatal lesions with ingrowth in the glans spongy tissue, and in large glandular T2 lesions and minimal T3 lesions with only tunical corporal involvement. In glansectomy, the glans is completely removed and a neo-glans can be reconstructed on the tips of the corpora cavernosa using a split-thickness skin graft. This results in excellent cosmetic and functional results [28, 29]. For cases of extensive carcinoma in situ, which is either non-responsive to a topical therapy or not amenable for topical therapy and/or circumcision, a *glans resurfacing* can be executed. In this kind of surgery, the skin covering the glans is removed from of the underlying spongy tissue. This tissue of the corpus spongiosum is then covered as is done in the glansectomy technique with a split-thickness skin graft, which is often harvested from the thigh. In cases of large lesions involving the glans and cases with suspicion of distal corporal involvement, a *distal partial penectomy* can be performed. While this is often done in a classical fashion with anastomosis of the urethra do the shaft skin, this can also be done with reconstructive techniques. For example in a technique conceived by Malone, the urethra is centralized and the corporal tips are covered by a skin graft to achieve an esthetical near-normal aspect of the penile glans [30].

Outcomes of Organ-Sparing Surgery

To report on outcome after OSS, there is a difficulty in coming to unified conclusions as there is considerable heterogeneity in terms of techniques in reported series as well as in terms of risk factors (grade, stage).

In large series such as Kamel et al., Baumgarten et al., and Djajadiningrat et al., mixed organ-sparing surgical techniques, including laser therapy, report on local recurrence rates ranging up from 20 to 27.7% [9, 25, 26]. Series reporting mixed "cold-knife" techniques, and in which no patients treated with laser ablation were included (i.e., Philippou et al., Parnham et al., and Sri et al.,), significantly lower local recurrence rates are reported ranging from 4 to 9.3% [5, 23, 29]. On the other hand, in series with glansectomy only, such as Parnham et al., 2017, recurrence rates are slightly higher. This problem probably reflects a patient selection including a higher portion of T2, T3 and grade 3 tumors than in mixed series which employ all techniques including circumcision and wide local excision (WLE) of tumor, and possibly have a higher proportion of lower grade, lower stage tumors and CIS cases. This hypothesis is further supported by the fact that risk factors for local recurrence have been described and these include higher local stage [5, 23], high grade [7, 23], concomitant carcinoma in situ, perineural invasion [7], lymphovascular invasion [23], positive section margins [7, 9] and clear margins lower than 1mm [5]. Protective against local recurrence seems to be the routine adoption of intraoperative frozen section assessment [26], which is therefore advocated.

It is known that overall survival and disease-specific survival in penile cancer are determined by the clinical and pathological lymph node state. Particularly by the number of lymph nodes involved, the presence for extracapsular extension (ENE) and the presence of pelvic lymph node involvement. Overall survival is not determined by the choice of surgery or by local recurrence. In large population based series, it has been shown that OSS results in similar overall survival data as partial penectomy. This is probably partially due to patient selection in which lower stages are selected for OSS in the population, but it also reflects the fact that local recurrence after OSS does not impact overall survival significantly [26].

Alternatives for Organ-Sparing Surgery

Non-surgical treatment modalities (i.e., topical therapy, laser ablation and radiotherapy) can be used for tumors with low risk for metastasis. These consist of Tis, Ta, and select T1 tumors [9].

Topical Therapy

When a patient is encountered with carcinoma in situ, aside from surgical options such as glans resurfacing, topical therapies can alternatively be employed. For this goal, 5-fluorouracil (5-FU) and Imiquimod have been retrospectively investigated. 5-FU blocks the action of thymidylate synthase, and should be applied twice daily for 4 to 6 weeks. The largest series are retrospective and report complete response of 57%, partial response of 13.6% and a non-response rate of 29.5%. Local toxicity and adverse event occur in 10 to 12% of cases [31]. Imiquimod activates the adaptive immune system via activation of Toll-like receptor 7. It should be applied 3 times a week for a total treatment duration of 12 weeks, although there is no clear data on optimal treatment protocols. A pooled review on in total 48 cases revealed a complete response rate of 62.5%, partial response of 13.6% and a non-response rate of 29% [32]. These numbers are comparable for Imiquimod and 5-FU. Imiquimod is further characterized by local toxicity, where skin irritation may be important and can be outspoken. Important to realize is, that an insufficient response to topical therapy may signify underlying invasive disease (20%). In those cases, surgery is needed and topical re-treatment should not be recommended.

Radiotherapy

The rationale for using radiotherapy for penile cancer is that most other squamous cell carcinoma primary sites (i.e., anal, uterine cervix, head and neck and esophagus) and their involved nodal basins are highly radiosensitive. Nevertheless, radiotherapy is applied rather infrequently for the treatment of penile cancer. It is only used in about 1.5% of the T1 lesions, and the main purpose is local control [33]. Both brachytherapy and external beam radiotherapy (EBRT) have been employed for the treatment of penile cancer. For brachytherapy, an amputation-free survival of about 73% at 8 to 10 years has been noted, with a 5-years local control rate of 81% between 5 and 10 years [34]. This treatment option is characterized by necrosis rates of 0 to 26%, and meatal stenosis rates of 9 to 45%. EBRT is associated with inferior efficacy, the 5-years amputation-free survival rate is about 43% and local control rates amounts to 62% at 5 years out. Necrosis has been observed in 1 to 3% of the cases and meatal stenosis in 7 to 28% of cases [34]. In our opinion, the disadvantage of employing radiotherapy for local control is that incisional biopsy should be carried out, and that a circumcision should be performed to prevent the occurrence of paraphimosis. An incisional biopsy may lead to understaging of the local tumor, which can lead to understaging of the regional lymph nodes. Furthermore, local follow-up can be difficult due to scarring and aberrant aspect of the glans after radiotherapy.

Laser

The concept of laser therapy of penile tumors is that it treats tumor with minimal morbidity and cosmetically acceptable outcomes. Most reports have been on lower stage lesions (CIS, T1, T2), with an extension not deeper than 2 to 2.5 mm. However, some series have used neo-adjuvant chemotherapy to downstage the bigger local tumors and this seems to be a feasible approach [35]. Laser therapy consists of laser dissection and/or laser ablation. Laser dissection often is done with a carbon dioxide (CO_2) laser, which provides limited thermal damage to surrounding tissue. Photocoagulation can be performed with a neodymium:yttrium-aluminium-garnet (Nd:YAG) laser, when a 3-10mm tissue penetration depth is more suitable [1, 35]. High local recurrence rates have been reported ranging from 10 to 26%, and in certain cases even 43% [1, 36]. A recent multi-center study further showed that the treatment of carcinoma in situ with laser therapy can result in 58.3% local recurrence rate [37]. And as for topical therapy and radiotherapy, incisional biopsies should to be taken before commencement of laser ablation which has an inherent risk of understaging. Furthermore, series of OSS including laser surgery display higher local recurrence rates than series in which local surgery is reported as pure surgical series without the employment of laser therapy [38].

Quality of Life Sexuality and Urinary Function Following Organ-Sparing Surgery for Penile Cancer

It has been shown that partial and total penectomy have profound effect on sexual function, urinary function, overall well-being and masculinity [8, 39]. Urinary function is often damaged after OSS. Meatal stenosis and spraying are common adverse events of all organ-sparing surgical techniques, but voiding standing up can often be preserved. In terms of esthetic appearance, it has been demonstrated that neo-glans reconstruction results in esthetically satisfying glans cosmesis [40]. This is the case for glansectomy, glans resurfacing as well as for distal partial penectomy in which a skin graft is employed to create a neo-glans. Surgery for penile cancer causes distress in a significant number of patients. Dräger and colleagues have published a narrative systematic review on 309 patients on the psychosocial aspects of penile cancer surgery [41]. They have shown that, compared to conventional techniques such as partial penectomy and total penectomy, organ-sparing interventions have a positive impact on Quality of Life and sexual function. Furthermore, it has been shown by Yang and colleagues in 135 cases that glans preservation results in a better performance in 4 of the 5 domains of the International Index of Erectile Dysfunction (Erectile Function, Orgasmic Function, Intercourse Satisfaction and Overall Satisfaction) [42]. They demonstrated a better tip rigidity at rigiscan measurements as well. There was a higher appearance satisfaction in cases where the glans could at least partially be preserved. Intercourse acceptability in both patients and partners was better when the glans could be preserved versus partial and total penectomy cases.

Regional Staging in Stage 1 and Stage 2 Disease

In clinically lymph node negative intermediate and high-risk local disease, as illustrated above, surgical staging is very important as these patients have a high risk of harboring micrometastatic disease. We know that CT or PET-CT scan are unreliable to detect inguinal basin micrometastases. Therefore, the EAU and NCCN guidelines illustrate that staging using imaging techniques is not needed if surgical staging is negative [1, 10]. The importance of immediate surgical staging is demonstrated by a series in which Kroon and colleagues report that immediate resection of occult lymph node positive disease results in 3 year disease specific survival of 84%, which drops down to 35% when inguinal lymph node dissection is performed at the moment that nodes become palpable [43]. However, due to the initial fear of staging-related morbidity, the use of surgical staging in this phase of the disease is underused, even in academic and referral hospitals [3]. There has been shown that centralization of care for penile cancer results in higher numbers of surgical staging in clinical node negative high-risk disease

[44]. This is an argument that a rare disease such as penile cancer may be considered an excellent candidate for centralized healthcare, as we know that both treatment becomes less invasive and staging becomes more accurate.

In the United States (US), modified inguinal lymph node dissection (mILND) is often the staging examination of choice. It was initially described by Catalona in 1988 [45]. The procedure employs a shorter incision (about 6 to 8 cm) compared to radical inguinal lymphadenectomy, and preserves the vena saphena magna and the area lateral to the arteria femoralis. Frozen section examination of the resected lymph nodes should be carried out to determine rather a radical inguinal lymph nodes dissection should be done in the same setting. This surgery is burden by a false negative rate of 0 to 5.5% and a complication rate of 10 to 36%, in which lymphedema and lymphocele are the most prevalent complications [46]. To overcome these complications of regional lymph node staging, Cabanas described in 1977 for the first time the use of the dynamic sentinel node biopsy (DSNB) procedure in penile cancer [47]. This technique was further optimized by Watkin in London and Horenblas in Amsterdam. In a series described by Lam and colleagues, the technical sensitivity per inguinal basin of DSNB was 92%, and the clinical sensitivity per patient was 91% [48]. Complication rates were much lower than conventional mILND with lymphocoele in about 3.4% and lymphedema in 0.8% of cases. When ultrasound screening of the groins is added to DSNB, the technical sensitivity of the combined biopsy approach is about 95%. Again, it should be mentioned that the low false negative numbers observed after DSNB combined with ultrasound of the groins is only observed in series that have been reporting on outcomes in centralized healthcare systems. In a recent systematic review the pooled sensitivity of DSNB was 88% [49]. When the use of patent blue was employed, the pooled sensitivity was 90% (15). DSNB has not been universally adopted in the US, but it has been adopted in the high-volume centers in Europe. Nonetheless, surgeons should perform at least about 20 DSNB cases with acceptable results before abandoning routine lymph node dissection [50]. It should be noted however, that the last statement is derived from data in breast cancer surgery, and no such data are available for penile cancer.

Clinical Stage 3: Inguinal Lymph Node Metastasis without Extracapsular Extension (N1-N2)

Diagnosis and Staging

Clinically palpable inguinal lymph nodes in a patient with penile cancer are highly suggestive of lymph node metastases. The idea that those lymph nodes may be inflammatory and that antibiotics should be prescribed to assess responses before performing further staging, has been abandoned and will delay correct treatment in a large majority of cases [1]. Physical examination should include the number of palpable lymph nodes on each side, and whether these are fixed or mobile. Additional imaging in cN1/cN2 cases should be done by CT scan or ^{18}FDG-PET/CT scan before embarking on surgical staging to rule out pelvic and distant metastasis and avoid potentially unnecessary surgery [1].

Prospective studies, although involving a small number of patients, have shown high sensitivity (88-100%) and specificity (98-100%) for detecting metastatic lymph nodes in cases with palpable lymph nodes using positron emission tomography (PET) combined with CT scan [51, 52]. Nonetheless, current data does not support a role for PET/CT as a diagnostic procedure in cases with impalpable lymph nodes [1]. Leijte and colleagues showed metastatic deposits of less than 10 mm could not be detected [53]. Furthermore, Dräger et al., showed in a group of 41 patients that PET-CT cannot replace invasive nodal staging due its limited sensitivity and specificity [54]. Compared with CT scan, PET-CT provides more precise inguinal lymph node assessment [52, 55].

Treatment Options

Radical Inguinal Lymphadenectomy (rILND)

For patients with metastatic disease in the groin, the lymph nodes should be surgically removed, ideally following confirmation by fine needle aspiration or trough-cut biopsy. Radical inguinal lymphadenectomy (rILND) remains the keystone of the treatment [1, 10]. In cases with 1 or 2 metastatic inguinal lymph nodes, rILND is curative in approximately 80% [56].

In rILND, an incision is made a few cm below and parallel to the inguinal ligament. The external oblique, the external inguinal ring, the spermatic cord and the inferior border of the inguinal ligament are exposed. The long saphenous vein can be revealed at the apex of the femoral triangle. This femoral triangle is bordered by the anterior superior iliac spine and pubic tubercle superiorly, the medial border of the sartorius laterally, and the lateral border of the adductor longus medially. In patients with minimal metastatic disease, it can be possible to preserve the saphenous vein in an attempt to minimize lower extremity lymphedema. A complete femoral triangle dissection is carried out. The preservation or resection of the fascia lata is a matter of debate.

Due the impaired lymph drainage from the legs and scrotum, morbidity can be as high as 50% after rILND [57]. The most common issues reported are lymphedema (5-13.9%), lymphocele formation (2.1-4%), wound infections (1.2-1.4%) and skin flap necrosis (0.6-4.7%) [58, 59]. Therefore, closed suction drains are placed to prevent seroma and lymphocele formation. Lymphatic vessels should be ligated, since these vessels do not contain smooth muscle and are therefore not reliable closed by electrocautery. As an alternative to open surgery and in an attempt to minimize complications, minimally-invasive techniques have been described which include video-endoscopic inguinal lymphadenectomy (VEIL) and robotic assisted video-endoscopic inguinal lymphadenectomy (RAVEIL). Kumar et al., showed in a prospective study of 42 patients that the wound complication rate was significantly lower compared to open rILND (6% vs 68%) [60]. Lymphocele rates were similar in both groups [60]. Matin and colleagues demonstrated in a phase 1 study that RAVEIL allowed adequate dissection in 18 of 19 inguinal fields [61]. If adequate oncological control and lower morbidity can indeed be confirmed, these techniques may become a standard treatment option for patients requiring inguinal lymph node dissection.

Pelvic Lymphadenectomy (PLND)

Lughezzani and colleagues showed in 2014 that the rates of positive pelvic nodes were 23% in cases with more than 2 positive inguinal nodes, and 56% in those with more than 3 positive inguinal nodes or extracapsular extension [62]. Therefore, the guidelines recommend to carry out pelvic lymph node dissection in all patients with more than two unilateral metastatic inguinal lymph nodes, bilateral positive inguinal lymph nodes, or in the presence of extracapsular lymph node extension [1]. Pelvic lymph node dissection should be only carried out at the inguinally affected side in unilateral regional metastatic disease.

PLND can be performed either by a lower abdominal midline incision or a unilateral muscle splitting incision. For bilateral PLND, it can be carried out through a midline suprapubic extraperitoneal incision. The borders of PLND are defined by the iliac bifurcation proximally, the ilioinguinal nerve laterally and the obturator nerve medially. An excision of the obturator, internal and extern iliac nodes should be performed, and the clinically positive nodes outside these confined regions should be resected as well. PLND may be performed simultaneously with rILND or as a separate procedure, although it is important to avoid delay if these procedures are indicated [63]. Robotic-assisted PLND is a common procedure in prostate and bladder cancer, and is widely employed for staging purposes in penile cancers as well. A direct comparison with open surgery has however not been made, so no conclusions can be made on superiority of either technique.

Due to the small patient population with advanced disease, there is a lack of data on the outcome of patients who underwent PLND. A survival benefit of prophylactic PLND in absence of macrometastasis has never been demonstrated. Nelson and colleagues demonstrated in a study of 40 patients an overall complication rate of 45% [64]. Most commonly occurring complication was lymphedema, which was mild to moderate in nature. Other complications are lymphocele, wound infection, wound dehiscence and flap necrosis.

Adjuvant Therapy

In penile cancer patients with a low metastatic burden, a cure can be achieved without adjuvant therapies chemotherapy and radiotherapy (see above). In more advanced cases, combined modality therapy could potentially provide benefit in terms of local control and survival. However, as the disease is rare and randomized data are lacking, the use of adjuvant therapy is subject of ongoing debate at the time of writing this chapter.

There is a paucity of clinical data on chemotherapy, and there are no prospective studies on adjuvant chemotherapy (AC). Based on retrospective data, the current EAU guidelines recommend adjuvant chemotherapy after lymphadenectomy in patients with pN2/pN3 disease [1]. Furthermore, the optimal timing for chemotherapy and radiotherapy in relation to LND remains conflicting [65]. In a retrospective study, Pizzocaro et al., demonstrated a long-term disease-free (DFS) survival of 84% in node-positive patients treated with AC, compared with 39% in cases without AC [66]. The patients were treated with vincristine, bleomycin and methotrexate (VBM). More recently in 2015, Sharma and colleagues showed in a study of 84 patients that adjuvant chemotherapy is associated with improved overall survival in cases with positive pelvic lymph nodes [67]. In another study by the Milan Cancer Institute, 52% of the patients treated with T-PF chemotherapy (i.e., taxane, cisplatin, and 5-FU) were still disease-free after a median follow up of 22 months, this difference in a small cohort however, could not reach statistical significance [68]. EAU guidelines state that adjuvant inguinal radiotherapy (AIRT) is not recommended outside of clinical studies [1]. In a recent systematic review regarding AIRT -selected studies including a total of 1605 men- this recommendation was confirmed [69]. However, in a recent retrospective study of 93 patients in 2018, Johnstone and colleagues demonstrated that ARIT had a significant impact on disease-specific survival [70]. This appeared to be limited to those with inguinal lymph nodes with extranodal extension. The latter study proposes that AIRT may have a role in advanced cases and these data combined may shift the debate back in the direction of the application of AIRT for certain subgroups. In our centre, we have multidisciplinary agreed on offering patients with inguinal nodes with extracapsular extension and pelvic disease adjuvant radiation therapy with the use of a radiosensitizer (cisplatinum). This is a deviation of EAU guidelines but it is supported by NCCN guidelines and we feel a subset of patients may indeed benefit from this strategy.

Vulvar squamous cell carcinoma (vSCC) has many parallels to penile carcinoma. Both diseases have similar anatomy, histology and risk factors, so it is believed that the evidence available in vulvar cancers offers valuable lessons to improve the management of penile cancer [71]. Compared to penile cancer, the level of evidence in vSCC seems to be more robust. Regarding adjuvant therapy, the efficacy of adjuvant radiation and chemotherapy has been tested in controlled trials and meta-analyses. The Gynecologic Oncology Group (GOG) enrolled 114 patients with groin node-positive vSCC [72].

Patients were randomly allocated to postoperative radiation or to ipsilateral pelvic node resection after radical vulvectomy and ILND. The cancer related death rate was significantly higher for PLND only compared with PLND+radiation (51% vs 29%). In another RCT, GOG found that preoperative chemoradiation for advanced VC for advanced VC could reduce the need for more radical surgery including pelvic exenteration [73].

The prospective worldwide study InPACT (International Penile Advance Cancer Trial) is currently ongoing. Patients with inguinal lymph node metastases are allocated to one of three initial treatments: standard surgery (ILND), neoadjuvant chemotherapy followed by ILND or chemoradiotherapy followed by ILND. Until results from InPACT are available, clinical recommendations may be, as illustrated above, extrapolated from other SCC sites such as vulvar/anal/cervical cancer. The data of these other anogenital malignancies would support the combination of radiation therapy and concurrent cisplatinum for definitive treatment or for surgical down-staging.

Stage 4: Locally Advanced Tumors, Advanced Regional Lymph Node Metastasis and Distant Metastasis (T4, N3, M1)

Diagnosis and Staging

In lymph nodes positive cases, EAU guidelines recommend to perform systemic staging using CT or PET-CT [1]. A bone scan should be obtained in patients with systematic disease and with relevant bone-related symptoms.

To evaluate the diagnostic accuracy of FDG-PET/CT, Graafland et al. showed in a study of 18 patients with proven inguinal metastasis that PET/CT scanning appears to be promising for detecting pelvic lymph nodes metastases [74]. Analysis revealed a sensitivity of 91% and a specificity of 100%. The diagnostic accuracy amounted to 96%. Furthermore, 5 patients were diagnosed with distant metastasis. Four of the cases were confirmed either CT or histopathology. In another study, Zhang and colleagues demonstrated a good sensitivity (85%) and specificity (86%) of FDG-PET/CT in the detection of metastatic disease in patients with advanced penile cancer [55, 75]

This data suggest that PET/CT is useful for accurate M-staging, which can be crucial for decision making. When distant metastases are found in patients, this changes their treatment to systemic or palliative regimens.

Treatment Options

Neoadjuvant Chemotherapy

In patients with bulky or fixed inguinal lymph nodes, presurgical systemic therapy is currently recommended [1]. If the patient responds to this therapy, this may technically facilitate radical lymphadenectomy and improve completeness of the resection.

A retrospective study in the Netherlands suggested that neoadjuvant chemotherapy is a valuable option for patients with irresectable primary penile cancer [76]. They demonstrated an objective tumor response in 12 out of 19 patients, of which 8 patients were long-term survivors (5 years). In multicenter analysis, Necchi summarized the results for men who underwent perioperative chemotherapy and lymphadenectomy. [77] This study demonstrated a moderate activity after chemotherapy. However, the combination chemotherapy was associated with a 2-yr overall survival of only +- 36%.

In a prospective phase 2 trial published in 2010, thirty patients with bulky adenopathies received neoadjuvant paclitaxel, ifosfamide and cisplatin chemotherapy [78]. Fifteen patients experienced an objective response, and 22 underwent surgery afterwards. Improved overall survival was significantly associated with a response to chemotherapy. The estimated time to progression (TTP) was 8.1 months, and the median OS was 17.1 months. Furthermore, absence of bilateral residual tumor, absence of extranodal extension and skin involvement had a significant impact on OS. Another phase 2 study in the UK of 2013 investigated the impact of the combination of docetaxel, cisplatin and 5FU (TPF) in patients with locally advanced or metastatic penile carcinoma [79]. Although in 10 of the 26 cases an objective response was achieved, in 19 patients (65.5%) grade 3-4 adverse advents were reported. They concluded that, based on the significant toxicity, this combination should not be recommended. Djajadiningrat and colleagues confirmed that TPF was poorly tolerated in a retrospective study in 2015 [80]. Despite good response percentage, survival rates were disappointed as well. They suggested that other treatment options should be considered. In conclusion, upfront cisplatin-based chemotherapy should be considered in patients with fixed inguinal lymphadenopathy. Treatment of choice is a cisplatin- and taxane based triple combination. Nevertheless, there is substantial need for additional data on combined treatment approaches in penile cancer.

Palliative Chemotherapy

The combination of cisplatin and irinotecan was assessed in a prospective phase 2 trial by the European Organisation for the Research and Treatment of Cancer (EORTC) in 2008, including 26 eligible patients [81]. Overall response rate was only 30.8%, survival estimates were not available. A more recent second phase 2 study of docetaxel, cisplatin and fluoracil displayed moderate responses (38,5%, 15 out of 39 patients) in M1 cases [82]. Overall survival was only 7 months in this patient group. In a retrospective study of 25 M+ patients treated with 5-FU and cisplatin, the overall response rate was 32% with an OS of 8 months [83]. A study of 1989 showed a modest activity of cisplatin alone [84]. There were 4 partial responses out of 26 patients, median survival was only 4.7 months. Another study including 140 patients receiving systemic therapy, displayed that visceral metastases and ECOG PS ≥ 1 were poor prognostic factors [85]. Cisplatin-based regimens had better outcomes than non-cisplatin-based. There are basically no data on second-line chemotherapy in penile cancer. In conclusion, triplet systemic chemotherapy including taxane and cisplatin are recommended. Prolongation of survival can be achieved. Nevertheless, the median survival with these regimens is approximately in the 8- to 9-month range and the treatment-related toxicity is high. The potential benefit should be weighed against the remaining quality of life.

New Horizons

Given the poor outcomes and toxicities of currently used therapies for patients with advanced disease, novel treatments are desperately needed.

Anti-epidermal growth factor receptor (EGFR) targeted therapies have been used as second-line treatment in refractory cases. Research demonstrated an over-expression of EGFR in the majority of penile cancer [86, 87]. Panitumumab, an anti-EGFR monoclonal antibody, showed to be active and safe in highly pretreated cases of penile cancer. However, this seemed to be without long-term response [88]. Dacomitinib is an irreversible, pan-epidermal growth factor receptor (HER) inhibitor. A recently published phase 2 study of Necchi and colleagues included 28 patients with advanced PSCC treated with dacomitinib [89]. An overall response rate of 32.1% and a 1-year OS of 54.9% was observed. They observed that dacomitinib was active and well tolerated. The authors highlighted the importance patient selection for such targeted compounds, based on the downstream effector of EGFR signaling.

Hopefully, penile cancer will benefit from the advent of immunotherapy in genitourinary oncology. Immune checkpoint inhibition of the PD-1/PD-L1 pathway could play an important role in penile cancer. Several studies reported the expression of PD-L1 in PSCC [90, 91]. Additionally, PD-L1 expression was positively correlated with lymph node metastasis and decreased CSS. An interesting ongoing phase 1 trial demonstrated objectives responses of the combination of cabozantinib and nivolumab in squamous cell genitourinary tumors, including penile cancer [92]. Cabo-Nivo seems to be well tolerated with no dose-limiting toxicity. Another ongoing phase 2 trial investigates the use of pembrolizumab for advanced PSCC following failure of chemotherapy.

Penile cancer is an oncological field of enquiry that is nearly completely devoid of basic and translational research into the mechanisms of the disease, and the mechanisms of resistance against current therapies. Animal models including nude mice with patient-derived xenografts as well as primary cell lines can aid in increasing our understanding of the disease and in the development of new therapies. The European Association of

Urology Research Foundation and eUROGEN are currently co-working on developing those research lines in Europe and hopes are high that these endeavours will ultimately lead to improved therapy for advanced and metastatic penile cancer, for which we contemporarily have no highly effective therapeutic options to resort to.

CENTRALIZATION OF CARE

Penile cancer is a rare and complex disease. Recent advances in surgical management of the primary tumor and dynamic sentinel node biopsy may improve survival and limit morbidity in the future. Since the disease is uncommon in Western societies, it is often managed in a community where required specific expertise may be lacking. The low operative volume and limited training may prevent adoption of these techniques in clinical practice. This is displayed in an observational study by Woldu et al., in 2018, which investigated 1,689 men diagnosed with intermediate to high risk clinically localized PSCC in the US [3]. They showed that only 25.3% of the patients underwent surgical lymph node staging, which is recommended by the guidelines. Furthermore, surgical staging seemed to be an independent predictor of overall mortality. Particularly the nonacademic institutions were less likely to adhere the recommendations for surgical lymph node staging. Linked with this data, Cindolo and colleagues demonstrated that guidelines adherence was associated with improved overall survival [93].

The rarity of the disease has resulted in nonuniform management despite the presence of treatment guidelines. Unstandardized care leads to over- or undertreatment, which can have significant functional, psychological and oncologic outcomes. The expected benefits of centralization, providing specialized multidisciplinary teams, are improved patient care with more appropriate management, and better subsequent outcomes. In the UK, penile cancer was centralized in 2002 based on the National Institute of Health and Care Excellence (NICE) guidelines [94]. Specialist services at a supra-network were set up, with the expectation of managing at least 25 new penile cancer cases per year. Bayles and colleagues showed that centralization in the UK results in improved outcomes both in terms of organ preservation and improved survival [4]. In case of histopathology, Tang et al., displayed that centralization has increased exposure to penile cancer and thereby increased diagnostic accuracy [95]. Governments and health care providers should therefore be encouraged to follow the lead of the UK, and other regions such as Scandinavia and The Netherlands and centralize healthcare for rare tumors such as penile squamous cell carcinoma.

Conclusion

Penile cancer is a rare but devastating disease. Clinical trial evidence on which to base treatment decisions is limited. This chapter aimed to overview the management options for the different stages of penile cancer, and highlight where we are currently failing to adequately tackle this malignancy. We refer the reader to dedicated chapters in this volume to gain a more detailed insight in the various aspects of penile cancer diagnosis, staging, and management.

Key Points

- Penile cancer remains is a rare disease, which makes it a diagnostic and therapeutic challenge for physicians. Recommendations are mainly based on retrospective data, and the rare encounter frequently results in suboptimal management.
- Organ-sparing techniques should be used for low-stage penile cancer whenever possible, as margins of a few millimeters suffice for adequate local cancer control and local recurrence does not impact survival. These techniques allow better cosmetic and functional results.
- The management the lymph nodes in penile cancer is crucial for prognosis. Even if there are no palpable lymph nodes, it is possible that micrometastatic disease has already occurred. For this reason, surgical lymph node staging should be carried out in cases of intermediate and high-risk localized penile cancer without palpable lymph nodes.
- In patients with inguinal lymph node metastasis, radical inguinal lymphadenectomy remains the keystone of the treatment. A pelvic lymph node dissection should be performed in patients with more than two metastatic inguinal lymph nodes, bilateral positive lymph nodes, or in the presence of extracapsular lymph node extension.
- The use of adjuvant chemotherapy is recommended in pN2/pN3 disease. Although adjuvant inguinal radiotherapy is currently only advised in clinical studies, recent data propose that ARIT could have a significant impact on disease-specific survival in cases with positive inguinal lymph nodes with extranodal extension.
- Upfront cisplatin-based chemotherapy should be considered in patients with fixed inguinal lymphadenopathy. In cases that respond, complete surgical treatment is possible.

- EGFR targeted therapies and immunotherapy are proposed second-line treatment modalities in advanced penile cancer. The role of these therapies should be further determined in the future.
- Centralization of penile cancer with providing specialized multidisciplinary teams should improve patient care with more appropriate management, and better subsequent outcomes.

REFERENCES

[1] Hakenberg OW, Compérat EM, Minhas S, Necchi A, Protzel C, Watkin N. EAU guidelines on penile cancer: 2014 update. *European Urology*. 2015;67(1):142–50.

[2] Cindolo L, Bada M, Varga J, Nyirady P, Battaglia M, Boccasile S, et al., The adherence to the eau guidelines on penile cancer treatment could influence the survival: Multicenter, retrospective, european study. *Journal of Urology*. 2017;197(4):976.

[3] Woldu SL, Ci B, Hutchinson RC, Krabbe L-M, Singla N, Passoni NM, et al., Usage and survival implications of surgical staging of inguinal lymph nodes in intermediate- to high-risk, clinical localized penile cancer: A propensity-score matched analysis. Urologic Oncology: *Seminars and Original Investigations*. 2018;36(4):159.e7-159.e17.

[4] Bayles AC, Sethia KK. The impact of Improving Outcomes Guidance on the management and outcomes of patients with carcinoma of the penis. *The Annals of The Royal College of Surgeons of England*. 2010;92(1):44–5.

[5] Sri D, Sujenthiran A, Lam W, Minter J, Tinwell BE, Corbishley CM, et al., A study into the association between local recurrence rates and surgical resection margins in organ-sparing surgery for penile squamous cell cancer. *BJU International*. 2018;122(4):576–82.

[6] Djajadiningrat RS, van Werkhoven E, Meinhardt W, van Rhijn BWG, Bex A, van der Poel HG, et al., Penile Sparing Surgery for Penile Cancer—Does it Affect Survival? *The Journal of Urology*. 2014;192(1):120–6.

[7] Albersen M, Parnham A, Joniau S, Sahdev V, Christodoulidou M, Castiglione F, et al., Predictive factors for local recurrence after glansectomy and neoglans reconstruction for penile squamous cell carcinoma. *Urologic Oncology*. 2018;36(4):141–6.

[8] Sosnowski R, Kuligowski M, Kuczkiewicz O, Moskal K, Wolski JK, Bjurlin MA, et al., Primary penile cancer organ sparing treatment. *Central European journal of urology*. 2016;69(4):377–83.

[9] Baumgarten AS, Fisher JS, Lawindy SM, Pavlinec JG, Carrion RE, Spiess PE. Penile sparing surgical approaches for primary penile tumors : preserving function and appearance. *Transl Androl Urol*. 2017;6(5):809–19.

[10] Clark PE, Spiess PE, Agarwal N, Biagioli MC, Eisenberger MA, Greenberg RE, et al., Penile cancer: Clinical Practice Guidelines in Oncology. Journal of the National Comprehensive Cancer Network : *JNCCN*. 2013;11(5):594–615.

[11] Van Poppel H, Watkin NA, Osanto S, Moonen L, Horwich A, Kataja V, et al., Penile cancer: ESMO Clinical Practice Guidelines for diagnosis, treatment and follow-up. *Annals of Oncology*. 2013;24(suppl 6):vi115-vi124.

[12] American Joint Committee on Cancers. Penis. In: AJCC Cancer Staging Manual. 8th ed. New York, NY. Springer. 2017;701–14.

[13] Zhou X, Qi F, Zhou R, Wang S, Wang Y, Wang Y, et al., The role of perineural invasion in penile cancer: a meta-analysis and systematic review. *Bioscience reports*. 2018;38(5).

[14] Kayes O, Minhas S, Allen C, Hare C, Freeman A, Ralph D. The Role of Magnetic Resonance Imaging in the Local Staging of Penile Cancer. *European Urology*. 2007;51(5):1313–9.

[15] O'Brien JS, Perera M, Manning T, Bozin M, Cabarkapa S, Chen E, et al., Penile Cancer: Contemporary Lymph Node Management. *Journal of Urology*. 2017;197(6):1387–95.

[16] Hughes B, Leijte J, Shabbir M, Watkin N, Horenblas S. Non-invasive and minimally invasive staging of regional lymph nodes in penile cancer. *World Journal of Urology*. 2009;27(2):197–203.

[17] Hughes BE, Leijte JAP, Kroon BK, Shabbir MA, Swallow TW, Heenan SD, et al., Lymph Node Metastasis in Intermediate-Risk Penile Squamous Cell Cancer: A Two-Centre Experience. *European Urology*. 2010;57(4):688–92.

[18] Kirrander P, Andrén O, Windahl T. Dynamic sentinel node biopsy in penile cancer: initial experiences at a Swedish referral centre. *BJU International*. 2013;111(3b): E48–53.

[19] Graafland NM, Lam W, Leijte JAP, Yap T, Gallee MPW, Corbishley C, et al., Prognostic Factors for Occult Inguinal Lymph Node Involvement in Penile Carcinoma and Assessment of the High-Risk EAU Subgroup: A Two-Institution Analysis of 342 Clinically Node-Negative Patients. *European Urology*. 2010;58(5): 742–7.

[20] Hoffman MA, Renshaw AA, Loughlin KR. Squamous cell carcinoma of the penis and microscopic pathologic margins: how much margin is needed for local cure? *Cancer*. 1999;85(7):1565–8.

[21] Agrawal A, Pai D, Ananthakrishnan N, Smile SR, Ratnakar C. The histological extent of the local spread of carcinoma of the penis and its therapeutic implications. *BJU International*. 2000;85(3):299–301.

[22] Minhas S, Kayes O, Hegarty P, Kumar P, Freeman A, Ralph D. What surgical resection margins are required to achieve oncological control in men with primary penile cancer? *BJU International.* 2005;96(7):1040–3.

[23] Philippou P, Shabbir M, Malone P, Nigam R, Muneer A, Ralph DJ, et al., Conservative Surgery for Squamous Cell Carcinoma of the Penis: Resection Margins and Long-Term Oncological Control. *The Journal of Urology.* 2012; 188(3):803–8.

[24] Leijte JAP, Kirrander P, Antonini N, Windahl T, Horenblas S. Recurrence Patterns of Squamous Cell Carcinoma of the Penis: Recommendations for Follow-Up Based on a Two-Centre Analysis of 700 Patients. *European Urology.* 2008;54(1):161–9.

[25] Djajadiningrat RS, van Werkhoven E, Meinhardt W, van Rhijn BWG, Bex A, van der Poel HG, et al., Penile Sparing Surgery for Penile Cancer—Does it Affect Survival? *The Journal of Urology*. 2014;192(1):120–6.

[26] Kamel MH, Bissada N, Warford R, Farias J, Davis R. Organ Sparing Surgery for Penile Cancer: A Systematic Review. *The Journal of Urology*. 2017;198(4):770–9.

[27] Burnett AL. Penile preserving and reconstructive surgery in the management of penile cancer. *Nature Reviews Urology*. 2016;13(5):249–57.

[28] Bracka A. Glans resection and plastic repair. *BJU International*. 2010;105(1):136–144.

[29] Parnham AS, Albersen M, Sahdev V, Christodoulidou M, Nigam R, Malone P, et al., Glansectomy and Split-thickness Skin Graft for Penile Cancer. *European urology.* 2018;73(2):284–9.

[30] Kranz J, Parnham A, Albersen M, Sahdev V, Ziada M, Nigam R, et al., Zentralisierung der Harnröhre und Pseudoglansbildung nach partieller Penektomie. *Der Urologe.* 2017;56(10):1293–7. [Centralization of the urethra and pseudo-glans formation after partial penectomy. The Urologist. 2017;56(10):1293-7].

[31] Alnajjar HM, Lam W, Bolgeri M, Rees RW, Perry MJA, Watkin NA. Treatment of Carcinoma In Situ of the Glans Penis with Topical Chemotherapy Agents. *European urology.* 2012;62:923–8.

[32] Deen K, Burdon-Jones D. Imiquimod in the treatment of penile intraepithelial neoplasia: An update. *Australasian Journal of Dermatology.* 2017;58(2):86–92.

[33] Burt LM, Shrieve DC, Tward JD. Stage Presentation, Care Patterns, and Treatment Outcomes for Squamous Cell Carcinoma of the Penis. *Radiation Oncology Biology.* 2014;88(1):94–100.

[34] Tward J. The case for nonsurgical therapy of nonmetastatic penile cancer. *Nature Reviews Urology*. 2018;15(9):574-584

[35] Bandieramonte G, Colecchia M, Mariani L, Lo S, Pizzocaro G, Piva L, et al., Peniscopically Controlled CO_2 Laser Excision for Conservative Treatment of In Situ and T1 Penile Carcinoma : Report on 224 Patients. *European urolgoy.* 2008;54:875–84.

[36] Tang DH, D M, Yan S, D M, Ottenhof SR, D M, et al., Laser ablation as monotherapy for penile squamous cell carcinoma : A multi-center cohort analysis. *Urologic Oncology*. 2018;36(4):147-152

[37] Chipollini J, Yan S, Ottenhof SR, Zhu Y, Baumgarten AS, Tang DH, et al., Surgical Management of Penile Carcinoma in Situ: Results from an International Collaborative Study and Review of the Literature. *BJU Int.* 2018;121(3):393-398.

[38] Leijte JAP, Kroon BK, Valdés Olmos RA, Nieweg OE, Horenblas S. Reliability and Safety of Current Dynamic Sentinel Node Biopsy for Penile Carcinoma. *European Urology.* 2007;52(1):170–7.

[39] Yu C, Hequn C, Longfei L, Minfeng C, Zhi C, Feng Z, et al., Sexual Function after Partial Penectomy: A Prospectively Study From China. *Scientific Reports.* 2016;6(1):21862.

[40] O'Kelly F, Lonergan P, Lundon D, Nason G, Sweeney P, Cullen I, et al., A Prospective Study of Total Glans Resurfacing for Localized Penile Cancer to Maximize Oncologic and Functional Outcomes in a Tertiary Referral Network. *The Journal of Urology.* 2017;197(5):1258–63.

[41] Dräger DL, Milerski S, Sievert KD, Hakenberg OW. Psychosoziale Auswirkungen bei Patienten mit Peniskarzinom. *Der Urologe.* 2018;57(4):444–52. [Psychosocial effects in patients with penile cancer. The Urologist. 2018;57(4)444-52].

[42] Yang J, Chen J, Wu X, Song N, Xu X, Li Q, et al., Glans preservation contributes to postoperative restoration of male sexual function: a multicenter clinical study of glans preserving surgery. *The Journal of urology*. 2014;192(5):1410–7.

[43] Kroon BK, Horenblas S, Lont AP, Tanis PJ, Gallee MPW, Nieweg OE. Patients with penile carcinoma benefit from immediate resection of clinically occult lymph node metastases. *Journal of Urology.* 2005;173(3):816–9.

[44] Matulewicz RS, Flum AS, Helenowski I, Jovanovic B, Palis B, Bilimoria KY, et al., Centralization of Penile Cancer Management in the United States: A Combined Analysis of the American Board of Urology and National Cancer Data Base. *Urology.* 2016;90:82–8.

[45] Catalona WJ. Modified inguinal lymphadenectomy for carcinoma of the penis with preservation of saphenous veins: technique and preliminary results. *The Journal of urology.* 1988;140(2):306–10.

[46] d'Ancona CAL, de Lucena RG, Querne FA de O, Martins MHT, Denardi F, Netto NR. Long-term followup of penile carcinoma treated with penectomy and bilateral modified inguinal lymphadenectomy. *The Journal of urology.* 2004;172(2):498–501; discussion 501.

[47] Cabañas R. an Approach for the Treatment of Penile. *Cancer.* 1977;39:456–66.

[48] Lam W, Alnajjar HM, La-Touche S, Perry M, Sharma D, Corbishley C, et al., Dynamic sentinel lymph node biopsy in patients with invasive squamous cell carcinoma of the penis: A prospective study of the long-term outcome of 500

inguinal basins assessed at a single institution. *European Urology*. 2013;63(4):657–63.

[49] Sadeghi R, Gholami H, Zakavi SR, Kakhki VRD, Tabasi KT, Horenblas S. Accuracy of Sentinel Lymph Node Biopsy for Inguinal Lymph Node Staging of Penile Squamous Cell Carcinoma: Systematic Review and Meta-Analysis of the Literature. *The Journal of Urology*. 2012;187(1):25–31.

[50] McMasters KM, Wong SL, Chao C, Woo C, Tuttle TM, Noyes RD, et al., Defining the optimal surgeon experience for breast cancer sentinel lymph node biopsy: a model for implementation of new surgical techniques. *Annals of surgery*. 2001;234(3):292-9; discussion 299-300.

[51] Schlenker B, Scher B, Tiling R, Siegert S, Hungerhuber E, Gratzke C, et al., Detection of inguinal lymph node involvement in penile squamous cell carcinoma by 18F-fluorodeoxyglucose PET/CT: A prospective single-center study. *Urologic Oncology: Seminars and Original Investigations*. 2012;30(1):55–9.

[52] Souillac I, Rigaud J, Ansquer C, Marconnet L, Bouchot O. Prospective Evaluation of 18F-Fluorodeoxyglucose Positron Emission Tomography-Computerized Tomography to Assess Inguinal Lymph Node Status in Invasive Squamous Cell Carcinoma of the Penis. *The Journal of Urology*. 2012;187(2):493–7.

[53] Leijte JAP, Graafland NM, Valdés Olmos RA, van Boven HH, Hoefnagel CA, Horenblas S. Prospective evaluation of hybrid ^{18}F-fluorodeoxyglucose positron emission tomography/computed tomography in staging clinically node-negative patients with penile carcinoma. *BJU International*. 2009;104(5):640–4.

[54] Dräger DL, Heuschkel M, Protzel C, Erbersdobler A, Krause BJ, Hakenberg OW, et al., [18F]FDG PET/CT for assessing inguinal lymph nodes in patients with penile cancer - correlation with histopathology after inguinal lymphadenectomy. *Nuklearmedizin* 2018;57(1):26–30.

[55] Ottenhof SR, Vegt E. The role of PET/CT imaging in penile cancer. *Translational andrology and urology*. 2017;6(5):833–8.

[56] Pandey D, Mahajan V, Kannan RR. Prognostic factors in node-positive carcinoma of the penis. *Journal of Surgical Oncology*. 2006;93(2):133–8.

[57] Stuiver MM, Djajadiningrat RS, Graafland NM, Vincent AD, Lucas C, Horenblas S. Early Wound Complications After Inguinal Lymphadenectomy in Penile Cancer: A Historical Cohort Study and Risk-factor Analysis. *European Urology*. 2013;64(3):486–92.

[58] Koifman L, Hampl D, Koifman N, Vides AJ, Ornellas AA. Radical Open Inguinal Lymphadenectomy for Penile Carcinoma: Surgical Technique, Early Complications and Late Outcomes. *The Journal of Urology*. 2013;190(6):2086–92.

[59] Yao K, Tu H, Li Y-H, Qin Z-K, Liu Z-W, Zhou F-J, et al., Modified Technique of Radical Inguinal Lymphadenectomy for Penile Carcinoma: Morbidity and Outcome. *The Journal of Urology*. 2010;184(2):546–52.

[60] Kumar V, Sethia KK. Prospective study comparing video-endoscopic radical inguinal lymph node dissection (VEILND) with open radical ILND (OILND) for penile cancer over an 8-year period. *BJU International.* 2017;119(4):530–4.

[61] Matin SF, Cormier JN, Ward JF, Pisters LL, Wood CG, Dinney CPN, et al., Phase 1 prospective evaluation of the oncological adequacy of robotic assisted video-endoscopic inguinal lymphadenectomy in patients with penile carcinoma. *BJU International*. 2013;111(7):1068–74.

[62] Lughezzani G, Catanzaro M, Torelli T, Piva L, Biasoni D, Stagni S, et al., The Relationship between Characteristics of Inguinal Lymph Nodes and Pelvic Lymph Node Involvement in Penile Squamous Cell Carcinoma: A Single Institution Experience. *The Journal of Urology.* 2014;191(4):977–82.

[63] Graafland NM, van Boven HH, van Werkhoven E, Moonen LMF, Horenblas S. Prognostic Significance of Extranodal Extension in Patients With Pathological Node Positive Penile Carcinoma. *The Journal of Urology.* 2010;184(4):1347–53.

[64] Nelson BA, Cookson MS, Smith Ja, Chang SS. Complications of inguinale and pelvic lymphadenectomy for squamous cell carcinoma of the penis: a contemporary series. *The Journal of Urology.* 2004;172(2):494–7.

[65] Necchi A. Systemic Therapy for Penile Cancer. *European Urology Supplements.* 2018;17(6):160–3.

[66] Pizzocaro G, Piva L. Adjuvant and neoadjuvant vincristine, bleomycin, and methotrexate for inguinal metastases from squamous cell carcinoma of the penis. *Acta oncologica.* 1988;27(6b):823–4.

[67] Sharma P, Djajadiningrat R, Zargar-Shoshtari K, Catanzaro M, Zhu Y, Nicolai N, et al., Adjuvant chemotherapy is associated with improved overall survival in pelvic node–positive penile cancer after lymph node dissection: A multi-institutional study. Urologic Oncology: *Seminars and Original Investigation*s. 2015;33 (11):496.e17-496.e23.

[68] Nicolai N, Sangalli LM, Necchi A, Giannatempo P, Paganoni AM, Colecchia M, et al., A Combination of Cisplatin and 5-Fluorouracil With a Taxane in Patients Who Underwent Lymph Node Dissection for Nodal Metastases From Squamous Cell Carcinoma of the Penis: Treatment Outcome and Survival Analyses in Neoadjuvant and Adjuvant Settings. *Clinical Genitourinary Cancer.* 2016;14(4):323–30.

[69] Robinson R, Marconi L, MacPepple E, Hakenberg OW, Watkin N, Yuan Y, et al., Risks and Benefits of Adjuvant Radiotherapy After Inguinal Lymphadenectomy in Node-positive Penile Cancer: A Systematic Review by the European Association of Urology Penile Cancer Guidelines Panel. *European Urology*. 2018;74(1):76–83.

[70] Johnstone PAS, Boulware D, Djajadiningrat R, Ottenhof S, Necchi A, Catanzaro M, et al., Primary Penile Cancer: The Role of Adjuvant Radiation Therapy in the Management of Extranodal Extension in Lymph Nodes. *European Urology Focus.* 2018 oct.

[71] Longpre MJ, Lange PH, Kwon JS, Black PC. Penile Carcinoma: Lessons Learned from Vulvar Carcinoma. *The Journal of Urology.* 2013;189(1):17–24.

[72] Kunos C, Simpkins F, Gibbons H, Tian C, Homesley H. Radiation Therapy Compared With Pelvic Node Resection for Node-Positive Vulvar Cancer. *Obstetrics & Gynecology.* 2009;114(3):537–46.

[73] Moore DH, Thomas GM, Montana GS, Saxer A, Gallup DG, Olt G. Preoperative chemoradiation for advanced vulvar cancer: a phase II study of the Gynecologic Oncology Group. *International journal of radiation oncology, biology, physics.* 1998;42(1):79–85.

[74] Graafland NM, Leijte JAP, Valdés Olmos RA, Hoefnagel CA, Teertstra HJ, Horenblas S. Scanning with 18F-FDG-PET/CT for Detection of Pelvic Nodal Involvement in Inguinal Node-Positive Penile Carcinoma. *European Urology.* 2009;56(2):339–45.

[75] Zhang S, Li W, Liang F. Clinical value of fluorine-18 2-fluoro-2-deoxy-D-glucose positron emission tomography/computed tomography in penile cancer. *Oncotarget.* 2016;7(30):48600–6.

[76] Leijte JAP, Kerst JM, Bais E, Antonini N, Horenblas S. Neoadjuvant Chemotherapy in Advanced Penile Carcinoma. *European Urology.* 2007;52(2): 488–94.

[77] Necchi A, Pond GR, Raggi D, Ottenhof SR, Djajadiningrat RS, Horenblas S, et al., Clinical Outcomes of Perioperative Chemotherapy in Patients With Locally Advanced Penile Squamous-Cell Carcinoma: Results of a Multicenter Analysis. *Clinical Genitourinary Cancer.* 2017;15(5):548–555.e3.

[78] Pagliaro LC, Williams DL, Daliani D, Williams MB, Osai W, Kincaid M, et al., Neoadjuvant Paclitaxel, Ifosfamide, and Cisplatin Chemotherapy for Metastatic Penile Cancer: A Phase II Study. *Journal of Clinical Oncology.* 2010;28(24):3851–7.

[79] Nicholson S, Hall E, Harland SJ, Chester JD, Pickering L, Barber J, et al., Phase II trial of docetaxel, cisplatin and 5FU chemotherapy in locally advanced and metastatic penis cancer (CRUK/09/001). *British Journal of Cancer.* 2013;109(10): 2554–9.

[80] Djajadiningrat RS, Bergman AM, van Werkhoven E, Vegt E, Horenblas S. Neoadjuvant Taxane-Based Combination Chemotherapy in Patients With Advanced Penile Cancer. *Clinical Genitourinary Cancer.* 2015;13(1):44–9.

[81] Theodore C, Skoneczna I, Bodrogi I, Leahy M, Kerst JM, Collette L, et al., A phase II multicentre study of irinotecan (CPT 11) in combination with cisplatin (CDDP) in metastatic or locally advanced penile carcinoma (EORTC PROTOCOL 30992). *Annals of Oncology*. 2008;19(7):1304–7.

[82] Zhang S, Zhu Y, Ye D. Phase II study of docetaxel, cisplatin, and fluorouracil in patients with distantly metastatic penile cancer as first-line chemotherapy. *Oncotarget.* 2015;6(31):32212–9.

[83] Di Lorenzo G, Buonerba C, Federico P, Perdonà S, Aieta M, Rescigno P, et al., Cisplatin and 5-fluorouracil in inoperable, stage IV squamous cell carcinoma of the penis. *BJU International.* 2012;110(11b):E661–6.

[84] Gagliano RG, Blumenstein BA, Crawford ED, Stephens RL, Coltman CA, Costanzi JJ. Cis-Diamminedichloroplatinum in the Treatment of Advanced Epidermoid Carcinoma of the Penis: A Southwest Oncology Group Study. *The Journal of Urology.* 1989141(1):66–7.

[85] Pond GR, Di Lorenzo G, Necchi A, Eigl BJ, Kolinsky MP, Chacko RT, et al., Prognostic risk stratification derived from individual patient level data for men with advanced penile squamous cell carcinoma receiving first-line systemic therapy. Urologic Oncology: *Seminars and Original Investigations.* 2014;32(4):501–8.

[86] Necchi A, Nicolai N, Colecchia M, Catanzaro M, Torelli T, Piva L, et al., Proof of Activity of Anti–Epidermal Growth Factor Receptor–Targeted Therapy for Relapsed Squamous Cell Carcinoma of the Penis. *Journal of Clinical Oncology.* 201129(22):e650–2.

[87] Gou H-F, Li X, Qiu M, Cheng K, Li L-H, Dong H, et al., Epidermal Growth Factor Receptor (EGFR)-RAS Signaling Pathway in Penile Squamous Cell Carcinoma. Viglietto G, editor. *PLoS ONE*. 2013;8(4):e62175.

[88] Necchi A, Giannatempo P, Lo Vullo S, Raggi D, Nicolai N, Colecchia M, et al., Panitumumab Treatment for Advanced Penile Squamous Cell Carcinoma When Surgery and Chemotherapy Have Failed. *Clinical Genitourinary Cancer.* 2016;14(3):231–6.

[89] Necchi A, Lo Vullo S, Perrone F, Raggi D, Giannatempo P, Calareso G, et al., First-line therapy with dacomitinib, an orally available pan-HER tyrosine kinase inhibitor, for locally advanced or metastatic penile squamous cell carcinoma: results of an open-label, single-arm, single-centre, phase 2 study. *BJU International.* 2018;121(3):348–56.

[90] Udager AM, Liu T-Y, Skala SL, Magers MJ, McDaniel AS, Spratt DE, et al., Frequent PD-L1 expression in primary and metastatic penile squamous cell carcinoma: potential opportunities for immunotherapeutic approaches. *Annals of Oncology.* 2016;27(9):1706–12.

[91] Ottenhof SR, Djajadiningrat RS, de Jong J, Thygesen HH, Horenblas S, Jordanova ES. Expression of Programmed Death Ligand 1 in Penile Cancer is of Prognostic Value and Associated with HPV Status. *The Journal of Urology*. 2017;197(3): 690–7.

[92] Apolo AB, Mortazavi A, Stein M, Pal SK, Davarpanah N, Parnes HL, et al., A phase I study of cabozantinib plus nivolumab (CaboNivo) in patients (pts)

refractory metastatic urothelial carcinoma (mUC) and other genitourinary (GU) tumors. *Annals of Oncology.* 2016;27(suppl_6).

[93] Cindolo L, Spiess PE, Bada M, Chipollini JJ, Nyirády P, Chiodini P, et al., Adherence to EAU guidelines on penile cancer translates into better outcomes: a multicenter international study. *World Journal of Urology.* 2018 Oct.

[94] Improving outcomes in urological cancers | Guidance and guidelines. *NICE.* Available from https://www.nice.org.uk/guidance/csg2.

[95] Tang V, Clarke L, Gall Z, Shanks JH, Nonaka D, Parr NJ, et al., Should centralized histopathological review in penile cancer be the global standard? *BJU Int.* 2014;114(3):340-3.

In: Penile Cancer: Challenges and Controversies
Editors: F. E. Martins and M. L. Djordjevic
ISBN: 978-1-53615-950-9

Chapter 17

Management of the Clinically Negative (cN0) Groin Patient: Timing for Intervention, Morbidity and Benefits

Mohamed Kamel[1,*], MD and Philippe E. Spiess[2], MD, MS
[1]Department of Urology, University of Arkansas for Medical Sciences, Little Rock, Arkansas, US
[2]Department of GU Oncology and Tumor Biology, Surgical Services, Moffitt Cancer Center, Professor of Oncology and Urology, University of South Florida, Tampa, Florida, US

Abstract

Inguinal lymph node metastasis is the single most important predictor of poor prognosis in penile cancer patient. One in every four patients with clinically negative groin exam (cN0) may still harbor metastasis. Inguinal lymph node dissection, though curative in many patients, is a morbid procedure. The ability to detect those PC patients, with occult inguinal lymph node metastasis is important. In this book chapter, we will focus on the management approach of the penile cancer patient with cN0 including the role of physical exam, imaging studies, molecular markers, risk stratification and intervention strategies.

Keywords: penile cancer, inguinal lymph nodes, groin, morbidity, penis; sentinel lymph node biopsy, lymphadenectomy, lymph node dissection, inguinal metastasis,

[*] Corresponding Author's E-mail: mkamel@uams.edu.

ABBREVIATIONS

CT	Computerized Tomography Scan
cN0	Clinically Negative Groin Lymph Node Involvement
DSLNB	Dynamic Sentinel Lymph Node Biopsy
EAU	European Association of Urology
FNAC	Fine Needle Aspiration Cytology
ILND	Inguinal Lymph Node Dissection
LN	Lymph Node
LNMRI	Lymphotropic Nanoparticle Enhanced Magnetic Resonance Imaging
MRI	Magnetic Resonance Imaging
NCCN	National Comprehensive Cancer Network
Pca	Penile Cancer
SLNB	Sentinel Lymph Node Biopsy
SPECT	Single Photon Emission Computerized Tomography
US	Ultrasound

INTRODUCTION

The presence or absence of inguinal lymph node (LN) metastasis is the most important predictor of survival in penile cancer (Pca). The 5 years survival rate in patients without inguinal LN metastasis is 85% versus 59% in patients with positive inguinal LN metastasis [1]. Consequently, the ability to accurately identify patients with Pca destined to develop inguinal LN metastasis is crucial. The natural history of penile cancer is characterized by a prolonged loco- regional phase before distant metastasis; this gives an opportunity to cure the patient with excision of the primary tumor and performing a regional inguinal LN dissection (ILND) [2]. Also it is widely accepted that inguinal LN involvement occurs before ipsilateral pelvic LN involvement and with no reported skip lesions [3]. Patients developing pelvic lymph node metastasis carried a very poor prognosis [4].

However, ILND is a morbid procedure. Contemporary literature revealed a complication rate of 19% and 27% for minor and major complications, respectively in diagnostic ILND in patients with clinically negative groin LN involvement (cN0) and a complication rate of 7% in Dynamic Sentinel Lymph Node Biopsy (DSLNB) [5]. These complications include skin necrosis; wound dehiscence, infection, and lymphedema. Therefore, subjecting the patient with cN0 to an ILND as well as the extent of lymph node dissection should be carefully considered. The clinical decision of whether to proceed with groin dissection or not in cN0 patient is further compounded by the fact that early ILND carries a significantly better survival than delayed ILND. Kroon et al. compared the survival and pathological findings in 20 patients received ILND following a positive DSLNB vs 20 patients received delayed ILND. The authors reported a 3 years survival rate of 84% versus 35% in the early versus delayed ILND groups with extra nodal extension detected in 20% versus 95% in the early versus delayed group [6]. Also ILND in patients with minimal LN involvement (1-2 inguinal LN) can be curative in 75% of patients [7].

In this chapter, we will focus on the management approach of the patient with cN0 including the role of physical exam, imaging studies, molecular markers, risk stratification and intervention strategies.

Role of Physical Exam in the cN0 Patient

Physical exam of the groin should be performed in all Pca patients to detect clinically enlarged inguinal LN. Unfortunately, there are challenges to physical exam in the Pca patient. Many Pca patients are from lower socioeconomic status, and suffering from obesity, some may have previous inguinal surgery for hernia repair, all may make physical exam difficult [8, 9]. Also, enlarged inguinal LN secondary to infection of the primary tumor rather than metastasis can occur in up to 50% of patients while 20% of patients with clinically negative groin exam may have inguinal LN metastasis [10]. Hornablas et al. conducted a study on 102 patients with Pca. The authors reported 82% sensitivity and 79% specificity for clinical exam of the groin. The same authors reported an under staging in 10% and over staging in 16% of patients [11]. We recommend physical exam as an integral part in the assessment of the Pca patient, however the above-mentioned limitations should be considered.

Role of Tumor Markers in the cN0 Patient

Molecular markers have been investigated to some part to predict LN metastasis in cN0 patient. MYC is a proto-oncogene that encodes target genes controlling key cellular functions including cell growth, cell cycle progression and DNA replication. Derangement of MYC function, reported to occur with Pca, leads to carcinogenesis and is reported to be associated with aggressive Pca with increased risk of metastasis and poor outcome [12]. The prognostic significance of p53, Ki-67, PCNA, E-Cadherin and Matrix Metalloproteases-9 (MMP-9) was evaluated in Pca as possible predictors of aggressive disease with increased risk of metastasis [13]. The over- expression of p53 was an independent predictor of metastasis [14]. The expression of Ki67 and PCNA were associated with increased risk of LN metastasis [15, 16]. KAI1/CD82 downregulation was associated with increased risk of LN metastasis [17]. However, overall the evidence to support the routine use of tumor markers in patients with cN0 to predict LN metastasis is not strong enough for this indication. Also; likely a panel of these markers will be more useful than using individual marker. We summarized the tumor markers that may have prognostic significance in predicting LN metastasis in Table 1 and studies relating to the outcomes of using more than biological marker in Table 2.

Table 1. Individual tumor markers thought to predict increased risk of lymph node metastasis

Marker	Location	Function	Anomaly	HPV relation	Outcome in cN0
p 53 [14, 18]	17p13.1	Tumor suppressor gene	Mutation leads to uninhibited cell growth	P53+HPV DNA →worse cancer specific survival	Increased risk of LN+
Ki67 [13, 19, 20]	Nuclear matrix protein	Role in Cell cycle progression	Overexpression	N/A	Controversial: -Increased risk of LN+[19] -No increased risk of LN+[13, 20]
PCNA [16]	Nucleus	Role in Cell proliferation	Overexpression	N/A	Increased risk of LN+
C-reactive protein [21]	Produced in liver and present in serum	Produced in response to inflammation	Increased serum level	N/A	Increased risk of LN+
E-cadherin [22]	Trans-membrane Protein	Maintaining cellular adhesion and signal transduction	Low level	N/A	Increased risk of LN +
Squamous cell carcinoma antigen [23]	Serum	Serum Glycoprotein	Increased absolute level or continuous rise after penectomy	N/A	Increased risk of LN+
MYC [12]	8q 24	Protooncogene Regulate cellular proliferation	Numerical aberrations (gains) or expression in >30% of primary tumor cells	N/A	Increased risk of LN+
Matrix Metalloproteases-9 (MMP-9) [22]	Basement membrane	Group of enzymes that degrade type IV collagen in the basement membrane and involved in invasion mechanism	Increased immunoreactivity	N/A	Increased risk of LN+

HPV: Human Papilloma Virus. PCNA: Proliferating Cell Nuclear Antigen. LN+: Lymph node metastasis. N/A: Not available data to document correlation or there may be no correlation at all.

Table 2. Studies combined more than one tumor marker to predict LN metastasis/survival

Study	Combination	End points	Outcome
*Zhu et al. [13]	-p53, Ki-67, E-cadherin and MMP-9	- CSS - LN+	-p53 overexpression was associated with ↓survival and ↑ risk of LN+
↓Gunia et al. [18]	-p53,p21 and Cyclin D1	- CSS	-p53 overexpression was associated with ↓survival
¶Campos et al. [22]	MMP-2, MMP-9 and E-cadherin	- CSS - LN+	-↓E-cadherin was associated with↑ risk of LN+ - ↑MMP-9 was associated with ↓survival
•Guimaraes et al. [16]	PCNA and MIB-1/Ki-67	- CSS - LN+	- Overexpression of PCNA and MIB-1/Ki-67 was associated with ↑ risk of LN+ - No effect of these markers on survival
×Protzel et al. [17]	KAI1/CD82	- CSS - LN+	- Low expression was associated with ↑ risk of LN + and ↓ survival

CSS: Cancer specific survival.CD82: Cluster of differentiation 82. KAI: Kang ai protein LN: Lymph node. LN+: Lymph node metastasis. MMP-9: Matrix Metalloproteases-9. MMP-2: Matrix Metalloproteases-2. PCNA: Proliferating Cell Nuclear Antigen.

*on univariate analysis Ki-67 was associated with increased risk of LN metastasis but on multivariable analysis this effect was not demonstrated.

↓CyclinD1 and p21 expression were not associated with worse survival. However adding p21 to the multivariable model improved the predictability of the model to survival.

¶ On multivariable analysis neither E-cadherin predicted LN metastasis nor MMP-9 predicted poor survival.

• On multivariable analysis, PCNA continued to predict LN metastasis but not MIB-1/Ki-67.

× the presence of HPV-DNA was associated with low expression of KAI1/CD82 and consequently poor survival

ROLE OF IMAGING IN THE CN0 PATIENT

Unlike other genitourinary cancers were imaging can accurately detect metastasis in patients with low stage disease, Pca represents a challenge for imaging modalities commonly used in clinical practice in the cN0 patient. The situation is compounded by the rarity of the disease which does not allow clinical studies on large group of patients, testing new imaging modalities that were proven useful in other cancers. In this section we will discuss the different imaging modalities tried in the cN0 patient as well as indications, outcomes and limitations.

Groin Ultrasound

Groin ultrasound (US) uses a high resolution 7.5 or 10 MHZ probe. It relies on the detection of a distortion in the normal architecture of the involved LN. Such changes in the LN cortical and hilar morphology are detected prior to the LN enlarges [24]. However, because of the overlap between benign and malignant features of distorted LN architecture, groin US is usually combined with Fine Needle Aspiration Cytology

(FNAC) of the sonographically abnormal LN. If the FNAC returns positive, ILND dissection is indicated with excision of the needle track to avoid the potential risk of seeding of malignant cells. Kroon et al. studied US+FNAC in 83 clinically negative groins as an initial investigation prior to DSLNB. 49/83 groins were negative on US and underwent DSLNB. 34/83 groins were suspicious on US exam and consequently all had FNAC. 9/34 were positive on FNAC. The reported sensitivity and specificity were 39% and 100% respectively. In this report US+FNAC reduced the need for DSLNB by 11%. [25] However, groin US has several limitations that make it unreliable if used as a single diagnostic modalityin the cN0 patient. The sensitivity is low (39%), FNAC can only detect metastasis > 2mm and it is reported to have a false negative rate of 29% [26, 27].

Abdominal and Pelvic Computerized Tomography (CT)Scan/ Magnetic Resonance Imaging (MRI)

Conventional CT or MRI scan can rarely detect micrometastasis in patients with cN0 disease [28, 11]. These imaging modalities, in the cN0 patient, are indicated if the physical exam is difficult as in the obese patients or in patients with previous inguinal surgery.[29] The National Comprehensive Cancer Network (NCCN) guidelines would recommend MRI as the investigation to be performed, should assessment of the depth of primary tumor invasion together with groin assessment are warranted simultaneously [30]. Though CT and MRI have limited role in the cN0 patient, these imaging modalities are indicated in patients with cN0 who are intermediate or high risks for lymph node metastasis, as discussed later, and consequently will be offered prophylactic ILND, but this will be for staging purposes [30, 31]. Also it is hoped that modifications to both the CT and MRI techniques, as discussed later, will improve the sensitivity and specificity of these imaging modalities in the cN0 patients.

Positron Imaging Tomography (PET)/CT

PET/CT combines functional information derived from the uptake of 18F-fluorodeoxyglucose (FDG) by the abnormal LN with the anatomical information provided with the low dose CT scan. However, its role in the cN0 patient is not well established. Souillac et al. prospectively evaluated the role of PET/CT in the cN0 patient. The authors investigated the outcome of PET/CT in 44 inguinal LN basins in 22 cN0 patients. The reported sensitivity and specificity were 75% and 87.5%. The test however had a dismal positive predictive value of only 37.5% in this group of patients [32]. Similarly, Sadeghi et al. conducted a meta-analysis on the role of PET/CT and the pooled sensitivity in the cN0 patients was 56.5%. The authors concluded PET/CT routine use in the cN0 is not justified [33]. Also the technique has the limitations of difficulty to identify metastatic disease <10 mm and to differentiate between inflammation and metastatic deposits [34]. In summary, there is likely a minimal to no role of PET/CT among penile cancer patients with cN0 disease unless a suspicious nodal area is seen on CT and/or MRI and is not amenable to image guided biopsy or there is suspicion of recurrence in the subsequent surveillance of such patients.

Single Photon Emission Computerized Tomography (SPECT)-CT

In this imaging technique, ^{99m}technetium nano-colloid is injected directly into the primary tumor or just proximal to the surgical scar in 4 points and can drain to the inguinal LN. A gamma camera is used to detect the photon emission from the "sentinel" LN in the groin using both dynamic (20 minutes) and early and delayed static images (5 and 120 minutes) post injections are taken. This functional information is overlapped with conventional CT imaging to provide a 3D CT image to identify the first drainage basin and to facilitate SLNB [35]. Preliminary data are encouraging. Lutzen et al. studied 25 patients with clinically inconspicuous inguinal LN who underwent SPECT/CT to facilitate SLNB. The authors reported a sensitivity and specificity of 88.8% and 86.7% respectively and a false negative rate of 4.5%. The same authors reported the technique shortened the duration of the SLNB [36].

Lymphotropic Nanoparticle Enhanced Magnetic Resonance Imaging (LNMRI)

The technique is meant to enhance the sensitivity and specificity of MRI in detecting micro metastasis. The concept of this new imaging modality relies on the presence of macrophages in the normal LN that engulf the injected nanoparticles and will appear dark on T2 weighted MRI. Metastatic LN lacks these macrophages and consequently the nanoparticles are not concentrated in the malignant LN that will appear bright on T2-weighted MRI. In brief, the technique involves the intravenous injection of Nano-particles of ferumoxtran-10 (iron oxide) and MRI imaging is performed before and 24 hours after injection. LN that are dark on T2 images or may have a central bright area (hilar LN fat) on T1-weighted images are considered normal. Tabatabaei et al. correlated the LNMRI and pathological LN findings in 113 LN excised from 7 patients. Of these patients 5 were cN0. Overall 13/113 LN were positive and reported a sensitivity, specificity, positive and negative predictive values of 100%, 97%, 81.2% and 100% respectively [37]. The results reported by the author are good, however the study population is small and there is no long term follow up. Nevertheless, nanotechnology is promising in the field of staging genitourinary cancers [38].

Lymphoscintigraphy and Sentinel Lymph Node Biopsy (SLNB)

Lymphoscintigraphy is usually discussed in the context of performing DSLNB. Based on in the initial lymphangiographic studies by Cabanas, anatomically, the sentinel LN is located close to the superficial epigastric vein [39]. The Sentinel LN area is comprised of ≤ 7 LN [40]. The SLN is the first lymph drainage area to the penis and consequently if it is negative, further LN dissection is discouraged.

Static SLNB is performed by making a 5 cms incision 2 finger breadths lateral and inferior to the pubic tubercle. This is followed by inserting a finger in an upward and medial direction towards the public tubercle to excise all the lymphatic tissue that comprises the SLN area. However, historical reports showed that the technique of Static SLNB is associated with a high false negative rate. Though most of these reports were case reports or small study series, the technique of static SLNB has been largely abandoned [41, 42].

In attempt to reduce the high false negative rate of Static SLNB, lymphoscintigraphy was used to combine functional and anatomic information to better identify the SLN area in penile cancer. In DSLNB, intradermal injection of hybrid tracer of ^{99m}technetium nano-colloid around the tumor is performed; this is followed by acquiring dynamic images at 10 minutes after injection on a coronal view, 30 min then 2 hours by dual-head gamma camera. A gamma probe is used to detect the SLN and at the beginning of the surgical procedure, patent blue dye is injected that will be up taken by the SLN to add visualization. The SLN are then removed and if positive radical ILND is performed. Using this standard technique for DSLNB, Spiess et al. reported a false negative rate of 25% [43]. A few modifications to the standard technique involved the use of hybrid radioactive and fluorescence tracer indocyanine green- ^{99m}technetium nano-colloid instead of the traditional patent blue-^{99m}technetium nano-colloid hybrid. In one study the new hybrid with this near infrared fluorescence showed better tissue penetration and visualization than patent blue and detected 95% of SLN compared to 54% using traditional patent blue [44]. Using the modifications to the dynamic technique for SLNB, and in centers that perform a minimum of 20 DSLNB per year, the contemporary, reported false negative rate is only 4.8% and complication rate of 5.7% in the cN0 patient [45].

Role of Nomograms in the cN0 Patient

Nomograms have been designed to predict LN metastasis in the cN0 patient and to aid in the clinical decision. Ficarra et al. proposed a nomogram using eight clinical and pathological variables derived from 175 patients from 11 institutions. These variables were clinical stage of LN, microscopic growth pattern, histologic grade, vascular invasion and invasion of corpus spongiosum, corpus cavernosum and urethra [46]. Kattan et al. proposed a second nomogram using the same criteria [47]. A third nomogram was proposed based on histological grade and the presence or absence of perineural invasion in tumors that are 5-10 mm in thickness [48]. However, these nomograms were not externally validated and there use in clinical practice is not popular and cannot be recommended as a standalone tool to predict LN metastasis in the cN0 patient.

Risk Stratification for Inguinal LN Metastasis in the cN0 Patient and Indications for Intervention

In the absence of validated nomograms, reliable imaging modalities, molecular markers together with the limitations of groin exam to predict inguinal LN metastasis in the cN0, pathological findings in the primary tumor are of paramount importance in the decision making on performing ILND or not in this group of patients. Slaton et al. studied the impact of pathological primary tumor stage, the presence of vascular invasion and the percentage of poorly differentiated tumor in the primary tumor as predictors of inguinal LN metastasis. The investigators reported the risk of inguinal LN metastasis to be 64% in pathological stage ≥ T2, 55% in the setting of vascular invasion and 61% in tumors exhibiting more than 50% of the poorly differentiated tumor grade. [49] In another study, Solsona et al. classified patients into three risk groups for developing inguinal LN metastasis based on tumor stage and grade [50]. These risk groups were 1) *Low risk* comprising patients with tumors that are T1 and G1 and the incidence of positive ILN metastasis was 0% in this group. 2) *Intermediate risk* comprising T 1 and G2-G3 or T2-3 and G1 tumors and the incidence of ILN metastasis was 36.4%. 3) *High risk* comprising patients with T2-3 and G2-3 tumors and the incidence of positive ILN metastasis was 80%. The work of the previous investigators as well as the work by others[51] had important implications on the management of Pca. The most recent (8th edition, 2016) Tumor Node Metastasis (TNM) staging for Pca was modified to reflect the increased risk of metastasis in patients with lymphovascular invasion and poorly differentiated cancer as stageT1b. Also, the European Association of Urology (EAU) classified patients with non-palpable inguinal LN into 3 risk categories for developing inguinal LN metastasis. These risk groups are 1) *Low risk* for inguinal LN metastasis comprising tumors that are

Tis (in situ), Ta (noninvasive tumors) and T1a (tumor invades dermis, lamina propria and dartos fascia and no lymphovascular invasion or poorly differentiated tumor grade). 2) *Intermediate risk* for inguinal LN metastasis comprising tumors that are T1b (lymphovascular invasion). 3) *High risk* for inguinal lymph node metastasis and this includes any G3 tumors or stage ≥T2 Pca [31].

Similarly, the NCCN guidelines on Pca identified certain pathological features as high risk for inguinal LN metastasis and consequently warrant prophylactic ILND in patients who are cN0. These features are 1) Presence of lymphovascular invasion. 2) T1 G3. 3) ≥ T2 any grade. 4) > 50% poorly differentiated tumors [31]. After examining these 2 major guidelines one can conclude that the presence of the high-risk features mentioned in the North American Guidelines coincides with the intermediate and high-risk groups of the EAU guidelines. The presence of these high risk pathological features warrants ILND. In the absence of these high-risk pathological features active surveillance is recommended.

However, despite the clear-cut criteria offered by these guidelines on when to offer active surveillance versus proceeding with prophylactic ILND; there remains one particular situation that is debatable regarding decision making. This will be the patient who presents with T1 tumor that is G2 [52]. Obviously if this T1G2 tumor exhibits lympho-vascular invasion, according to the latest American Joint Committee on Cancer (AJCC) penile cancer staging, this will be stage T1b disease and prophylactic ILND is recommended following appropriate imaging investigations to stage the cancer. However, the guidelines are not clear in the T1 G2 tumor that does not exhibit lymphovascular invasion; stage T1aG2. Thuret et al. studied the cancer specific mortality of T1 Pca patients using the Surveillance, Epidemiology and End Results (SEER) data base in patients who had excision of the primary tumor and without ILND. The authors reported a 5 years cancer specific mortality of 2.6%, 10% and 15.9% for T1G1, T1G2 and T1G3 tumors respectively ($P<0.05$) [53]. However, owing to the limitations of the data set used pathological tumor criteria as lymphovascular invasion and or invasion into perineural spaces could not be counted for. Consequently, it is reasonable in the situation of T1aG2 to individualize the decision based on the overall general health of the patient and in patients with coexisting morbidities that can increase the risks of developing complications following ILND. Another approach in this situation is to perform a DSLNB, in centers experienced in performing this procedure (>20 procedures/year), or to perform superficial ILND with intraoperative frozen section to reduce the morbidity of the ILND surgery.

In patients of the intermediate and high-risk group for inguinal lymph node metastasis, modified ILND with excision of lymphatic tissue of the central and superior areas of Dressler triangle is recommended. Another approach is to proceed with DSLNB and to be followed by superficial and deep ILND if LN is positive for metastasis. Also performing superficial ILND with intraoperative frozen section and if the frozen section is positive for metastasis, bilateral superficial and deep ILND is performed, is another acceptable option [29, 54].

Bilateral versus Unilateral ILND in the cN0 Patient

Kroon et al. studied the lymphatic drainage in Pca patients using lymphoscintigraphy [55]. In 20 patients studied, 18 (90%) patients demonstrated bilateral inguinal lymph node drainage and in 1 (5%) patient drainage to the prepubic area were noted. Consequently, bilateral ILND, when decided in the cN0 patient should be the norm. Similarly in patients in whom one groin is demonstrating an enlarged inguinal lymph node while the other groin is clinically negative for an enlarged lymph node, the risk of harboring micrometastasis could be as high as 30% in this groin and consequently bilateral ILND is indicated [56]. Regarding performing concomitant pelvic lymph node dissection with ILND in the cN0 patient, it is not indicated unless a frozen section exam showed ≥2 inguinal lymph nodes that are positive for metastasis [57].

Role of Prophylactic Inguinal LN Radiation Therapy in cN0 patients

Radiation therapy for the clinically negative groin patient has not been evaluated in a rigorous manner in the contemporary peer reviewed literature. Historical reports revealed the risk of recurrence is 25% in cN0; similar to the reported incidence of micro-metastasis in the cN0 patient [58]. Consequently, prophylactic radiation to the patient with cN0 is not indicated [54]. Perhaps in the high-risk patient for inguinal LN metastasis who is not fit for or unwilling to undergo ILND, prophylactic External Beam Radiation Therapy may be considered.

Special Histological Considerations

Patients with Pca are classified into 3 groups depending on the histological type of the penile cancer [31]. The low risk group and this includes verrucous, warty and papillary types. The intermediate risk group and this includes the common squamous cell carcinoma and mixed forms. The high-risk group and this includes the basaloid, sarcomatoid, adenosquamous and poorly differentiated/undifferentiated types. Guimaraes et al. studied the risk of inguinal LN metastasis in 333 patients from Brazil [59] . In those patients who developed inguinal lymph node metastasis (overall 24%) such incidence classified by histological type was for, common squamous cell carcinoma type 28%, verrucous type 0%, warty type 17%, papillary type 12%, basaloid type 50%, sarcomatoid type 75% and adenosquamous type 50%. Based on these results, it is recommended that patients with the low grade verrucous type Pca offered active surveillance while in patients with high risk histological types, prophylactic ILND should be considered.

Follow-Up Protocols Following Treatments in cN0 Patients

The follow-up for patients with cN0 will depend on the 1) choice of treatment of the groin whether active surveillance was elected for the patient and 2) the pathological findings in patients who had an ILND.

In patients received active surveillance, examination of the groin every 3 months for 1-2 years then every 6 months for 3-5 years then annually thereafter. In patients underwent ILND with N0 and N1 disease, the follow up protocol is groin exam every 6 months for the first 2 years then yearly afterwards. For N2-N3 disease, the follow up protocol is groin exam every 3-6 months for the first 2 years then every 6-12 months afterwards. For N2-N3 disease, in addition to the groin exam, chest imaging with chest X-ray and abdominal/Pelvic CT or MRI are added [60].

Conclusion

Management of the groin in the cN0 Pca patient represents a decision challenge to the treating urologic-oncologist. Risks of performing ILND should be weighed against potential benefits. Physical exam has limitations in detecting enlarged ILN in particular in the obese patients and patients received prior groin surgery or radiation and even in-patient normal groins, may still harbor micrometastasis in the groin LN. Tumor markers as predictors of LN metastasis in the cN0 are currently lacking necessary sensitivity and specificity to be reliably used in this situation. Nomograms are not popular for use in the cN0 patients and are not externally validated. Overall imaging modalities are not sensitive or specific enough in order to reliably rely on it as a sole investigation to rule out ILN micrometastasis. However combing groin US+FNAC in patients with sonographically suspicious LN has better sensitivity and specificity than groin US alone. Also conventional CT or MRI are not recommended as initial investigation in the cN0 patient except in patients in whom groin exam is challenging or as a staging investigations in patients with high risk for groin LN metastasis. Incorporating nanotechnology to conventional CT scan or MRI is promising in detecting micrometastasis in groin LN but still under investigation. The routine use of PET/CT in patients with cN0 is not justified. Static SLN is abandoned because of its high false negative rate. DSLNB, in centers with the infrastructure and experience (>20 procedures/year) in performing the technique is more reliable than SLNB in detecting micrometastesis and represents a useful diagnostic tool in this regard. Pathological criteria in the primary tumor remain the key parameters that will determine if a cN0 patient to be offered active surveillance or prophylactic ILND. These adverse pathological features include the presence of high-grade tumor (>50% of tumor), stage ≥ T2, lymphovascular invasion and rare aggressive histopathological variants warrants prophylactic ILND which should be performed bilateral. Prophylactic groin radiation therapy in patient with cN0 is not indicated except in patients with high risk for ILN metastasis or those who are unfit or unwilling to undergo ILND.

We have illustrated a proposed algorithm for the management of the patient with cN0 based on the best available evidence in Figure 1.

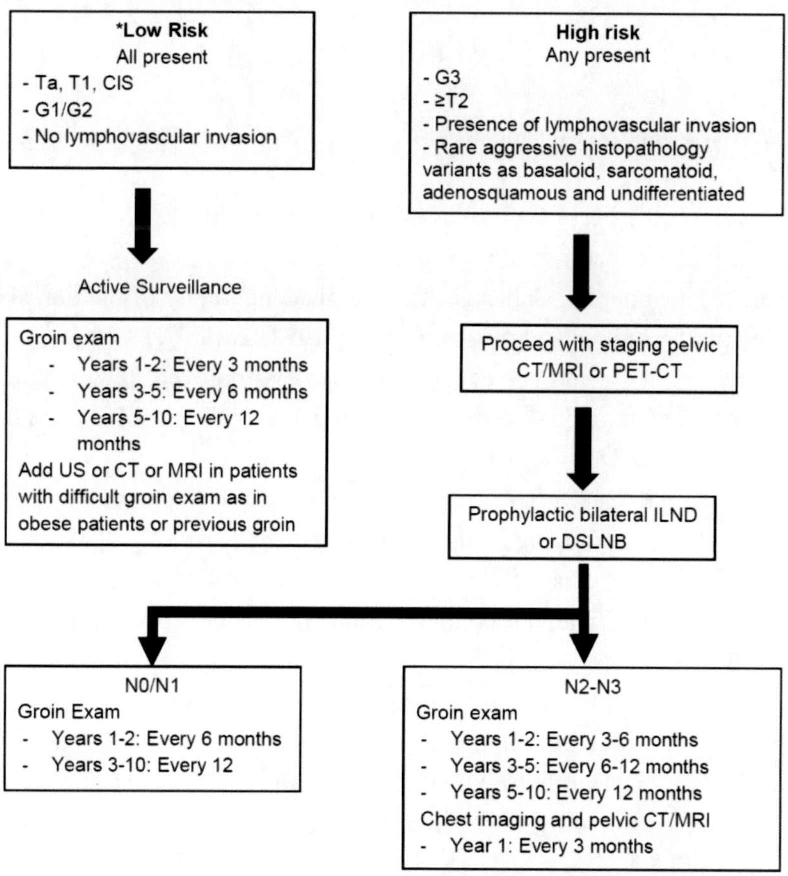

*T1G2 without LVI consider DSLNB or bilateral superficial ILND with intraoperative frozen section versus active surveillance

Figure 1. Management of the cN0 patient.

Key Points

- Physical exam has limitations in the obese patient and in patients with previous groin surgeries or irradiation.
- Conventional CT scan and MRI scan usually fail to detect micro metastasis in the inguinal lymph nodes and routine PET/CT in patients with cN0 is not indicated.
- DSLNB is more reliable than SLNB, provided the necessary infrastructure and experience exists.
- Pathological criteria in the primary tumor is the most important predictor of micro- metastasis in the inguinal LN.
- The presence of ≥T2 disease, G3 (≥50% of tumor volume), LVI and rare aggressive histology, in the primary tumor warrants prophylactic ILND.
- No role for prophylactic groin irradiation in cN0 penile cancer patient.

References

[1] https:// www.cancer.org/cancer/penile-cancer/detection-diagnosis-staging/survival-rates.html.

[2] Pow-Sang, M. R., Ferreira, U., Pow-Sang, J. M. et al.: Epidemiology and natural history of penile cancer. *Urology*, **76:** S2, 2010.

[3] Riveros, M., Garcia, R., Cabanas, R.: Lymphadenography of the dorsal lymphatics of the penis. Technique and results. *Cancer,* **20:** 2026, 1967.

[4] Graafland, N. M., van Boven, H. H., van Werkhoven, E. et al.: Prognostic significance of extranodal extension in patients with pathological node positive penile carcinoma. *J Urol,* **184:** 1347, 2010.

[5] Spiess, P. E., Hernandez, M. S., Pettaway, C. A.: Contemporary inguinal lymph node dissection: minimizing complications. *World J Urol*, **27:** 205, 2009.

[6] Kroon, B. K., Horenblas, S., Lont, A. P. et al.: Patients with penile carcinoma benefit from immediate resection of clinically occult lymph node metastases. *J Urol,* **173:** 816, 2005.

[7] Horenblas, S.: Lymphadenectomy for squamous cell carcinoma of the penis. Part 2: the role and technique of lymph node dissection. *BJU Int,* **88:** 473, 2001.

[8] Hernandez, B. Y., Barnholtz-Sloan, J., German, R. R. et al.: Burden of invasive squamous cell carcinoma of the penis in the United States, 1998-2003. *Cancer,* **113:** 2883, 2008.

[9] Barnes, K. T., Smith, B. J., Lynch, C. F. et al.: Obesity and Invasive Penile Cancer. *European Urology*, **63:** 588, 2013.

[10] Hegarty, P. K., Kayes, O., Freeman, A. et al.: A prospective study of 100 cases of penile cancer managed according to European Association of Urology guidelines. *BJU Int*, **98:** 526, 2006.

[11] Horenblas, S., Van Tinteren, H., Delemarre, J. F. et al.: Squamous cell carcinoma of the penis: accuracy of tumor, nodes and metastasis classification system, and role of lymphangiography, computerized tomography scan and fine needle aspiration cytology. *J Urol*, **146:** 1279, 1991.

[12] Masferrer, E., Ferrandiz-Pulido, C., Lloveras, B. et al.: MYC copy number gains are associated with poor outcome in penile squamous cell carcinoma. *J Urol,* **188:** 1965, 2012.

[13] Zhu, Y., Zhou, X. Y., Yao, X. D. et al.: The prognostic significance of p53, Ki-67, epithelial cadherin and matrix metalloproteinase-9 in penile squamous cell carcinoma treated with surgery. *BJU Int,* **100:** 204, 2007.

[14] Lopes, A., Bezerra, A. L., Pinto, C. A. et al.: p53 as a new prognostic factor for lymph node metastasis in penile carcinoma: analysis of 82 patients treated with amputation and bilateral lymphadenectomy. *J Urol*, **168:** 81, 2002.

[15] Protzel, C., Knoedel, J., Zimmermann, U. et al.: Expression of proliferation marker Ki67 correlates to occurrence of metastasis and prognosis, histological subtypes and HPV DNA detection in penile carcinomas. *Histol Histopathol*, **22:** 1197, 2007.

[16] Guimaraes, G. C., Leal, M. L., Campos, R. S. et al.: Do proliferating cell nuclear antigen and MIB-1/Ki-67 have prognostic value in penile squamous cell carcinoma? *Urology,* **70:** 137, 2007.

[17] Protzel, C., Kakies, C., Kleist, B. et al.: Down-regulation of the metastasis suppressor protein KAI1/CD82 correlates with occurrence of metastasis, prognosis and presence of HPV DNA in human penile squamous cell carcinoma. *Virchows Arch*, **452:** 369, 2008.

[18] Gunia, S., Kakies, C., Erbersdobler, A. et al.: Expression of p53, p21 and cyclin D1 in penile cancer: p53 predicts poor prognosis. *J Clin Pathol,* **65:** 232, 2012.

[19] Berdjis, N., Meye, A., Nippgen, J. et al.: Expression of Ki-67 in squamous cell carcinoma of the penis. *BJU Int*, **96:** 146, 2005.

[20] Stankiewicz, E., Ng, M., Cuzick, J. et al.: The prognostic value of Ki-67 expression in penile squamous cell carcinoma. *J Clin Pathol,* **65:** 534, 2012.

[21] Steffens, S., Al Ghazal, A., Steinestel, J. et al.: High CRP values predict poor survival in patients with penile cancer. *BMC Cancer,* **13:** 223, 2013.

[22] Campos, R. S., Lopes, A., Guimaraes, G. C. et al.: E-cadherin, MMP-2, and MMP-9 as prognostic markers in penile cancer: analysis of 125 patients. *Urology,* **67:** 797, 2006.

[23] Laniado, M. E., Lowdell, C., Mitchell, H. et al.: Squamous cell carcinoma antigen: a role in the early identification of nodal metastases in men with squamous cell carcinoma of the penis. *BJU Int*, **92:** 248, 2003.

[24] Vassallo, P., Wernecke, K., Roos, N. et al.: Differentiation of benign from malignant superficial lymphadenopathy: the role of high-resolution US. *Radiology,* **183:** 215, 1992.

[25] Kroon, B. K., Horenblas, S., Deurloo, E. E. et al.: Ultrasonography-guided fine-needle aspiration cytology before sentinel node biopsy in patients with penile carcinoma. *BJU Int,* **95:** 517, 2005.

[26] Chaux, A., Cubilla, A. L.: Diagnostic problems in precancerous lesions and invasive carcinomas of the penis. *Semin Diagn Pathol,* **29:** 72, 2012.

[27] Hughes, B., Leijte, J., Shabbir, M. et al.: Non-invasive and minimally invasive staging of regional lymph nodes in penile cancer. *World J Urol,* **27:** 197, 2009.

[28] Singh, A. K., Gonzalez-Torrez, P., Kaewlai, R. et al.: Imaging of penile neoplasm. *Semin Ultrasound CT MR*, **28:** 287, 2007.

[29] Hakenberg, O. W., Comperat, E. M., Minhas, S. et al.: EAU guidelines on penile cancer: 2014 update. *Eur Urol*, **67:** 142, 2015.

[30] Spiess, P. E.: New treatment guidelines for penile cancer. *J Natl Compr Canc Netw,* **11:** 659, 2013.

[31] Hakenberg, O. W., Comperat, E. M., Minhas, S. et al.: EAU guidelines on penile cancer: 2014 update. *Eur Urol*, **67:** 142, 2015.

[32] Souillac, I., Rigaud, J., Ansquer, C. et al.: Prospective evaluation of (18)F-fluorodeoxyglucose positron emission tomography-computerized tomography to assess inguinal lymph node status in invasive squamous cell carcinoma of the penis. *J Urol,* **187:** 493, 2012.

[33] Sadeghi, R., Gholami, H., Zakavi, S. R. et al.: Accuracy of 18F-FDG PET/CT for diagnosing inguinal lymph node involvement in penile squamous cell carcinoma: systematic review and meta-analysis of the literature. *Clin Nucl Med,* **37:** 436, 2012.

[34] O'Brien, J. S., Perera, M., Manning, T. et al.: Penile Cancer: *Contemporary Lymph Node Management. J Urol,* **197:** 1387, 2017.

[35] Saad, Z. Z., Omorphos, S., Michopoulou, S. et al.: Investigating the role of SPECT/CT in dynamic sentinel lymph node biopsy for penile cancers. *European Journal of Nuclear Medicine and Molecular Imaging,* **44:** 1176, 2017.

[36] Lützen, U., Naumann, C. M., Marx, M. et al.: A study on the value of computer-assisted assessment for SPECT/CT-scans in sentinel lymph node diagnostics of penile cancer as well as clinical reliability and morbidity of this procedure. *Cancer Imaging,* **16:** 29, 2016.

[37] Tabatabaei, S., Harisinghani, M., McDougal, W. S.: Regional lymph node staging using lymphotropic nanoparticle enhanced magnetic resonance imaging with ferumoxtran-10 in patients with penile cancer. *J Urol*, **174:** 923, 2005.

[38] Mouli, S. K., Zhao, L. C., Omary, R. A. et al.: Lymphotropic nanoparticle enhanced MRI for the staging of genitourinary tumors. *Nature Reviews Urology*, **7:** 84, 2010.

[39] Cabanas, R. M.: Anatomy and biopsy of sentinel lymph nodes. *Urol Clin North* Am, **19:** 267, 1992.

[40] Kroon, B. K., Horenblas, S., Nieweg, O. E.: Contemporary management of penile squamous cell carcinoma. *J Surg Oncol,* **89:** 43, 2005.

[41] Bouchot, O., Auvigne, J., Peuvrel, P. et al.: Management of regional lymph nodes in carcinoma of the penis. *Eur Urol,* **16:** 410, 1989.

[42] Perinetti, E., Crane, D. B., Catalona, W. J.: Unreliability of sentinel lymph node biopsy for staging penile carcinoma. *J Urol,* **124:** 734, 1980.

[43] Spiess, P. E., Izawa, J. I., Bassett, R. et al.: Preoperative lymphoscintigraphy and dynamic sentinel node biopsy for staging penile cancer: results with pathological correlation. *J Urol,* **177:** 2157, 2007.

[44] Brouwer, O. R., van den Berg, N. S., Matheron, H. M. et al.: A hybrid radioactive and fluorescent tracer for sentinel node biopsy in penile carcinoma as a potential replacement for blue dye. *Eur Urol*, **65:** 600, 2014.

[45] Leijte, J. A., Kroon, B. K., Valdes Olmos, R. A. et al.: Reliability and safety of current dynamic sentinel node biopsy for penile carcinoma. *Eur Urol,* **52:** 170, 2007.

[46] Ficarra, V., Zattoni, F., Artibani, W. et al.: Nomogram predictive of pathological inguinal lymph node involvement in patients with squamous cell carcinoma of the penis. *J Urol,* **175:** 1700, 2006.

[47] Kattan, M. W., Ficarra, V., Artibani, W. et al.: Nomogram predictive of cancer specific survival in patients undergoing partial or total amputation for squamous cell carcinoma of the penis. *J Urol,* **175:** 2103, 2006.

[48] Velazquez, E. F., Ayala, G., Liu, H. et al.: Histologic grade and perineural invasion are more important than tumor thickness as predictor of nodal metastasis in penile squamous cell carcinoma invading 5 to 10 mm. *Am J Surg Pathol*, **32:** 974, 2008.

[49] Slaton, J. W., Morgenstern, N., Levy, D. A. et al.: Tumor stage, vascular invasion and the percentage of poorly differentiated cancer: independent prognosticators for inguinal lymph node metastasis in penile squamous cancer. *J Urol*, **165:** 1138, 2001.

[50] Solsona, E., Iborra, I., Rubio, J. et al.: Prospective validation of the association of local tumor stage and grade as a predictive factor for occult lymph node micrometastasis in patients with penile carcinoma and clinically negative inguinal lymph nodes. *J Urol*, **165:** 1506, 2001.

[51] Cubilla, A. L., Reuter, V., Velazquez, E. et al.: Histologic classification of penile carcinoma and its relation to outcome in 61 patients with primary resection. *Int J Surg Pathol*, **9:** 111, 2001.

[52] Chaux, A., Cubilla, A. L.: Optimal management of T1G2 penile cancer remains unclear. *Nature Reviews Urology*, **10:** 9, 2012.

[53] Thuret, R., Sun, M., Abdollah, F. et al.: Competing-risks analysis in patients with T1 squamous cell carcinoma of the penis. *BJU Int,* **111:** E174, 2013.

[54] Spiess, P. E., National Comprehensive Cancer, N.: New treatment guidelines for penile cancer. *J Natl Compr Canc Netw*, **11:** 659, 2013.

[55] Kroon, B. K., Valdes Olmos, R. A., van Tinteren, H. et al.: Reproducibility of lymphoscintigraphy for lymphatic mapping in patients with penile carcinoma. *J Urol,* **174:** 2214, 2005.

[56] Grabstald, H.: Controversies concerning lymph node dissection for cancer of the penis. *Urol Clin North Am*, **7:** 793, 1980.

[57] Lont, A. P., Kroon, B. K., Gallee, M. P. et al.: Pelvic lymph node dissection for penile carcinoma: extent of inguinal lymph node involvement as an indicator for pelvic lymph node involvement and survival. *J Urol,* **177:** 947, 2007.

[58] Murrell, D. S., Williams, J. L.: Radiotherapy in the Treatment of Carcinoma of the Penis. *Br J Urol,* **37:** 211, 1965.

[59] Guimaraes, G. C., Cunha, I. W., Soares, F. A. et al.: Penile squamous cell carcinoma clinicopathological features, nodal metastasis and outcome in 333 cases. *J Urol*, **182:** 528, 2009.

[60] Clark, P. E., Spiess, P. E., Agarwal, N. et al.: Penile cancer: Clinical Practice Guidelines in Oncology. *J Natl Compr Canc Netw*, **11:** 594, 2013.

In: Penile Cancer: Challenges and Controversies
Editors: F. E. Martins and M. L. Djordjevic
ISBN: 978-1-53615-950-9

Chapter 18

MINIMALLY INVASIVE TECHNOLOGY IN GROIN LYMPH NODE DISSECTION: IMPACT ON MORBIDITY

Luis G. Medina**, Akbar Ashrafi and Rene Sotelo
University of Southern California, Institute of Urology,
Los Angeles, California, US

ABSTRACT

Penile cancer is a rare but debilitating cancer affecting older males. After treatment of the primary tumor, management of the regional inguinal lymph nodes is a cornerstone of surgical management. Open inguinal lymph node dissection has traditionally been associated with significant morbidity which can be physically disfiguring and pose significant psychological burden on patients. In this chapter, we review some of the concepts that have been explored to reduce the morbidity burden of inguinal lymph node dissection including improvements in patient selection for lymph node dissection, sentinel node biopsy, dynamic sentinel node biopsy, modified dissection templates and minimally invasive surgical approaches to inguinal lymph node dissection. In particular, we will focus on robotic-assisted and purely endoscopic inguinal lymph node dissection which may improve the complication rate without compromising oncological outcomes.

Keywords: penile cancer, minimally invasive, endoscopic, groin dissection, lymph node dissection, morbidity, complications, outcomes

* Corresponding Author's E-mail: L.medinanavarro@gmail.com; luis.medina@med.usc.edu.

INTRODUCTION

Penile cancer is a rare yet potentially devastating disease. Its incidence is associated to geographical region, race, age, and social factors. In Europe and in the US, the prevalence of penile squamous cell carcinoma (SCC) is estimated to be less than 0.5% of all malignancies in men [1]. However, in other regions of the world such as South America, South East of Asia and Africa, the prevalence can be as high as 2% of the malignancies. Penile SCC is more commonly seen in Hispanics, Alaskans, Native American and African Americans and is usually diagnosed in older men, although it may be seen in younger adults [2].

These regional trends may be explained by the social risk factors associated with penile cancer which include poverty, promiscuity, human papillomavirus infection, lower socioeconomic status, and bad hygiene. Further, a significant portion of patients seek medical attention late in the disease course and not immediately after identifying the primary penile lesion due to social stigma, misconceptions and embarrassment [3].

The primary landing site for penile SCC metastasis is the inguinal lymph nodes. Overall 5-year survival ranges from 19.3-53% in patients with regional metastasis to the inguinal lymph nodes [4]. A clinically palpable inguinal lymph node is a useful surrogate with pathological lymph node metastasis. Further, micrometastatic disease can be identified in 1 out of each 4 patients with clinically non-palpable inguinal nodes [5]. The presence and extent of inguinal lymph node metastasis is the most valuable predictor of long-term survival in patients with this uncommon, yet devastating cancer [6, 7]. Overall 5-year survival for patients with less than three positive nodes for penile cancer after they undergo inguinal lymphadenectomy is about 75.6%. On the other hand, 5-year survival is as low as 8.4% in patients with four or five positive nodes on pathological analysis [4]. Hence, surgical management of the inguinal nodes is of paramount importance in the prognostication and treatment of patients with penile cancer.

Bilateral inguinal lymph node dissection (ILND) is recommended in patients with intermediate or high-risk tumors after initial management of the primary tumor. Also, it should be performed in any patient with non-bulky palpable nodes less than 4cm in size and those with pathologically confirmed penile SCC on fine needle aspiration or node biopsy [8]. Despite these indications, recent data shows poor adherence to clinical guidelines by surgeons in USA when compared with Europe (27.2 vs 70%) despite the unquestionable evidence demonstrating an important survival advantage with ILND. This study also showed that, after analyzing the National Cancer Database of the American College of Surgeons, the patients that were more likely to undergo ILND were younger, presented with palpable adenopathy and were treated in academic facilities [9]. The risk of overtreatment together with the morbidity of the procedures may be the main reasons why urologists are hesitant or reluctant to perform ILND when indicated [5, 7, 9].

Historically, ILND has been linked with high morbidity rates. Gopman et al. reported the largest study assessing postoperative complications based on a retrospective multicenter study of 327 patients who underwent ILND and reported an overall complication rate of 55.4%. Moreover, other authors reported complication rates as high as 70% [10]. The most common and significant complications associated with ILND are skin flap necrosis, seroma, infection, lymphoceles, lymphorrhea and lymphedema. Further, these complications can have significant impact on quality of life.

Over the last decades, efforts have been made to improve patient selection and to reduce the morbidity derived from ILND by refining the technique or proposing new surgical approaches. The growing enthusiasm and utilization of minimally invasive surgery have led to the introduction of this approach in an effort to decrease morbidity and improve the quality of life in these patients without compromising oncological outcomes.

Herein, we will review the historical context, uptake and impact of minimally invasive techniques for inguinal lymph node dissection in penile cancer. We will describe initiatives to improve patient selection, and contemporary techniques with particular focus on minimally invasive endoscopic ILND.

Improvements in Patient Selection

Palpation of the inguinal region is not always reliable in identifying nodal metastasis in patients with penile cancer. In 1977, Cabanas et al. proposed the concept of sentinel lymph node biopsy for penile cancer, based on the assumption that the lymphatic spread of cancer cells follows a predictable pattern. The first group of nodes affected are the nodes in the superficial group, followed by the ones in the deep group and then the pelvic region, respectively [11]. It was proposed that a negative sentinel node biopsy would avoid unnecessary ILND and its associated morbidity, while only those with a positive sentinel node biopsy would proceed to ILND reducing overtreatment. The sentinel node biopsy technique involved the removal of a node found superomedial to the fossa ovalis. Nevertheless, this technique failed to gain widespread acceptance due to concerns regarding its false-negative rates [11, 12].

Later on, an extended sentinel node dissection was described arguing that false-negative results may improve by removing all the lymphatic tissue located between the inguinal ligament, the medial border of the saphenous vein and the superior external pudendal vein. This technique was abandoned as well after false-negative rates of 25% were reported in the initial series [6]. These techniques did not take into account an important principle: the lymphatic drainage of the inguinal area is dynamic, varies between patients and is not necessarily predictable in each and every patient.

Dynamic sentinel node biopsy (DSNB) was reported as an alternative following on from the lack of success of sentinel node biopsy together with the advent of lymphoscintigraphy that could potentially aid in the identification of patients in need of an ILND more efficiently, especially those with clinically negative groins, and avoid overtreatment [13]. To perform a DSNB, technetium-99m nanocolloid and blue dye injection are used for further imaging guidance with lymphoscintigraphy to identify a specific sentinel lymph node for each individual patient rather than excise in a specific anatomical location. However, false negatives still occurred using this technique. However, modifications of technique, improved experience and mastery of the procedure, and the addition of the preoperative ultrasound and intraoperative palpation have improved the false negative rate from 19.2% to 4.8% [14]. A comprehensive systematic review on DSNB reported a cumulative sensitivity and specificity of 84.4% and 99.4%, respectively [6]. Expertise in performing this procedure is crucial, particularly given other studies have reported false-negative rates as high as 22% [15]. The main disadvantage of the technique is that achieving expertise with this uncommon pathology is troublesome. The learning curve required to achieve proficiency, estimating 50 cases, is not that easy to do in rare diseases such as penile cancer. The National Comprehensive Cancer Network (8) has incorporated this aspect into its penile cancer guidelines and recommends that that DSNB should be done only when performed by expert hands [8, 14, 16].

Finally, some other patient characteristics have been studied to identify predictors of regional lymph node involvement. Based on these characteristics some nomograms and predictive models have already been proposed. The factors most commonly used are tumor stage, tumor grade, the presence of lymphovascular invasion, p53 mutations, and the expression of some molecular factors like Ki-67 or cadherins [17-19].

REFINING THE LYMPH NODE DISSECTION TEMPLATE

Parallel to the efforts made on patient selection described in the previous section, strategies to decrease the morbidity of the ILND were also proposed and evaluated to optimize the outcomes of traditional radical ILND. One of the first modifications to the technique was to perform a superficial dissection only in the first instance (superficial inguinal lymph node dissection). The superficial package includes the nodes located above to the fascia lata. These nodes are evaluated by the pathologist using frozen section. If superficial nodes are positive for malignancy, a deep inguinal lymph node dissection should be undertaken [20]. The rationale is that if the lymph nodes in the superficial compartment are negative, there should be no metastatic involvement of the nodes in the deep package. In a retrospective series reported by Spiess et al., none of the

31 patients with no nodal involvement after undergoing superficial lymph node dissection only reported recurrences after a median of follow-up of three years [21].

Nevertheless, some concern has been raised on the accuracy of this technique in properly identifying nodes affected by cancer. Chipollini et al, in a retrospective series of 84 patients, calculated the sensitivity and specificity of frozen section pathological analysis for penile SCC to be 74% and 100%, respectively. This implies that while this technique is specific, it does miss some positive nodes resulting in an incomplete resection, and thus compromising the patient's oncological care [22]. Hence some surgeons argue that both superficial and deep nodal packets should be removed to avoid undertreatment. Others are of the opinion of waiting for the final pathological evaluation of the superficial package and, if metastasis is confirmed, proceeding to the deep nodal dissection in a second stage procedure. The main disadvantage of this approach is that the patient is required to have a second procedure for complete inguinal node dissection. Further, the initial superficial dissection may make the subsequent second deep dissection more challenging and increased the risk of morbidity.

The limits of the traditional ILND dissection template are the sartorius muscle laterally, the inguinal ligament superiorly, and the adductor longus muscle medially. In the late 1980s, Catalona et al. proposed a modification of the dissection template and surgical approach to decrease the burden of morbidity while maintaining the same oncological outcomes. This modified template omits the field lateral to the femoral artery and distal to the saphenofemoral junction from the traditional dissection template, and promotes the preservation of the saphenous vein to decrease the lymphatic-related complication and avoid interposition of the Sartorius muscle [23].

Subsequent studies reported on outcomes using this technique showed worrisome results with regards to recurrence rates which reached values as high as 15%, this may suggest that the nodes located in the lateral quadrants should not be discarded from the dissection template. Additionally, mapping studies have found that positive nodes can be found in 10% and 23% of the cases in the superolateral and inferolateral quadrants, respectively [24, 25].

ENDOSCOPIC LYMPH NODE DISSECTION

Eventually, minimally invasive surgery (MIS) was introduced in penile cancer surgical management as in many other fields in urologic oncology to decrease length of stay, reduce recovery time and improve the morbidity from skin-related and lymph-related postoperative complications, The theoretical advantages of this approach are that it reduces interruption of the blood supply to the skin provided by the branches of the femoral artery and preserves the collateral lymphatic channels that made their way up through Camper's fascia. It has been proposed that the incidence of skin-related and lymph-related complications will be improved by preserving the skin and subcutaneous vascular and lymphatic channels.

The first report of an endoscopic ILND (EILND) was published in 2003 in cadavers and humans [26]. Subsequently, Tobias-Machado et al. reported the first series from Brazil on EILND that consisted of 15 consecutive patients of which ten patients underwent open ILND in one side and EILND on the other and another five patients had bilateral EILND. No differences were found in terms of number of nodes removed (9.7 vs. 10.8; p = 0.4). EILND was associated with longer operative times (120 vs. 92 min; p = 0.0002), shorter times to reach a drain tube output of <50 mL per day (4.9 vs. 6.4; p = 0.008), and a significant lower complication rates (70 vs. 20%; p = 0.01), which was probably driven by the marked difference in skin-related complications in favor of EILND (5 vs. 50%; p = 0.009) [27].

In 2007, Sotelo et al. reported another series on 14 inguinal endoscopic ILNDs in eight patients with an average node yield of 9 nodes [4-15]. No wound-related complications were seen on these cases and only three lymphoceles were reported [28]. For the endoscopic approach, overall minor and major complications occur 27, and 14.6% of the cases, respectively [29]. Wang et al. reported a series comparing sixteen and eighteen patients who underwent EILND and traditional open ILND, respectively [30].When baseline characteristics were compared, the only difference found was a higher node size in the open group (2.66 vs. 1.66 cm; p = 0.03). No differences were seen between the endoscopic and open arms regarding operative time (169.8 vs. 139.5 min; p = 0.08), total lymph node yield (10.78 vs. 12.60; p = 0.24), or hospital stay (10.43 vs. 12.50 days; p = 0.15). EILND was associated with less intraoperative blood loss (22.50 vs. 68.44 ml, p = 0.00), shorter drainage tube removal time (7.23 vs. 11.4 days; p = 0.00). Additionally, the overall complication rate (21.05 vs. 61.90; p = 0.01), skin necrosis rate (5.3 vs. 28.6; p = 0.04), and lymphocele rate (0 vs. 4.8; p = 0.02) were all in favor of EILND. Saphenous vein preservation was not performed in any of these cases [30].

The first robotic ILND (RILND) was published later in 2009 using the Si Da Vinci Surgical System [31]. No complications were reported with this initial patient. Potential advantages of robotic surgery were the tridimensional view, improved ergonomics, elimination of the tremor, greater magnification and range of motion in a limited working space leading to greater dexterity and a shorter learning curve. However, it was an unpractical procedure at the moment because it needed to be performed in a staged manner because of the operative room configuration needed with the robotic system. In order to overcome this difficulty, the first simultaneous bilateral ILND without robot repositioning was described by Sotelo et al. [32]. Bilateral dissections when an ILND is performed is a basic principle of the surgical management of penile cancer. The lymphatic drainage of the penis converges at the root of the penis below the pubic symphysis. Importantly, the lymphatic circulation can crossover here which makes it possible to have contralateral and bilateral lymph node metastasis from a single unilateral primary penile cancer lesion.

At present, MIS ILND seemed a feasible, safe procedure with lower complications rates that the standard ILND based on retrospective studies. Yet, it was not until the study by Matin et al. from the M.D Anderson Cancer Center that oncological equivalence was demonstrated. In this phase 1 prospective study, 10 patients with T1-3 N0 penile cancer underwent RILND and an expert open surgical oncologist would inspect the surgical field looking for residual nodes after a robotic ILND was performed. No differences in the number of positive nodes was found when both procedures were compared. The verifying surgeon confirmed two residual lymph nodes in only one out of 19 fields evaluated and none of these nodes were positive for cancer [33]. In summary, data to date leads us to infer that the morbidity of an endoscopic ILND is lower than what has been stated for the standard open series with equivalent oncological outcomes. A systematic review on RILND for melanoma, penile cancer and vulvar cancer reported that the most frequent complications of this procedure are lymphoceles (13.7%), cellulitis (7.8%), lymphedema (7.8%), skin breakdown/infection (3.9%), abscess (3.9%), seromas (3.9%), sepsis (1.9%) and skin complications (1.9%). No intraoperative complications were recorded [34].

Different studies evaluating differences between MIS approaches and open ILND have been reported. Preliminary results from a series from the MD Anderson Cancer Center reported a retrospective series comparing 36 groins that underwent RILND versus 34 open superficial ILND cases. No differences were found in terms of lymph node yield (26.7 vs. 25.8), overall complication rate per patient (27.8 vs. 35%), wound complications (19.4 vs. 23.5%). RILND was associated with significantly longer operative times (372.2 vs. 261.6 min; $p = <0.01$) [35].

Singh et al. published a comparative study based on a retrospective series of 51 patients who underwent RILND and 100 patients who received open ILND. Baseline characteristics were comparable between groups except the RILND patients were significantly older when compared to the open group (58 vs. 54 years; $p = 0.04$). With regards to postoperative and oncological outcomes, RILND was associated with longer median operative time (75 vs. 60 minutes; $p = <0.0001$), shorter hospital stay (3 vs. 4 days, $p = 0.0008$), lower duration of surgical drain (12 vs. 15 days; $p = <0.0001$), lower major complications rate (2 vs. 17%; $p = 0.006$), lower skin edge necrosis (9.8 vs. 23%; $p = 0.04$), lower flap necrosis (2 vs. 13%; $p = 0.03$) and lower severe lymphedema (0 vs. 9%; $p = 0.02$). No differences were seen in terms of intraoperative complications, intraoperative blood loss, lymphocele rate, surgical site infections and early or late limb edema. A multivariable analysis was also performed to select variables associated with major complications, and found that pathological nodal stage and open ILND were independent risk factors for the occurrence of major complications [36].

To our knowledge, there is only one study comparing EILND with RILND. Russel et al. published a retrospective comparative series of comprised of 27 and 7 patients who underwent the robotic and laparoscopic approaches, respectively. No differences were found regarding the depth of the dissection, number of nodes resected, number of positive nodes identified, pathological node status, operative time, time to drain removal or estimated blood loss. RILND had equivalent overall complication rates when compared with EILND (11 vs. 43%; p = 0.09). Saphenous vein preservation was more common in the robotic cohort (100 vs. 57%; p = <0.01). Interestingly, significant lower complication rates were seen in patients with saphenous sparing procedures (p = 0.02). This could explain why the RILND had a clear trend towards lower complications compared to the purely laparoscopic approach [37]. However, more studies are required in this regard. The choice of minimally invasive approach to ILND will also largely depend on surgeon preference and equipment/robot availability.

Surgical Technique

The patient is placed in lithotomy position. This position allows access to both groins and allows the surgeon and assistant surgeon to easily switch positions to facilitate bilateral EILND. For the right EILND, the surgeon stands lateral to the right lower extremity and the assistant surgeon stands between the legs. For the left EILND, the surgeon stands between the legs, and the assistant stands lateral to the left lower extremity. A urethral Foley catheter is placed. The surgical field is prepared and draped in a traditional fashion ensuring full exposure form the anterior superior iliac spine down to the knees bilaterally. Anatomic landmarks are palpated and recognized on the skin surface and an inverted triangle is marked out which includes the inguinal ligament, the sartorius muscle laterally, and the adductor longus muscle medially. Identification of the anatomy at this point is crucial in ensuring correct port placement and complete dissection of the whole anatomical template.

We describe three-port three-step technique for pure endoscopic EILND which is simple and reproducible. A 2-cm vertical incision is made 3 cm inferior to the apex of the triangle (which is approximately 25 cm below the inguinal ligament) (Figure 1). Scarpa's fascia is recognized as a white subcutaneous layer below the subcutaneous tissue. The index finger is used in a sweeping manner to dissect this plane and create a space underneath the Scarpa's plane. The index finger is used to guide the initial dissection of the skin flap. A 10mm camera port is placed is placed at the initial incision site. A purse string suture is placed to approximate the camera port skin incision and prevent gas leak during insufflation. The skin flap is further extended with the endoscope by sweeping the space within the inverted triangle with one hand with simultaneous palpation with the other hand to ensure skin flap thickness. This step strives to generate a subcutaneous flap beneath the plane of Scarpa's fascia.

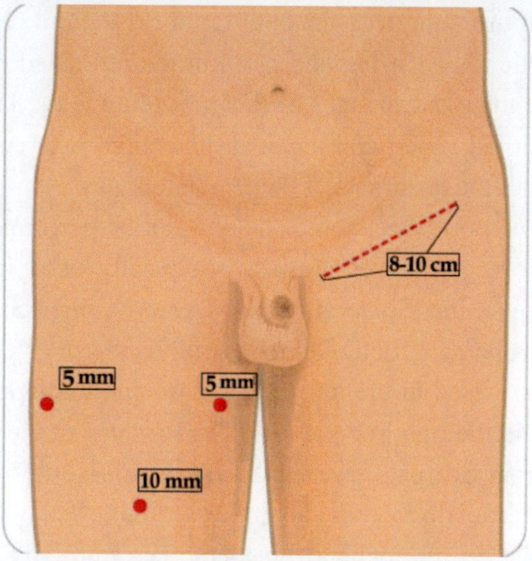

Figure 1. Representation of the surgical wounds after open inguinal lymph node dissection (right side) and inguinal lymph node dissection with the tri-port technique (left).

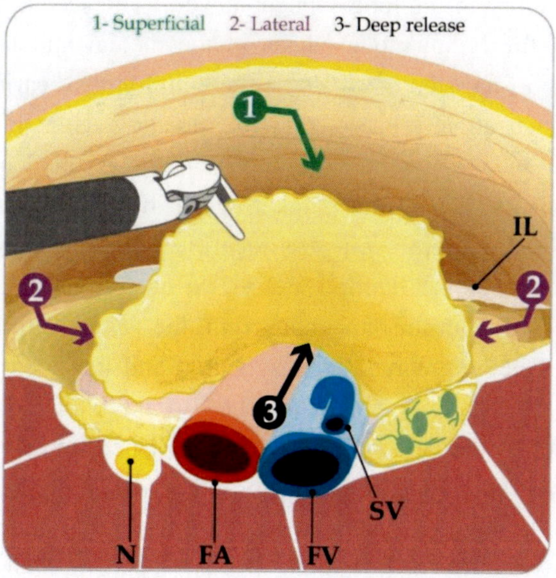

Figure 2. Superficial package being removed along with saphenous vein preservation. N: femoral nerve; SV: saphenous vein; FV: femoral vein; FA: femoral artery. Superficial, lateral and deep release are shown.

Once the skin flap is created, insufflation pressure is fixed at 20 mm Hg for 10 minutes to establish the working field. Insufflation pressure is reduced to 15 mm Hg after that, and a 0-degree 10 mm endoscope. Two 5mm trocars are placed laterally and medially, respectively, cranial to the camera port to facilitate triangulation. For robotic EILND, two 8mm robotic ports are placed. An additional 5mm assistant port may be placed between the camera and right-sided port if required. For robotic EILND, the robot is can be docked from the same side for both groin dissections. Typically, we dock the robot lateral to the patient's right leg and perform the left sided dissection followed by the right side. One the many advantages of this procedure is the fact that the template is not limited to the modified superficial inguinal dissection, with endoscopic ILND nodes will be removed from all the quadrants of the template.

The simplified three-port three-step technique can be performed with a camera port and two additional ports. A bowel grasper is typically used in the left arm and a Harmonic device (Ethicon Inc. Somerville, New Jersey, United States) in the right hand during EILND. For robotic EILND, bipolar Maryland, or PK forceps® (Olympus, Hamburg, Germany) are used in the left robotic arm, and monopolar scissors or robotic ultrasonic instruments in the right robotic arm. The first step of the three-step is to release the fibrofatty tissue from Scarpa's fascia (superficial release) (Figure 2). The fibrofatty tissue is dissected superficially across the entire anatomic template beginning caudally and continuing cephalad to the inguinal ligament. The fibrofatty tissue is continuously rolled or retracted inferiorly during this step. The tissue is dissected from the inguinal ligament, the spermatic cord and the external oblique aponeurosis cranially. Care is taken to avoid inadvertent injury to the long saphenous vein. The second step is to release the lateral attachment of the lymph node packet at the medial and lateral borders of the template. The third and final step is to release the lymph node-bearing tissue from fascia lata (deep release) from an inferior to superior direction using both, sharp and blunt dissection (Figures 3 and 4). The nodal tissue is initially rolled or retracted cranially using blunt dissection. Particular care is taken when dissecting in the femoral triangle. The femoral artery and femoral vein are identified and preserved during the deep dissection. The pulsation of the femoral artery is a useful anatomical reference. If the tissue cannot be released from the saphenous vein, the vein is clipped using Hem-o-lok clips (Weck clips®, Teleflex, Wayne, Pennsylvania) and ligated at the saphenofemoral junction. When the lymphatic tissue is attached to the saphenous arch, the venous tributaries are clipped. Any other prominent feeding or perforated vessels are dissected, clipped and ligated as required. The dissection continues cranially and any remaining deep attachments to the inguinal ligament are divided. At this point, the nodal tissue is rolled inferiorly to provide maximal traction. The left hand can be used to hold the tissue away and provide counter-traction while the deeper dissection is performed with the Harmonic scalpel. Visualization of the fascia of the adductor and sartorius muscles and further correlating the internal dissection with the previously made skin marks aids in the delineating the external and medial borders of the resection. If a deep inguinal node dissection is carried out, the fascia lata medial to the saphenous arch is incised to reveal the saphenofemoral junction. Inferomedial dissection around the femoral vein facilitates resection of the deep package [29]. Dissection should follow the femoral canal until the pectineus muscle is revealed to ensure proper dissection. The superficial and deep nodal packets are removed en-bloc. A 5mm camera is used and the specimen is placed into a

10mm Endocatch bag passed through the main 10mm port. At the end of this dissection, the inguinal ligament is recognized as a transverse array of white fibers and the spermatic cord can be seen at the superomedial limit of the dissection.

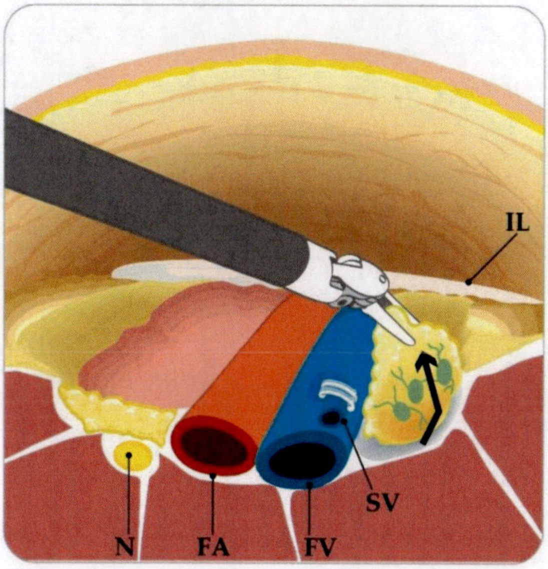

Figure 3. Deep lymph node dissection resection. N: femoral nerve; SV: saphenous vein; FV: femoral vein; FA: femoral artery; IL: Inguinal Ligament.

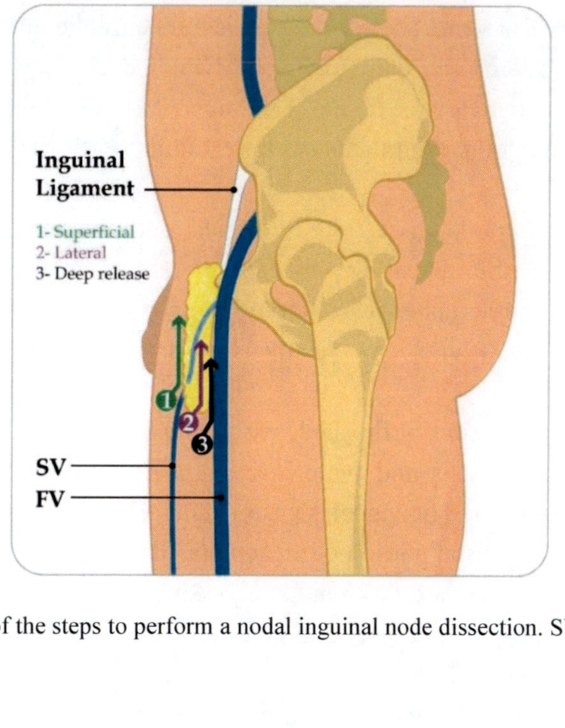

Figure 4. Lateral view of the steps to perform a nodal inguinal node dissection. SV: saphenous vein; FV: femoral vein.

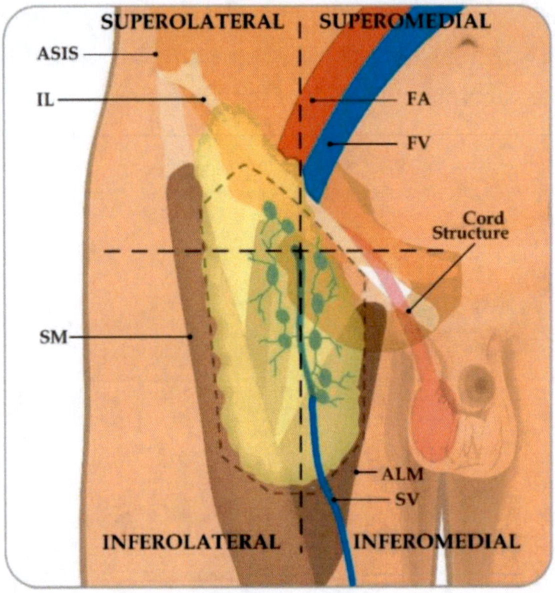

Figure 5. Graphic representation of the inguinal groin anatomy plus limits of the dissections. IL: inguinal ligament; FA: femoral artery; FV: femoral vein; ASIS: Anterior superior iliac spine; SM: Sartorius muscle; SV: Saphenous vein; ALM: Adductor longus muscle.

An alternative approach to this technique is to release the lymph node-bearing tissue from the deeper layers as the first step, again proceeding in an inferior to superior direction to the inguinal ligament Particular care is taken to dissect the fibrofatty tissue off the femoral artery and vein. The second step is to release the lateral attachments at the limit of the anatomic template, and finally the lymph node-bearing tissue is dissected superficially away from Scarpa's fascia. The superficial and deep nodes are similarly removed en-bloc through the central camera port. Limits of the dissection are depicted in Figure 5.

If a deep inguinal node dissection is carried out, the fascia lata medial to the saphenous arch is incised to reveal the saphenofemoral junction. Inferomedial dissection around the femoral vein facilitates resection of the deep package [29]. Dissection should follow the femoral canal until the pectineus muscle is revealed to ensure proper dissection.

When the node dissection is finished, we lower the insufflation to 5 mm Hg and ensure appropriate hemostasis and lymphatic channels which is critical to avoid the formation of hematomas and lymphoceles postoperatively. A closed Jackson Pratt suction drain is positioned in the distal portion of the template via one of the 5mm ports. Surgical incisions are closed in a standard fashion. Compressive dressing is applied. The patient is allowed to ambulate the day of surgery and given a regular diet. Oral antibiotics are given until the drains are removed. Drains are removed with the output becomes less than 50 mL per day. Thromboembolism prophylaxis is provided to all patients with unfractionated heparin or low-molecular-weight heparin during the hospital stay. Compressive garments are used for three months after surgery.

ROBOTIC VERSUS ENDOSCOPIC ILND

Nowadays, there are no studies comparing robotic versus purely endoscopic ILND. No advantage has been demonstrated of the robotic approach over the endoscopic one so far. In our experience, the purely endoscopic procedure is simple, has a lower operating time, can be performed routinely with three ports only and uses smaller 5mm ports. On the other hand, ergonomics and the 3D view are potential advantages with the robotic approach.

For both MIS ILND, the creation of the working space is performed in a similar way. However, the size of the ports is different between techniques. The two approaches use rigid ultrasonic instruments which can be troublesome if a specific angulation of the instrument is required for lymph vessel sealing.

The new Xi robotic platform has several benefits over the Si system. First, the system can be repositioned easily. Second, it allows intraoperative rotation of the camera and the camera can be used from any of the ports. Enthusiasm has been raised as well with the new single port robotic platform by perhaps reducing skin complications at its maximum without increasing the complexity of the procedure. Single-site video endoscopic ILND was also described. This technique proposes a three-port technique to decrease even more cutaneous complications [38]. However, extreme interference of the instruments in the working field is one of the difficulties with this technique.

ADJUNCT PROCEDURES

The robotic platform also allows the capacity to use indocyanine green (ICG) during groin dissection. There is some data that ICG can facilitate the identification of lymphatics leaks and possibly bypass these complications [39]. A study published by Bjurlin in 2017 described and reported a very successful experience using this technology. Intradermal ICG is administer at the base of the phallus, visualization of the lymphatic circulation should be evident after 15 minutes. A total of 10 RILND were performed on this series with mean node yield of 7 [5-13], mean operative time 207 min (164-258), mean estimated blood loss was 38 ml [25-50], mean hospital stay 1.8 days (0-4) [39]. They report complete identification of the lymphatic drainage pattern from the superficial package towards the deep one in all the patients. Not a single complication in this series with a median follow up of 10 months was reported whilst the pathologically involved nodes were visualized using the near infrared fluorescence imaging.

INGUINAL LYMPH NODE DISSECTION MORBIDITY

ILND is a staging and therapeutic procedure which saves lives. However, it is considered a morbid procedure which adds considerably distress to patients that suffer from an already disfiguring initial management of the primary lesion. This is why efforts have been made to improve patient selection, refine the surgical technique for open ILND and proposing new minimally invasive approaches to decrease rates of overtreatment and morbidity associated with it.

There is no standardization in the reporting methods for postoperative complications after ILND in the literature, compromising the adequacy of the analysis and comparisons made on several papers within the literature. Further, another important factor is that penile cancer is a rare disease and it is not easy to perform big prospective randomized studies.

Using Clavien-Dindo classification Gopman et al. reported the overall complication rate for open ILND to be 55.4%. The majority of those complications (65.7%) were deemed to be minor. The number of nodes removed was identified as an independent predictor for complications, which supports the proposal of limiting the dissection templates or performing deep package dissection only when necessary to try and reduce significant morbidity [10]. Other predictors for complications were Sartorius interposition and increased age. Interposition of the sartorius muscle is unnecessary with EILND which may confer some of the benefits in morbidity seen with this approach.

Skin complications are mainly infectious or associated to ischemia (0.6-43% of all the complications) [10, 40, 41]. One factor that may impact infectious complications is the proper antibiotic usage targeting for gram negative rods as well as gram positive cocci (i.e., Diphterioids, staphylococcus). Further, in the past, it was thought that up to 50% of the clinically palpable nodes were linked to inflammatory or infective lymphadenitis rather than metastatic involvement. Current guidelines however do not recommend delay in lymph node management for empirical treatment with antibiotics. There is no good evidence of benefit with bowel preparation or enemas prior the procedure. However, caution should be taken of not prolonging the time for ILND given that there is evidence that late ILND (defined as an ILND performed 3 months after the management of the primary lesion) is associated with poorer oncological outcomes, specifically increased recurrences and decreased survival. The most frequent causes for the delay were referral to a tertiary center and neoadjuvant treatments prior to the groin dissection [42].

Preservation of the blood supply of the skin that goes through the subcutaneous plane of Campers fascia and a meticulous postoperative care are critical to avoid ischemic skin complications. Theoretically, endoscopic techniques address this specific complication for ILND by limiting the amount of skin affected during the surgery. A prospective study showed that endoscopic ILND may retrieve a higher number overall and positive nodes and a significant decrease on major complications (5 vs 68%). However, the two populations were very heterogeneous [43, 44]. On the other hand, preoperative anticoagulation may play a role on the appearance of skin complications. It has been said that heparin may pose a risk for wound hematomas [45]. However, most authors still recommend low molecular weight heparin subcutaneously pre- and post-operatively to decrease the risk of deep vein thrombosis. Early ambulation is also recommended in this regard although there are conflicting opinions with some physicians suggesting early ambulation may increase lymphatic leak as the lymphatic channels have not had enough time to regenerate themselves. They recommend bed rest for a week after the procedure ([44]). Another aspect to take into consideration is the use of compressive garments. If they are used, they should be used from the ankles all the way up until few centimeters below the umbilicus. The use of elastic garments can be used for about 6 months after the procedure, care should be taken of using them in cases were the flap was deemed to be too thin may cause or exacerbate skin necrosis by reducing the skin blood flow.

Another concept is that if the fascia lata is preserved during the ILND postoperative complications may be reduced by ensuring enough pressure in the anterior muscle compartment of the thigh allowing a better flow of blood of lymphatic fluid though the collateral vessels within the muscle ([46]. Omental flap pediculoplasty was also proposed to decrease the lymphedema rates. This was first reported by Benoit et al. in combined pelvic and open approaches during which the omental flap is mobilized and passed below the inguinal ligament to the surgical field [46]. The initial report was based on seven patients of which none of them reported lymphedema, skin necrosis or infectious complications. Obviously, the main disadvantage that additional extraperitoneal access is needed in these cases which has its own potential morbidity and sequelae.

Seromas and lymphatic complications occur in up to 26.5% of the patients (2.4-26.5%). [10, 40]. Historically, drains are left in place until the measured output of the drain goes below 50 cc per day, which is usually two weeks after the procedure. Some surgeons see the time to drain removal as a surrogate of a good surgery and may remove drains before it is advisable to do so. If fluid accumulates in the area after early drain removal the patient may need to go through multiple needle aspirations to treat a lymphatic collection with increased risk of infections complications. On the other hand, excessive drain time can also increase the risk of complications due to colonization of the drains. One of the other considerations with regards to drain management is whether to use bulb suction or not. In our experience, we believe that suctioning systems may lengthen and increase the inflammatory reaction on the surgical area which could prolong the closing of lymphatic channels in the postoperative period. Surgically, saphenous vein preservation was proposed by Catalona et al. to decrease lymphatic complications by improving the lymph circulation of the region [23]. A study performed in patients undergoing ILND for vulvar cancer showed a 30% decreased in overall complication rate when saphenous vein is spared [47]. In the same manner, a randomized comparison published in 2016 also identify that sparing of the saphenous vein diminished the lymphedema rates by more than 25% [9, 44].

The energy mechanism used for the intraoperative management of the lymph vessels may be important. Some authors argue that ultrasonic energy may be superior to electrocautery [48, 49]. Our experience also suggests that the ultrasonic devices are effective in controlling lymphatic channels during ILND. Fibrin sealants haven also been proposed to seal leaking lymphatic capillaries or fill dead spaces in the surgical area, avoiding accumulation of other fluids in the area [44]. Yet, more data on the impact of the energy used or the application of fibrin sealants on postoperative complications are needed.

Conclusion

The presence and extent of lymph node metastasis is the most important prognostic factor in penile cancer. Inguinal lymph node dissection is a cornerstone of surgical management in penile squamous cell carcinoma. The indications for inguinal lymph node dissection are clinically palpable lymph nodes and intermediate or high-risk primary tumors in patients with clinically non-palpable lymph node. Traditional open ILND is associated with significant morbidity which may explain the poor uptake of this important procedure in patients who would most benefit from it. Dynamic sentinel node biopsy for penile cancer is associated with significant false negative rates (approximately 5-19% with contemporary techniques). Minimally invasive inguinal lymph node techniques must be able to replicate the oncological principle of open dissection including bilateral groin dissection and dissection of both the superficial and deep nodes. Several studies have demonstrated that endoscopic ILND appears to offer similar lymph node yield while reducing post-operative pain, length of hospital stay and major post-operative complications compared to open ILND.

Key Points

- Lymph node metastasis is the most important prognostic factor in penile cancer.
- Lymph node dissection is thus of paramount importance in the diagnostic and therapeutic management of patients with penile cancer.

- The significant morbidity and adverse quality of life associated with traditional open inguinal lymph node dissection have led to several innovations to try and reduce the skin and lymphatic complications after inguinal lymph node dissection.
- Endoscopic inguinal lymph node dissection using a purely endoscopic or a robotic-assisted approach has been shown to be safe and feasible.
- The potential benefits of minimally invasive inguinal lymph node dissection with regards perioperative outcomes include improved cosmesis and scarring, reduced blood loss, improved pain control, shorter length of stay, faster recovery and reduced skin, lymphatic and infectious complications without compromising lymph node yield.
- Longer term data on oncological efficacy of endoscopic inguinal lymph node dissection will confirm the role of minimally invasive ILND within the urological landscape.

REFERENCES

[1] Christodoulidou M, Sahdev V, Houssein S, Muneer A. Epidemiology of penile cancer. *Curr Probl Cancer*. 2015;39(3):126-36.

[2] Chaux A NG, Rodríguez IM, Barreto JE, Oertell J, Ocampos S, Boggino H, Codas R, Xavier Bosch F, de Sanjose S, Muñoz N, Hildesheim A, Cubilla AL. Epidemiologic profile, sexual history, pathologic features, and human papillomavirus status of 103 patients with penile carcinoma. *World J Urol.* 2013;31(4):861-7.

[3] Torbrand C, Wigertz A, Drevin L, Folkvaljon Y, Lambe M, Hakansson U, et al. Socioeconomic factors and penile cancer risk and mortality; a population-based study. *BJU Int.* 2017;119(2):254-60.

[4] Pandey D, Mahajan V, Kannan RR. Prognostic factors in node-positive carcinoma of the penis. *J Surg Oncol.* 2006;93(2):133-8.

[5] Slaton JW, Morgenstern N, Levy DA, Santos MW, Jr., Tamboli P, Ro JY, et al. Tumor stage, vascular invasion and the percentage of poorly differentiated cancer: independent prognosticators for inguinal lymph node metastasis in penile squamous cancer. *J Urol.* 2001;165(4):1138-42.

[6] Pettaway CA, Pisters LL, Dinney CP, Jularbal F, Swanson DA, von Eschenbach AC, et al. Sentinel lymph node dissection for penile carcinoma: the M. D. Anderson Cancer Center experience. *J Urol*. 1995;154(6):1999-2003.

[7] Pizzocaro G, Algaba F, Horenblas S, Solsona E, Tana S, Van Der Poel H, et al. EAU penile cancer guidelines 2009. *Eur Urol*. 2010;57(6):1002-12.

[8] https://www.nccn.org/store/login/login.aspx?ReturnURL=https://www.nccn.org/professionals/physician_gls/pdf/penile.pdf. Accessed February 19, 2019. NCCNPCV.

[9] Correa AF, Handorf E, Joshi SS, Geynisman DM, Kutikov A, Chen DY, et al. Differences in Survival Associated with Performance of Lymph Node Dissection in Patients with Invasive Penile Cancer: Results from the National Cancer Database. *J Urol.* 2018;199(5):1238-44.

[10] Gopman JM, Djajadiningrat RS, Baumgarten AS, Espiritu PN, Horenblas S, Zhu Y, et al. Predicting postoperative complications of inguinal lymph node dissection for penile cancer in an international multicentre cohort. *BJU Int.* 2015;116(2):196-201.

[11] Cabanas RM. An approach for the treatment of penile carcinoma. *Cancer.* 1977;39(2):456-66.

[12] Srinivas V, Joshi A, Agarwal B, Mundhada U, Shah A, Phadke AG. Penile cancer--the sentinel lymph node controversy. *Urol Int.* 1991;47(2):108-9.

[13] Leijte JA, Kroon BK, Valdes Olmos RA, Nieweg OE, Horenblas S. Reliability and safety of current dynamic sentinel node biopsy for penile carcinoma. *Eur Urol.* 2007;52(1):170-7.

[14] Leijte JA, Hughes B, Graafland NM, Kroon BK, Olmos RA, Nieweg OE, et al. Two-center evaluation of dynamic sentinel node biopsy for squamous cell carcinoma of the penis. *J Clin Oncol.* 2009;27(20):3325-9.

[15] Tanis PJ LA, Meinhardt W, Olmos RA, Nieweg OE, Horenblas S. Dynamic sentinel node biopsy for penile cancer: reliability of a staging technique. *J Urol.* 2002;168(1):76-80.

[16] Neto AS, Tobias-Machado M, Ficarra V, Wroclawski ML, Amarante RD, Pompeo AC, et al. Dynamic sentinel node biopsy for inguinal lymph node staging in patients with penile cancer: a systematic review and cumulative analysis of the literature. *Ann Surg Oncol.* 2011;18(7):2026-34.

[17] Ficarra V, Zattoni F, Artibani W, Fandella A, Martignoni G, Novara G, et al. Nomogram predictive of pathological inguinal lymph node involvement in patients with squamous cell carcinoma of the penis. *J Urol.* 2006;175(5):1700-4; discussion 4-5.

[18] Zhu Y, Zhang HL, Yao XD, Zhang SL, Dai B, Shen YJ, et al. Development and evaluation of a nomogram to predict inguinal lymph node metastasis in patients with penile cancer and clinically negative lymph nodes. *J Urol.* 2010;184(2):539-45.

[19] Zhu Y, Zhou XY, Yao XD, Dai B, Ye DW. The prognostic significance of p53, Ki-67, epithelial cadherin and matrix metalloproteinase-9 in penile squamous cell carcinoma treated with surgery. *BJU Int.* 2007;100(1):204-8.

[20] Puras-Baez A R-HJ, Miranda G, et al. Role of superficial inguinal lymphadenectomy in carcinoma of the penis. *J Urol.* 1995;153(246A).

[21] Spiess PE, Izawa JI, Bassett R, Kedar D, Busby JE, Wong F, et al. Preoperative lymphoscintigraphy and dynamic sentinel node biopsy for staging penile cancer: results with pathological correlation. *J Urol.* 2007;177(6):2157-61.

[22] Chipollini J, Tang DH, Manimala N, Gilbert SM, Pow-Sang JM, Sexton WJ, et al. Evaluating the accuracy of intraoperative frozen section during inguinal lymph node dissection in penile cancer. *Urol Oncol.* 2018;36(1):14 e1- e5.

[23] Catalona WJ. Modified inguinal lymphadenectomy for carcinoma of the penis with preservation of saphenous veins: technique and preliminary results. *J Urol.* 1988;140(2):306-10.

[24] Bouchot O, Rigaud J, Maillet F, Hetet JF, Karam G. Morbidity of inguinal lymphadenectomy for invasive penile carcinoma. *Eur Urol.* 2004;45(6):761-5; discussion 5-6.

[25] d'Ancona CA, de Lucena RG, Querne FA, Martins MH, Denardi F, Netto NR, Jr. Long-term followup of penile carcinoma treated with penectomy and bilateral modified inguinal lymphadenectomy. *J Urol.* 2004;172(2):498-501; discussion

[26] Bishoff J, Basler JW, Teichman JM. Endoscopic subcutaneous modified inguinal lymph node dissection (ESMIL) for squamous cell carcinoma of the penis. *J Urol.* 2003;169(78).

[27] Tobias-Machado M, Tavares A, Ornellas AA, Molina WR, Jr., Juliano RV, Wroclawski ER. Video endoscopic inguinal lymphadenectomy: a new minimally invasive procedure for radical management of inguinal nodes in patients with penile squamous cell carcinoma. *J Urol.* 2007;177(3):953-7; discussion 8.

[28] Sotelo R, Sanchez-Salas R, Carmona O, Garcia A, Mariano M, Neiva G, et al. Endoscopic lymphadenectomy for penile carcinoma. *J Endourol.* 2007;21(4):364-7; discussion 7.

[29] Master VA, Jafri SM, Moses KA, Ogan K, Kooby DA, Delman KA. Minimally invasive inguinal lymphadenectomy via endoscopic groin dissection: comprehensive assessment of immediate and long-term complications. *J Urol.* 2012;188(4):1176-80.

[30] Wang S DP, Tang X, An C, Zhang N, Yang Y. Comparison of Efficiency of Video Endoscopy and Open Inguinal Lymph Node Dissection. *Anticancer Res.* 2017;37(8):4623-8.

[31] Josephson DY, Jacobsohn KM, Link BA, Wilson TG. Robotic-assisted endoscopic inguinal lymphadenectomy. *Urology*. 2009;73(1):167-70; discussion 70-1.

[32] Sotelo R, Cabrera M, Carmona O, de Andrade R, Martin O, Fernandez G. Robotic bilateral inguinal lymphadenectomy in penile cancer, development of a technique without robot repositioning: a case report. *Ecancermedicalscience*. 2013;7:356.

[33] Matin SF, Cormier JN, Ward JF, Pisters LL, Wood CG, Dinney CP, et al. Phase 1 prospective evaluation of the oncological adequacy of robotic assisted video-

endoscopic inguinal lymphadenectomy in patients with penile carcinoma. *BJU Int.* 2013;111(7):1068-74.

[34] Gkegkes ID ME, Iavazzo C. Robotic-assisted inguinal lymphadenectomy: a systematic review. *J Robot Surg.* 2018.

[35] McCormick B MM, Papadopoulos J, Matin S, Pettaway C. Robotic assisted inguinal lymph node dissection (RAIL) for clinical node negative penile squamous carcinoma: recent results from the MD Anderson cancer center (MDACC) experience and comparison to a contemporary open cohort. *J Urol*. 2018;199(4S).

[36] Singh A JJ, Goel A, Shah S, Bhardwaj R, Baidya S, Jain J, Jain C, Rawal S. Comparing Outcomes of Robotic and Open Inguinal Lymph Node Dissection in Patients with Carcinoma of the Penis. *J Urol*. 2018;199(6):1518-25.

[37] Russell CM SS, Niemann A, Weizer AZ, Tomlins SA, Morgan TM, Montgomery JS. Minimally Invasive Inguinal Lymphadenectomy in the Management of Penile Carcinoma. *Urology*. 2017;106:113-8.

[38] Tobias-Machado M, Correa WF, Reis LO, Starling ES, de Castro Neves O, Juliano RV, et al. Single-site video endoscopic inguinal lymphadenectomy: initial report. *J Endourol.* 2011;25(4):607-10.

[39] Bjurlin MA, Zhao LC, Kenigsberg AP, Mass AY, Taneja SS, Huang WC. Novel Use of Fluorescence Lymphangiography During Robotic Groin Dissection for Penile Cancer. *Urology.* 2017;107:267.

[40] Koifman L, Hampl D, Koifman N, Vides AJ, Ornellas AA. Radical open inguinal lymphadenectomy for penile carcinoma: surgical technique, early complications and late outcomes. *J Urol.* 2013;190(6):2086-92.

[41] Stuiver MM, Djajadiningrat RS, Graafland NM, Vincent AD, Lucas C, Horenblas S. Early wound complications after inguinal lymphadenectomy in penile cancer: a historical cohort study and risk-factor analysis. *Eur Urol.* 2013;64(3):486-92.

[42] Chipollini J, Tang DH, Gilbert SM, Poch MA, Pow-Sang JM, Sexton WJ, et al. Delay to Inguinal Lymph Node Dissection Greater than 3 Months Predicts Poorer Recurrence-Free Survival for Patients with Penile Cancer. *J Urol.* 2017;198(6):1346-52.

[43] Kumar V, Sethia KK. Prospective study comparing video-endoscopic radical inguinal lymph node dissection (VEILND) with open radical ILND (OILND) for penile cancer over an 8-year period. *BJU Int.* 2017;119(4):530-4.

[44] Pompeo AC HC, Abrams P. Management of the lymph nodes in penile cancer. In: CF H, editor. *Penile Cancer.* 1st ed. Santiago, Chile: Societe Internationale d' Urologie; 2009. p. 133-75.

[45] Tomic R, Granfors T, Sjodin JG, Ohberg L. Lymph leakage after staging pelvic lymphadenectomy for prostatic carcinoma with and without heparin prophylaxis. *Scand J Urol Nephrol.* 1994;28(3):273-5.

[46] Gupta MK PA, Master VA. Technical considerations to minimize complications of inguinal lymph node dissection. *Transl Androl Urol.* 2017;6(5):820-5.

[47] Zhang SH SA, Sorosky JI, Anderson B, Buller RE. Preservation of the saphenous vein during inguinal lymphadenectomy decreases morbidity in patients with carcinoma of the vulva. *Cancer.* 2000;89(7):1520-5.

[48] Sotelo R, Sanchez-Salas R, Clavijo R. Endoscopic inguinal lymph node dissection for penile carcinoma: the developing of a novel technique. *World J Urol.* 2009;27(2):213-9.

[49] Gallo Rolania FJ, Beneitez Alvarez ME, Izquierdo Garcia FM. The role of inguinal lymphadenectomy in epidermoid carcinoma of the penis. Use of Ligasure and analysis of the results. *Arch Esp Urol*. 2002;55(5):535-8.

In: Penile Cancer: Challenges and Controversies
Editors: F. E. Martins and M. L. Djordjevic
ISBN: 978-1-53615-950-9

Chapter 19

RISKS AND BENEFITS OF PENILE PRESERVATION

Clare O'Connell[1,*], Gregory Nason[1] and Paul Hegarty[1,2,3]
[1]Department of Urology, Mater Misericordiae University Hospital, Dublin, Ireland
[2]Department of Urology, Mater Private Hospital, Dublin, Ireland
[3]Department of Urology, Mater Private Hospital, Cork, Ireland

ABSTRACT

Penile cancer is a rare disease, accounting for <1% of all malignancies. It has a profound impact on affected men, with poor survival rates for those with metastatic disease, and with significant treatment-associated impairments for those fortunate enough to present with localised disease. Historically, men presenting with localised penile cancer would undergo radical surgery in the form of total amputation or aggressive partial penectomy. This has far-reaching consequences for both men and their partners. While this strategy is still required for very locally advanced lesions, the last 20 years has seen a shift in practice toward phallus-sparing management for penile cancer. It was previously thought that neoplastic penile lesions must be excised with a 2cm margin of normal tissue to produce oncologically robust results. Evidence to the contrary has allowed surgeons to safely excise invasive tumours while preserving more normal tissue than previously thought possible, in order to produce better functional and aesthetic outcomes. While phallus-preserving techniques are associated with higher recurrence rates than radical surgery, it has been shown that local recurrences do not adversely affect long-term survival, as long as patients are followed up closely and recurrences are managed in a timely fashion. A patient's lymph node status remains the single most important predictor of long-term survival.

There is now a large armamentarium available for tackling malignant lesions of the foreskin and glans penis. Each case should be examined separately, and a strategy agreed upon taking into consideration patient concerns and local expertise. Available techniques include topical therapy, photodynamic therapy, laser ablation, Mohs micrographic

* Corresponding Author's E-mail: oconnec2@tcd.ie.

surgery, wide local excision with or without reconstruction, glans resurfacing, partial and total glansectomy, and partial penectomy. Organ-sparing surgery has become the norm for other urological cancers, including kidney and bladder, and there is an ever-expanding body of evidence supporting the oncologic safety of organ-preserving techniques for penile cancer. The average Urologist will see a case of penile cancer only once every 1-2 years, therefore the importance of tertiary referral of cases to high volume centres cannot be understated. As is the case for other operations, outcomes in phallus-sparing surgery for penile cancer are improved when these cases are managed by expert surgeons, in institutions that are properly resourced to handle the level of complexity associated with their care.

Keywords: penile cancer, penile preservation, glansectomy, risks, benefits, complications, morbidity, outcomes, psychosexual impact, prognosis

INTRODUCTION

Penile cancer represents a devastating diagnosis for men and also for their partners (Figure 1). They are not only faced with the prospect of a cancer diagnosis and risk of mortality, but also the fear of undergoing life-altering surgery in the form of penile amputation. The traditional gold standard of penectomy produces good oncological outcomes, but the resultant deformity can be a hugely traumatising event and can lead to long-term functional deficits and psychosocial problems (Figure 2). Treatment for penile cancer has been shown to negatively impact patient psychological well-being, with 50% patients showing some degree of psychiatric symptoms or distress [1].

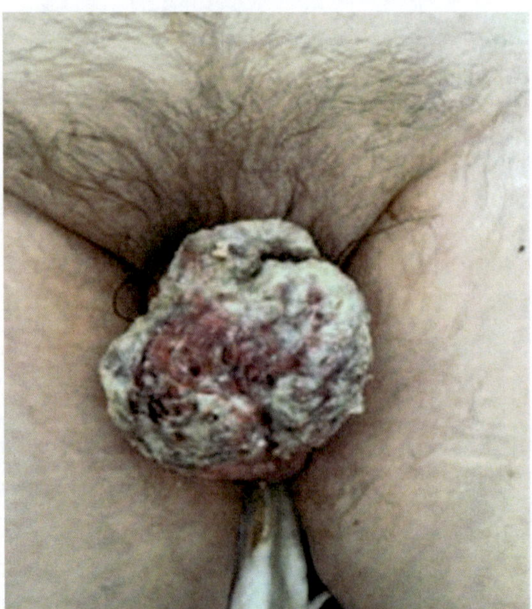

Figure 1. Fungating penile lesion.

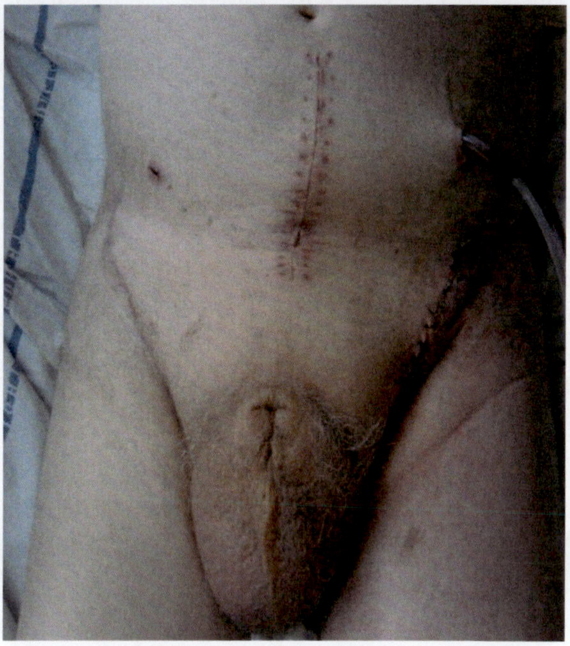

Figure 2. Post total penectomy and groin and pelvic node dissection.

Rationale for Phallus-Preserving Surgery

Until relatively recently, most men with penile cancer underwent aggressive surgical management of local disease, generally in the form of partial or total amputation. In the last 20 years there has been a drive to refine penile surgery to not only establish oncologically robust results, but to preserve as much of the native organ as possible in order to produce better functional and aesthetic outcomes. Practice is shifting toward penile-conservation, with many previously firmly-held beliefs being challenged. One of the most important shifts in practice has been the move away from the strict criteria of a 2cm margin that was thought to be required for an oncologically robust procedure. One of the first to challenge this paradigm was Hoffman et al. [2], who reported outcomes of 17 patients after total or partial penectomy with average resection margins of 14mm, including 7 patients with margins <10mm, none of whom developed a local recurrence at follow up. A key pathological study that allowed Urologists to push the boundaries of resection margins was by Agrawal et al. [3] they examined 64 total and partial penectomy specimens, graded according to the Broder classification, and found that no grade 1-2 tumour extended more than 10mm beyond the visible clinical lesion, and that three grade 3 lesions extended 10mm beyond the visible lesion, but none extended to 15mm. No discontinuous tumour extension was seen, and this study strongly suggested that a 10mm is adequate for grade 1-2 lesions. In patients undergoing phallus-preserving surgery, margins closer than the traditional 2cm have not been associated with high rates of local recurrence, with only 2 patients developing local recurrence on follow up in a study examining 102 surgical margins, in which 90% patients had a margin <20mm, and 48% had a margin <10mm [4]. Organ sparing surgery has become commonplace in other urological cancers including kidney [5], upper tract urothelial [6], bladder [7] and testis [8], and is now becoming the norm for many cases of penile cancer.

Moreover, there is evidence to suggest that local recurrence has little impact on long-term survival [9, 10], making organ-preserving strategies justifiable. The main determinant of longterm outcome and risk of metastatic disease is lymph node status, making accurate lymph node staging an essential step in diagnosis and management [10]. Invasive lymph node staging should be considered for patients with T stage pT1G2 and above [11, 12], and radical lymph node dissection may be required, but this does not preclude phallus-sparing surgery, and the primary tumour and lymph nodes can be managed in a staged fashion. Although there is a higher rate of local recurrence with phallus-sparing surgery, this does not appear to impact longterm survival, and rates of 5-year survival as high as 92% have been reported for patients with a local recurrence after penile-sparing surgery [10].

Advances in Penile Preservation Techniques

There are a wide variety of phallus-preserving modalities for the treatment of the primary lesion in penile cancer, and for pre-malignant lesions. There is a paucity of randomised control trial data in this area, and the optimum strategy for the management of penile cancer is not known. Cases are managed depending on the stage, structures involved by the tumour, patient preference, and surgeon expertise.

Topical Therapy

Topical chemotherapeutic agents are safe and effective for the initial treatment of carcinoma in situ of the glans penis. The most commonly used agents are 5-fluorouracil (5-FU) and imiquimod. 5-FU is an anti-metabolic chemotherapeutic which inhibits the action of thymidylate synthetase [13]. Imiquimod is an immunomodulatory drug which acts via toll-like receptor 7 (TLR-7) to lead to the release of several cytokines including TNF and interleukin-6 [14]. A study in 2012 retrospectively reviewed 42 patients treated with topical 5-FU for carcinoma in situ of the penis and observed a complete response (CR) in 21 cases (50%) [15], and a partial response (PR) in 13 cases. They also reported data on 9 patients who received imiquimod as second line therapy for failure or partial response after 5-FU; 4 patients had a CR and 5 patients had no response. Local toxicity was reported in 4 patients after treatment with 5-FU (10%). They identified five recurrences (20%) at mean follow up of 34 months, indicating the need for vigilant surveillance of patients treated with topical therapies. Most of the data for imiquimod comes from small studies and case series. The EAU guidelines recommend that if topical therapy fails it should not be repeated [16].

Photodynamic Therapy

Photodynamic therapy (PTD) involves application of a photosensitizing agent to a penile lesion, then exposing it to light from the red part of the light spectrum (600-730nm). Most of the data regarding this technique comes from small case series. One series of 10 patients reported outcomes when PTD was used to treat penile intraepithelial neoplasia (PIN) in 10 men, with clearance of PIN in 7 cases [17]. Superficial skin erosion was a common side effect but healed within days and there was no longterm deformity.

Laser Ablation and Excision

Laser therapy is a commonly used strategy for small focal lesions. There are two types of laser available: the CO_2 laser and the Nd:YAG laser. The CO_2 laser has a shallow depth of penetration and vaporizes tissues. The Nd:YAG laser is a coagulative laser and has a deeper penetration than the CO_2 laser. A retrospective review of 224 patients with penile lesions managed by CO_2 laser excision reported complete excision (negative margins) in 221 cases (98.7%), and a recurrence rate of 17% at 10 years [18]. One study examined a combined CO_2 and Nd:YAG laser and reported local recurrences rates of 19%, with 77% of those who had a recurrence successfully treated with further laser therapy [19]. Local recurrence rates of 15-30% are noted across several studies in the literature, emphasising the importance of diligent follow-up for patients treated with laser therapy [20, 21]. The EAU guidelines recommend re-biopsy after laser treatment to ensure disease eradication [16]. While laser therapy is generally used for small superficial lesions, a study by Meijer et al. in 2007 reported its use in 44 patients with carcinoma, T1 and T2 disease [21]. They reported a recurrence rate of 48%, and 10 cases of nodal metastases, 8 of which were originally staged T2. This strongly suggests that laser should be reserved for TiS and Ta tumours.

Mohs Micrographic Surgery (MMS)

Mohs micrographic surgery is a technique widely used for excision of skin cancers, developed by Dr Frederic Mohs in 1933 [22], based on sequential excision of tissues layers under microscopic guidance, thus aiming to preserve the maximum amount of normal tissue. The same operator resects the tissue and immediately examines it under the microscope. This technique can be used for small penile cancers and pre-malignant lesions and was first described by Mohs in 33 patients, with a cure rate of 74% at 5 years [23]. The most contemporary series examining this technique reports one recurrence in 19 patients with PIN treated with MMS, and no recurrences in 10 cases of primary invasive squamous cell carcinoma of the penis managed with MMS [24]. Despite this, it has not been widely adopted for management of localised penile cancer.

Wide Local Excision (WLE) with Circumcision

For small lesions limited to the foreskin, wide local excision and circumcision is often sufficient for a curative operation (Figure 3) [25]. This approach is associated with an excellent functional and aesthetic outcome, but this must be balanced with ensuring that adequate margins are achieved (Figure 4) [26]. Discrete T1 lesions located on the glans can be challenging to manage in this manner. Small lesions that are not close to the urethral meatus can often be excised and closed primarily without causing too much deformity of the glans, but larger lesions may require a skin graft to cover the defect [26]. As for the other glans-preserving methods discussed thus far, there is a high rate of local recurrence reported [27], meaning meticulous follow up is required. However, second operations for local recurrences are usually successful, and local recurrences do not adversely affect long-term survival, as long as close patient follow-up is observed [28].

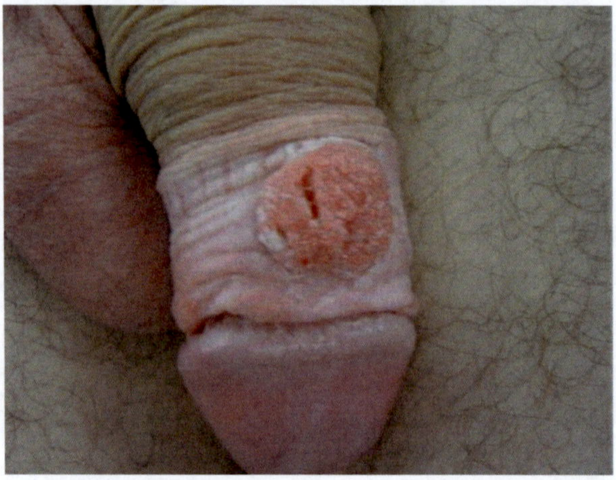

Figure 3. Malignant lesion of the foreskin.

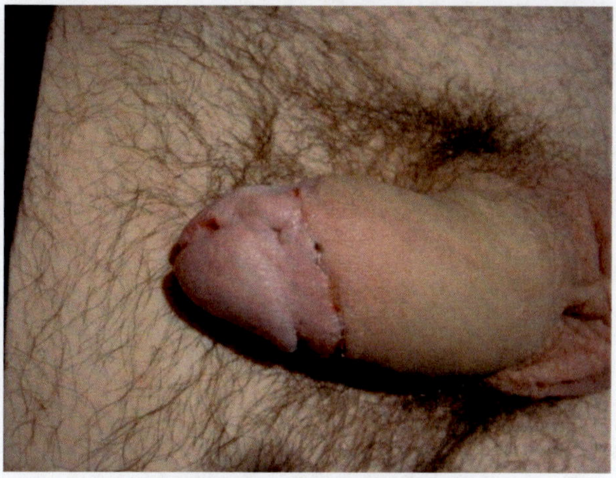

Figure 4. Lesion managed by WLE and circumcision.

Total Glans Resurfacing

First described by Bracka [29] in 2000 for the management of severe refractory balanitis xerotica obliterans (BXO), this technique is now commonly used for pre-malignant lesions of the glans penis, and early penile cancer. The technique involves sharply dissecting the glans epithelium and sub-epithelium off the glans spongiosus, using a tourniquet to control bleeding, either in a retrograde fashion in four quadrants starting at the meatus [30], or in an antegrade fashion beginning with a sub-coronal circumferential incision (Figure 5) [31]. The exposed glans surface is then 'resurfaced' with a split-thickness skin graft from the thigh, which is sutured in place with absorbable sutures. Quilting sutures are also used to prevent haematoma formation. Reported outcomes from this procedure are favourable. Hadway et al. [32] described initial outcome data from 10 patients who underwent total glans resurfacing for pre-malignant lesions of the penis. All 10 cases had clear surgical margins, complete graft take, and no disease recurrence had occurred at a median of 30-month follow-up. Shabbir et al. [30] reported outcomes of 15 cases of partial glans resurfacing (PGR) and 10 cases of total glans resurfacing (TGR) for CiS of the glans penis. At a mean of 29 month follow up, 24 of 25 patients had complete graft take, and 12 of 25 patients had positive margins, but only 7 required further surgery. Overall local recurrence rate was 4%, and there were no cases of progression of disease. A recent prospective series from O'Kelly et al. [33] described the oncological, functional and aesthetic outcomes of 19 patients who underwent glans resurfacing for suspected CiS or superficial disease (TiS/Ta). 94.7% patients had complete graft take, with a median score of 5 out of 5 for cosmesis on a visual analogue scale (Figure 6). Margins were clear in all but one patient, and one patient went on to develop a local recurrence, but there were no nodal recurrences at median follow up of 23 months. All 14 patients who had been sexually active pre-operatively had regained full activity within 6 months, there was no significant difference in median IIEF score, and 81% patients reported an improvement in their sex life after the operation. These results are hugely encouraging for the future of organ-preserving management of localised penile cancer.

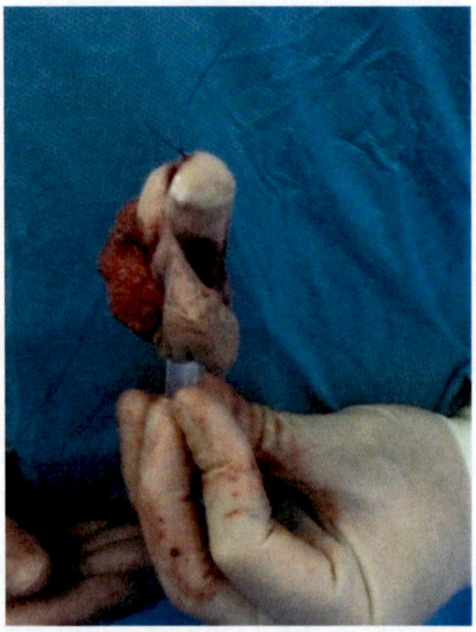

Figure 5. Specimen from total glans resurfacing.

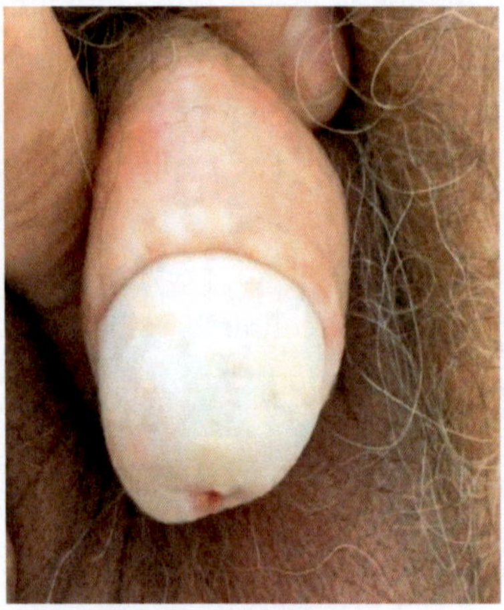

Figure 6. Total glans resurfacing at 3 months.

Glansectomy

Men with T2 tumours of the glans previously underwent radical surgery or radiotherapy. Austoni et al. were the first to report on glansectomy as an effective treatment for invasive penile cancer confined to the glans (Figures 7 and 8) [34]. Davis et al. reported on three distal penile tumours all managed with cavernosal-sparing glansectomy, two of whom had normal erections post operatively, and one of whom was able to have sexual intercourse with the aid of a vacuum device [35]. Hatzichristou et al. described a series of patients with verrucous carcinoma or giant condyloma acuminatum of the glans penis treated with glansectomy [36]. All patients returned to normal sexual activity within one month of their operation. One patient required further surgery due to local recurrence, and all were disease free at 18-65 month follow-up. One of the largest series to date is a report from Pietrzak et al. of 78 patients referred to their tertiary referral centre for management of penile cancer, 29 of whom underwent glansectomy, with no recurrence on follow up [37].

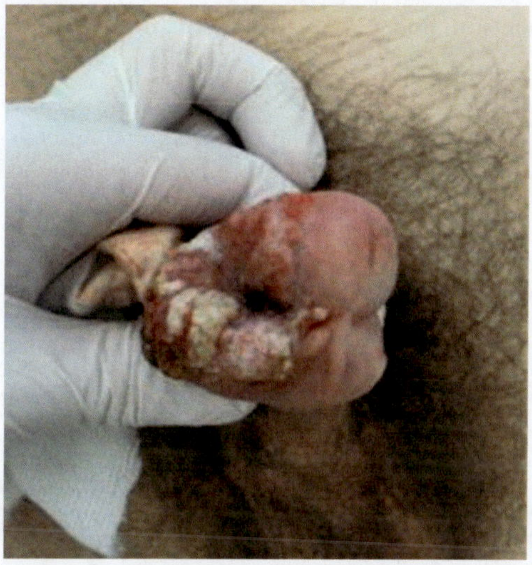

Figure 7. Malignant lesion of the glans penis.

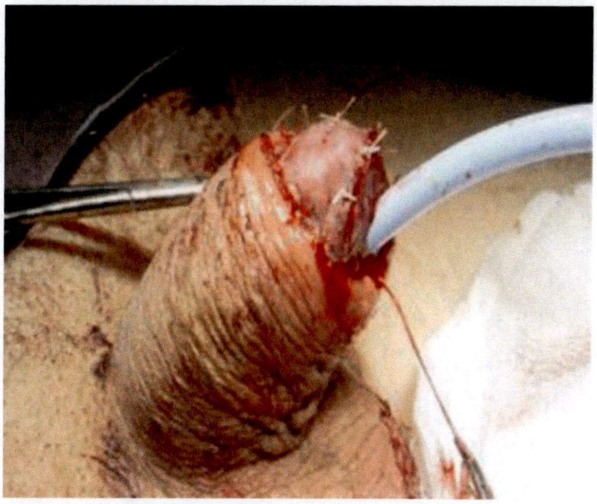

Figure 8. Skin graft covering glansectomy defect.

Partial Penectomy

Partial penectomy is warranted when a tumour extends into cavernosal bodies. Although there is generally significant loss of length, most men prefer this procedure to total amputation. Intraoperative frozen section is useful in this setting, to maximise the amount of normal tissue that can be left behind while ensuring tumour eradication. An extra 2cm of penile length can be gained by dividing the suspensory ligaments below the pubic arch [25]. A series from Korets et al. reported outcomes from 32 patients managed with partial penectomy with a 1cm surgical margin from palpable/visible tumour edge [38]. At mean follow up of 34 months, there was only one recurrence. 6 patients reported a decrease in erectile function, and 5 reported lower limb swelling.

Benefits of Phallus-Preserving Surgery

Urinary Function

Radical surgery in the form of total penectomy and aggressive partial penectomy can leave men with significantly altered voiding function. Total penectomy necessitates the formation of a perineal urethrostomy, and men who undergo this procedure must then sit to void. The rate of urethrostomy stenosis is 18% [39], with many men having to undergo multiple dilatations, and learn to perform self-dilatation to keep their tract patent. Length-preserving procedures such as wide local excision and glans-resurfacing have excellent rates of urethral patency [26, 33]. For more extensive procedures such as glansectomy and partial penectomy, the urethra should be left 10-15mm longer than the corpora, to allow for wide spatulation of the meatus, reducing the rates of urethral stenosis [25].

Sexual Function

Men who undergo partial penectomy have lower scores in all domains of the IIEF questionnaire post operatively when compared to pre-operative scores, including decreased erectile function, decreased sexual desire and a loss of overall satisfaction with their sexual function [40]. Most men report decreased frequency of sexual intercourse, with many reporting the reason for this being a sense of shame due to shortened penile length [40, 41]. During psychological interviews after surgery for penile cancer, men commonly report an altered sense of masculinity [42]. While there are no randomised control trials directly comparing partial penectomy to phallus-preserving surgery, most retrospective studies show worse self-reported sexual outcomes and higher rates of erectile dysfunction after partial penectomy [43, 41]. In one study of laser treatment of the primary lesion, 87% of patients who had been sexually active prior to treatment had resumed activity at interview post treatment, and 72% reported unaltered erectile function [44].

Psychological Wellbeing

Surgery for penile cancer is associated with significant psychological stress and impacts on quality of life for patients. There is good evidence supporting the negative psychological effect of surgery for penile cancer. When interviewed at the time of diagnosis, patients report significant fears about the prospect of undergoing potentially mutilating surgery and the risks to their future sexual function [45]. A study by Fiacarra et al. [46] showed impaired well-being, as measured by the General Health Questionnaire (GHQ) in 37.5% of patients who underwent partial penectomy and demonstrated that 53.5% patients showed signs of mental illness on assessment by a psychiatrist, with two patients in the group suffering from PTSD. Men whose primary tumour is managed with partial penectomy report higher rates of interference with quality of life, as measured by the IOC-2 questionnaire (Impact of Cancer, Version 2), and have more concerns regarding the appearance after surgery when compared to those who undergo phallus-sparing operations [43]. It is well documented that men with genitourinary cancers are at an increased risk of dying by suicide [47, 48].

RISKS OF PENILE PRESERVATION

Complications of Phallus-Sparing Techniques

Overall, the complication rate from penile-sparing surgery is low, and most of the morbidity associated with treatment for penile cancer comes from lymph node dissections [49], or more radical surgical techniques. Complications from laser treatment include bleeding in 8% cases, local infections in 2% and meatal stenosis in <1% cases. Most men regain their level of sexual activity post treatment [50, 51]. Mohs micrographic surgery also has low rates of complications, which include local infections in up to 3% cases and meatal stenosis in 6% cases [23, 24, 52]. Data for complications following glans-resurfacing is sparsely reported, but one can extrapolate from reconstructive techniques elsewhere in the body that due to the excellent blood supply of the glans penis, the rate of graft take is high.

Oncologic Safety and Overall Survival

The concern for any surgical technique that places form and function to the fore is the risk of sacrificing oncologic control. The rate of local recurrence is certainly higher for penile conserving strategies than for radical surgery, but with appropriate surveillance and repeat surgery if needed, there is no effect on long-term survival [53]. Local recurrences have been reported as far out as >10 years post initial resection [54], making the care for stringent long-term follow up. Men who are referred to tertiary centres for management penile cancer may have to travel long distances to access appointments, which may affect compliance with long-term follow-up.

Conclusion

Penile cancer is an uncommon disease, therefore the average Urologist in the UK & Ireland will only see a new case every 2 years [55]. For this reason, the management of penile cancer should be triaged to supra-regional centres which have a caseload of at least 25 cases per year, in order to maximise the potential oncologic and functional outcomes for patients [56, 57]. The reassuring oncological results from these studies have encouraged the development and refinement of new techniques in penile surgery, to maximise functional and aesthetic outcomes while maintaining the best oncologic results [59]. New techniques are allowing men to not only survive penile cancer, but to do so while preserving the best possible level of urinary and sexual function. We believe all men with penile cancer should be referred to a high-volume centre, where then can be afforded the best possible opportunity to undergo penile-sparing treatment, in order to have the best oncologic and functional outcome.

Key Points

- Radical surgery for penile cancer results in life-altering impairment for men and has a negative functional and psychological impact on men and their partners.
- Phallus-preserving surgery has been shown to have excellent outcomes in terms of sexual function and psychological wellbeing. Techniques such as laser ablation and glans resurfacing allow men to return to their pre-operative level of sexual function and have high satisfaction rates for patients.
- There is mounting evidence to support the oncologic safety of phallus-preserving strategies for penile cancer. While there are significant local recurrence rates with

many techniques, this has been found to have minimal impact on long-term survival; lymph node status remains the most important predictor of survival.

- A wide array of techniques is available to remove the offending lesion while preserving as much normal tissue as possible. As penile cancer is a rare disease, management should be individualised for each case.
- Outcomes are improved when men with penile cancer are managed in a supra-regional high-volume centre, which can offer tailored care to each patient.

REFERENCES

[1] Maddineni SB, Lau MM, Sangar VK. Identifying the needs of penile cancer sufferers: a systematic review of the quality of life, psychosexual and psychosocial literature in penile cancer. *BMC Urology*. 2009 Dec;9(1):8.

[2] Hoffman MA, Renshaw AA, Loughlin KR. Squamous cell carcinoma of the penis and microscopic pathologic margins. *Cancer*. 1999 Apr 1;85(7):1565-8.

[3] Agrawal A, Pai D, Ananthakrishnan N, Smile SR, Ratnakar C. The histological extent of the local spread of carcinoma of the penis and its therapeutic implications. *BJU international*. 2000 Feb;85(3):299-301.

[4] Minhas S, Kayes O, Hegarty P, Kumar P, Freeman A, Ralph D. What surgical resection margins are required to achieve oncological control in men with primary penile cancer? *BJU international*. 2005 Nov 1;96(7):1040-3.

[5] Volpe A, Blute ML, Ficarra V, Gill IS, Kutikov A, Porpiglia F, Rogers C, Touijer KA, Van Poppel H, Thompson RH. Renal ischemia and function after partial nephrectomy: a collaborative review of the literature. *European urology*. 2015 Jul 1;68(1):61-74.

[6] Seisen T, Nison L, Remzi M, Klatte T, Mathieu R, Lucca I, Bozzini G, Capitanio U, Novara G, Cussenot O, Compérat E. Oncologic outcomes of kidney sparing surgery versus radical nephroureterectomy for the elective treatment of clinically organ confined upper tract urothelial carcinoma of the distal ureter. *The Journal of urology*. 2016 May 1;195(5):1354-61.

[7] El-Achkar A, Souhami L, Kassouf W. Bladder Preservation Therapy: Review of Literature and Future Directions of Trimodal Therapy. *Current urology reports*. 2018 Dec 1;19(12):108.

[8] Bojanic N, Bumbasirevic U, Vukovic I, Bojanic G, Milojevic B, Nale D, Durutovic O, Djordjevic D, Nikic P, Vuksanovic A, Tulic C. Testis sparing surgery in the treatment of bilateral testicular germ cell tumors and solitary testicle tumors: a single institution experience. *Journal of surgical oncology*. 2015 Feb;111(2):226-30.

[9] Philippou P, Shabbir M, Malone P, Nigam R, Muneer A, Ralph DJ, Minhas S. Conservative surgery for squamous cell carcinoma of the penis: resection margins and long-term oncological control. *The Journal of urology.* 2012 Sep 1;188(3):803-8.

[10] Leijte JA, Kirrander P, Antonini N, Windahl T, Horenblas S. Recurrence patterns of squamous cell carcinoma of the penis: recommendations for follow-up based on a two-centre analysis of 700 patients. *European urology.* 2008 Jul 1;54(1):161-9.

[11] Alkatout I, Naumann CM, Hedderich J, Hegele A, Bolenz C, Jünemann KP, Klöppel G. Squamous cell carcinoma of the penis: predicting nodal metastases by histologic grade, pattern of invasion and clinical examination. In *Urologic Oncology: Seminars and Original Investigations* 2011 Nov 1 (Vol. 29, No. 6, pp. 774-781). Elsevier.

[12] Lonergan PE, Riogh AN, O'Kelly F, Lundon DJ, O'Sullivan D, O'Connell M, Hegarty PK. Dynamic sentinel node biopsy for penile cancer: an initial experience in an Irish Hospital. *Irish Journal of Medical Science* (1971-). 2017 Nov 1;186(4):841-5.

[13] Eaglstein WH, Weinstein GD, Frost P. Fluorouracil: Mechanism of action in human skin and actinic keratoses: I. Effect on DNA synthesis in vivo. *Archives of dermatology.* 1970 Feb 1;101(2):132-9.

[14] Manjunath A, Brenton T, Wylie S, Corbishley CM, Watkin NA. Topical Therapy for non-invasive penile cancer (Tis)—updated results and toxicity. *Translational andrology and urology.* 2017 Oct;6(5):803.

[15] Alnajjar HM, Lam W, Bolgeri M, Rees RW, Perry MJ, Watkin NA. Treatment of carcinoma in situ of the glans penis with topical chemotherapy agents. *European urology.* 2012 Nov 1;62(5):923-8.

[16] Hakenberg OW, Compérat EM, Minhas S, Necchi A, Protzel C, Watkin N. EAU guidelines on penile cancer: 2014 update. *European urology.* 2015 Jan 1;67(1):142-50.

[17] Paoli J, Bratel AT, Löwhagen GB, Stenquist B, Forslund O, Wennberg AM. Penile intraepithelial neoplasia: results of photodynamic therapy. *Acta dermato-venereologica.* 2006 Sep 1;86(5):418-21.

[18] Bandieramonte G, Colecchia M, Mariani L, Vullo SL, Pizzocaro G, Piva L, Nicolai N, Salvioni R, Lezzi V, Stefanon B, De Palo G. Peniscopically controlled CO2 laser excision for conservative treatment of in situ and T1 penile carcinoma: report on 224 patients. *European urology.* 2008 Oct 1;54(4):875-84.

[19] Windahl T, Andersson SO. Combined laser treatment for penile carcinoma: results after long-term follow up. *The Journal of urology*. 2003 Jun 1;169(6):2118-21.

[20] Van Bezooijen BP, Horenblas S, Meinhardt W, Newling DW. Laser therapy for carcinoma in situ of the penis. *The Journal of urology.* 2001 Nov 1;166(5):1670-1.

[21] Meijer RP, Boon TA, van Venrooij GE, Wijburg CJ. Long-term follow-up after laser therapy for penile carcinoma. *Urology.* 2007 Apr 1;69(4):759-62.

[22] Wong E, Axibal E, Brown M. Mohs Micrographic Surgery. *Facial Plastic Surgery Clinics.* 2019 Feb 1;27(1):15-34.

[23] Mohs FE, Snow SN, Larson PO. Mohs micrographic surgery for penile tumors. *The Urologic Clinics of North America.* 1992 May;19(2):291-304.

[24] Machan M, Brodland D, Zitelli J. Penile squamous cell carcinoma: penis-preserving treatment with Mohs micrographic surgery. *Dermatologic Surgery.* 2016 Aug 1;42(8):936-44.

[25] Hegarty PK, Shabbir M, Hughes B, Minhas S, Perry M, Watkin N, Ralph DJ. Penile preserving surgery and surgical strategies to maximize penile form and function in penile cancer: recommendations from the United Kingdom experience. *World journal of urology.* 2009 Apr 1;27(2):179-87.

[26] Bissada NK. Conservative extirpative treatment of cancer of the penis. *The Urologic Clinics of North America.* 1992 May;19(2):283-90.

[27] Horenblas S, Van Tinteren H. Squamous cell carcinoma of the penis. IV. Prognostic factors of survival: analysis of tumor, nodes and metastasis classification system. *The Journal of urology.* 1994 May 1;151(5):1239-43.

[28] Lont AP, Gallee MP, Meinhardt W, Van Tinteren H, Horenblas S. Penis conserving treatment for T1 and T2 penile carcinoma: clinical implications of a local recurrence. *The Journal of urology*. 2006 Aug 1;176(2):575-80.

[29] Depasquale I, Park AJ, Bracka A. The treatment of balanitis xerotica obliterans. *BJU international.* 2000 Sep 1;86(4):459-65.

[30] Shabbir M, Muneer A, Kalsi J, Shukla CJ, Zacharakis E, Garaffa G, Ralph D, Minhas S. Glans resurfacing for the treatment of carcinoma in situ of the penis: surgical technique and outcomes. *European urology.* 2011 Jan 1;59(1):142-7.

[31] Palminteri E, Berdondini E, Lazzeri M, Mirri F, Barbagli G. Resurfacing and reconstruction of the glans penis. *European urology.* 2007 Sep 1;52(3):893-900.

[32] Hadway P, Corbishley CM, Watkin NA. Total glans resurfacing for premalignant lesions of the penis: initial outcome data. *BJU international*. 2006 Sep;98(3):532-6.

[33] O'Kelly F, Lonergan P, Lundon D, Nason G, Sweeney P, Cullen I, Hegarty P. A prospective study of total glans resurfacing for localized penile cancer to maximize oncologic and functional outcomes in a tertiary referral network. *The Journal of urology.* 2017 May 1;197(5):1258-63.

[34] Austoni E, Fenice O, Kartalas YG, Colombo F, Mantovani F, Pisani E. New trends in the surgical treatment of penile carcinoma. *Archivio italiano di urologia, andrologia: organo ufficiale [di] Societa italiana di ecografia urologica e nefrologica.* 1996 Jun;68(3):163-8.

[35] Davis JW, Schellhammer PF, Schlossberg SM. Conservative surgical therapy for penile and urethral carcinoma. *Urology.* 1999 Feb 1;53(2):386-92.

[36] Hatzichristou DG, Apostolidis A, Tzortzis V, Hatzimouratidis K, Ioannides E, Yannakoyorgos K. Glansectomy: an alternative surgical treatment for Buschke-Löwenstein tumors of the penis. *Urology.* 2001 May 1;57(5):966-9.

[37] Pietrzak P, Corbishley C, Watkin N. Organ-sparing surgery for invasive penile cancer: early follow-up data. *BJU international.* 2004 Dec;94(9):1253-7.

[38] Korets R, Koppie TM, Snyder ME, Russo P. Partial penectomy for patients with squamous cell carcinoma of the penis: the Memorial Sloan-Kettering experience. *Annals of surgical oncology.* 2007 Dec 1;14(12):3614-9.

[39] Myers JB, Porten SP, McAninch JW. The outcomes of perineal urethrostomy with preservation of the dorsal urethral plate and urethral blood supply. *Urology.* 2011 May 1;77(5):1223-7.

[40] Romero FR, dos Santos Romero KR, de Mattos MA, Garcia CR, de Carvalho Fernandes R, Perez MD. Sexual function after partial penectomy for penile cancer. *Urology.* 2005 Dec 1;66(6):1292-5.

[41] Sansalone S, Silvani M, Leonardi R, Vespasiani G, Iacovelli V. Sexual outcomes after partial penectomy for penile cancer: results from a multi-institutional study. *Asian journal of andrology.* 2017 Jan;19(1):57.

[42] Bullen K, Edwards S, Marke V, Matthews S. Looking past the obvious: experiences of altered masculinity in penile cancer. *Psycho-oncology.* 2010 Sep;19(9):933-40.

[43] Kieffer, J.M., Djajadiningrat, R.S., van Muilekom, E.A., Graafland, N.M., Horenblas, S. and Aaronson, N.K., 2014. Quality of life for patients treated for penile cancer. *The Journal of urology*, *192*(4), pp.1105-1110.

[44] Windahl T, Skeppner E, Andersson SO, Fugl-Meyer KS. Sexual function and satisfaction in men after laser treatment for penile carcinoma. *The Journal of urology.* 2004 Aug 1;172(2):648-51.

[45] D'Ancona CA, Botega NJ, De Moraes C, Lavoura ND, Santos JK, Netto NR. Quality of life after partial penectomy for penile carcinoma. *Urology.* 1997 Oct 1;50(4):593-6.

[46] Ficarra V, Righetti R, D'amico A, Pilloni S, Balzarro M, Schiavone D, Malossini G, Mobilio G. General state of health and psychological well-being in patients after surgery for urological malignant neoplasms. *Urologia internationalis.* 2000;65(3):130-4.

[47] Klaassen Z, Jen RP, DiBianco JM, Reinstatler L, Li Q, Madi R, Lewis RW, Smith AM, Neal Jr DE, Moses KA, Terris MK. Factors associated with suicide in patients with genitourinary malignancies. *Cancer.* 2015 Jun 1;121(11):1864-72.

[48] Alanee S, Russo P. Suicide in men with testis cancer. *European journal of cancer care.* 2012 Nov;21(6):817-21.

[49] Horenblas S. Lymphadenectomy for squamous cell carcinoma of the penis. Part 2: the role and technique of lymph node dissection. *BJU international.* 2001 Sep 1;88(5):473-83.

[50] Colecchia M, Nicolai N, Secchi P, Bandieramonte G, Paganoni AM, Sangalli LM, Pizzocaro G, Piva L, Salvioni R. pT1 penile squamous cell carcinoma: a clinicopathologic study of 56 cases treated by CO2 laser therapy. *Analytical and quantitative cytology and histology.* 2009 Jun;31(3):153-60.

[51] Skeppner E, Windahl T, Andersson SO, Fugl-Meyer KS. Treatment-seeking, aspects of sexual activity and life satisfaction in men with laser-treated penile carcinoma. *European urology.* 2008 Sep 1;54(3):631-9.

[52] Shindel AW, Mann MW, Lev RY, Sengelmann R, Petersen J, Hruza GJ, Brandes SB. Mohs micrographic surgery for penile cancer: management and long-term followup. *The Journal of urology.* 2007 Nov 1;178(5):1980-5.

[53] Lindegaard JC, Nielsen OS, Lundbeck FA, Mamsen A, Studstrup HN, Von Der Maase H. A retrospective analysis of 82 cases of cancer of the penis. *British journal of urology.* 1996 Jun;77(6):883-90.

[54] Horenblas S, Newling DW. Local recurrent tumour after penis-conserving therapy. A plea for long-term follow-up. *British journal of urology.* 1993 Dec;72(6):976-.

[55] Mistry T, Jones RW, Dannatt E, Prasad KK, Stockdale AD. A 10-year retrospective audit of penile cancer management in the UK. *BJU international.* 2007 Dec;100(6):1277-81.

[56] Davis NF, Fitzgerald M, Burke JP, Breen KJ, Elamin S, Brady CM, Power DG, Hegarty PK, Sweeney P. Is there a role for the development of a supra-regional network for the management of penile cancer in the Republic of Ireland?. *The Surgeon.* 2016 Apr 1;14(2):82-6.

[57] Matulewicz RS, Flum AS, Helenowski I, Jovanovic B, Palis B, Bilimoria KY, Meeks JJ. Centralization of penile cancer management in the United States: a combined analysis of the American Board of Urology and National Cancer Data Base. *Urology.* 2016 Apr 1;90:82-8.

[58] Kumar P, Singh S, Goddard JC, Terry TR, Summerton DJ. The development of a supraregional network for the management of penile cancer. *The Annals of The Royal College of Surgeons of England.* 2012 Apr;94(3):204-9.

[59] Breen KJ, O'Connor KM, Power DG, Mayer NJ, Rogers E, Sweeney P. Penile cancer–Guideline adherence produces optimum results. *The Surgeon.* 2015 Aug 1;13(4):200-6.

In: Penile Cancer: Challenges and Controversies
Editors: F. E. Martins and M. L. Djordjevic
ISBN: 978-1-53615-950-9

Chapter 20

Reconstructive Surgery for Penile Cancer Survivor: When, How, and by Whom?

Marco Falcone[1,*], MD, PhD
and Giulio Garaffa[2], MD, PhD, FECSM, FRCS
[1]Urology Clinic, Molinette Hospital, Città della Salute e della Scienza,
University of Turin, Turin, Italy
[2]The Institute of Urology, Westmoreland Hospital,
University College of London Hospital, London, United Kingdom

Abstract

Traditionally, the surgical management of locally advanced penile cancer involves a partial or a total penectomy with groin and potentially pelvic lymph nodes dissection.

Although an aggressive demolitive approach might guarantee a better chance of cancer's clearance, it has a profound functional and psychological impact on the patients and their partners and may have a dramatical impact on their quality of life.

Following these leads, the extent of the demolitive surgery for penile cancer should be minimized as much as possible without jeopardizing the cancer control. Following these leads, various organ-sparing approaches have been proposed to manage localized penile cancer. However, an extended penile resection may be required in locally advanced cancers. In the case of an inadequate residual penile stump, different strategies can be considered to permit the patient to regain both sexual and urinary function. If various lengthening procedures aiming to maximize a residual penile stump may be considered as a first less invasive option, in selected cases a total phallic reconstruction (TPR) represents the only reconstructive option.

* Corresponding Author's E-mail: marcofalcone1986@gmail.com.

Due to the unique anatomy of the male genitalia and to the lack of tissue that may adequately replace the smooth muscle of the cavernosal bodies and the spongiosum, TPR still represents a real challenge for the reconstructive surgeon.

The main goals of a TPR are the creation of a cosmetically acceptable phallus with both tactile and erogenous sensation. Ideally, the phallus should have an incorporated neourethra, to allow the patient to void and ejaculate from the tip of the neoglans and adequate bulk to allow the insertion of an internal stiffener to guarantee the rigidity necessary to successfully engage in penetrative sexual intercourse.

The main types of phalloplasty to date are:

1. The radial artery phalloplasty, which is a free flap phalloplasty
2. The infraubilical phalloplasty also known as pubic phalloplasty, which is a pedicled phalloplasty
3. The anterolateral thigh flap, which can be performed either as a pedicled (if the pedicle is long enough) or as a free flap
4. The latissimus dorsi flap, which is a free flap

Despite the high incidence of postoperative complications and the possible need for multiple operations, TPR yields to excellent surgical and functional results.

Keywords: penile cancer, reconstructive surgery, phalloplasty, cancer survivorship

INTRODUCTION

Although penile cancer is quite a rare entity in Western countries, it constitutes a severe health problem in Eastern countries and Southern America where its incidence can be up to five times higher [1, 2]. Traditionally, the surgical management of locally advanced penile cancer involves a partial or a total penectomy with groin and potentially pelvic lymph nodes dissection. Although an aggressive demolitive approach might guarantee a better chance of cancer's clearance, it has a profound functional and psychological impact on the patients and their partners and may have a dramatical impact on their quality of life. If the vast majority of patients affected by a penile cancer are elderly and potentially not bothered by the risk of loss of sexual and urinary function, this is certainly not the case for younger men, who are keen to preserve an acceptable cosmesis and function of the external genitalia. When organ preserving surgery is contraindicated, total phallic reconstruction (TPR) may allow patients to resume sexual and urinary function with confidence.

In the era of minimally invasive surgical approaches, we highlight the need of reducing the extent of the demolitive surgery for penile cancer without compromising the clearance rates of the disease. Since this condition is relatively rare, it is paramount that penile cancer is treated in a tertiary referral center, large volume center where a multidisciplinary team approach can be offered to patients.

Organ Sparing Surgery and Multidisciplinary Approach for Penile Cancer

Traditionally, the primary tumor used to be excised leaving a 2 cm free margin as it was common believe that such a large margin was necessary to guarantee an adequate clearance of the disease [3]. This aggressive approach was certainly associated with satisfactory rates of clearance of the disease, but this was achieved at the cost of sacrificing completely sexual and urinary function. More recently, evidences have clearly shown that oncologic safety does not seem to be jeopardized when only a few millimeters of safe margins are preserved [4, 5]. Consequently, penile-sparing approaches have been increasingly employed, with excellent functional outcomes and a significant improvement in patients' quality of life, compared to the standard demolitive approaches.

At present, demolitive procedures (partial or total amputation) are only reserved for locally advanced tumors or for recurrence after organ-sparing surgery. On the other hand, conservative procedures such as glans resurfacing and glansectomy are considered the gold standard respectively for T1 and T2 tumors [6].

The most recent series have confirmed that with the organ-sparing approaches most patients can obtain satisfactory cosmetic and functional results without compromising the oncological clearance [6–8].

The reconstructive surgeon should be part of the multidisciplinary team from the start as he/she is then responsible of the reconstruction of the genitalia once the demolitive phase has been completed.

How to Select a Suitable Candidate for a Penile Reconstruction

While genital reconstruction after glans resurfacing or glansectomy is relatively easy, as it requires only the application of a split thickness skin graft to cover the denuded spongiosum or the corporeal heads to recreate a pseudo-glans [9], the situation changes dramatically in patient who have undergone partial or subtotal penectomy as they may require a TPR [10].

Most likely, the correct timing to discuss with a patient the possible reconstructive options is when discussing demolitive surgery as this may help the patient to better go through the surgeryss, as they are given a realistic hope of a possible deferred restoration of both sexual and urinary functions.

The early detection of possible candidates for penile reconstruction is extremely important as this may modify to a certain extent the approach in the demolitive phase. In particular, some anatomical considerations must be taken in account when a deferred total phallic reconstruction is considered. Preservation of some anatomical structures, when this does not interfere with oncological clearance, should be carefully planned by the oncological and reconstructive surgeon, as this may help in the subsequent stage of total penile reconstruction. In particular, efforts should be paid during groin dissection to preserve the branches of the long saphenous vein, because they may be needed for the vascular anastomosis in patients undergoing total phallic reconstruction with the use of a free flap. Similarly, in the rare event a pelvic node dissection becomes necessary, it is paramount to preserve the inferior epigastric arteries as they are usually anastomosed in an end to end fashion to the artery of the free flap. Additionally, the proximal urethral stump should be kept as long as possible to allow a primary tension free end to end anastomosis to the phallic neourethra at the time of the TPR.

Furthermore, as a general principle, when possible, efforts should be paid to preserve as much genital skin as possible, as its unique characteristics in terms of innervation, texture and pigmentation render it an ideal tissue to be utilized for the subsequent reconstruction. In case of subtotal penectomy, it is also advisable to preserve the crura. This portion of the corpora will prove extremely useful in the subsequent total phallic reconstruction as it will house the rear aspect of the penile implant thus obviating the need to fashion a windsock in vascular prosthesis materials such as Dacron and Goretex.

However, it is no doubt true that no compromises should ever be done during tumor resection to facilitate the desired phallic reconstruction. The oncological safety should be always considered as the primary goal.

FUTURE PERSPECTIVES : THE NEED OF SPECIFIC TRAINING FOR RECONSTRUCTIVE UROLOGISTS

As all other branches of urology, reconstructive urology is becoming more and more a super-specialized field. The widening of the number of pathologies treated by the reconstructive urologists as well as the increase of surgical procedures performed recall the need of setting-up a structured surgical training aiming to develop the specific skills to deal with all aspects of the genital reconstruction. In fact, differently from other branches of urology, reconstructive surgery of the male genitalia requires skills such as the use of skin grafts, of pedicled or free flaps and microsurgery, which are not generally included in a basic urology training. This consideration suggests that the creation of a structured specific training for reconstructive urology represents the first step towards the increase of the level of care for patients affected by penile cancer.

Considering that penile cancer is relatively rare, this condition should be treated in supra-regional tertiary referral centers by a dedicated multidisciplinary team formed by surgeons, clinical oncologists, radiation oncologists, radiologists and nurse specialists.

PENILE LENGTHENING STRATEGIES AFTER PENILE CANCER ABLATION

As discussed in the previous paragraphs, in the case of a locally advanced penile cancer or after recurrence of conservative treatments, a partial penectomy may be needed. According to the original length of the penis and to the extent of the corpora removed during the demolitive phase, the residual stump may be inadequate to guarantee adequate sexual and urinary function.

The following procedures may help to optimize the length of the penile stump:

1. *Prepubic V-Y plasty*

   The most common procedure is the prepubic V-Y plasty. It consists in an inverted "V" skin flap on the suprapubic area, which is mobilized caudally and sutured in a "Y" fashion in order to advance the prepubic and penile skin. The "V" incision allows to expose the fundiform and the suspensory ligament.
2. *Suspensory ligament division*

   Penile shaft has two different systems of fixation: the fundiform ligament, which represents a continuation of the abdominal Scarpa's fascia and the suspensory ligament, which is a strong fibrous ligament lying between the arch of the pubic and the penile shaft. Among them, the latter represents the main element of shaft's stability. The surgical division of these structures allows to increase the length of the exposed portion of the shaft. This can be achieved at the cost of an increased instability of the penis. Usually, at the time of surgery, a silicon buffer is interposed between the pubic bone and the corpora to prevent the divided ligament from reattaching and scarring down causing penile retraction.
3. *Scrotoplasty for webbed penis*

   This procedure consists in the excision of the penoscrotal web and allows the re-creation of a correct peno-scrotal angle.
4. *Skin grafts or local rotational flaps apposition to maximize penile shaft length*

   The combination of partial penectomy or excessive circumcision with excessive prepubic adiposity can lead to the condition known as "buried penis" (Figure 1). This condition may have a profound impact on patients' quality of life as both urinary and sexual function are completely compromised. The pooling of urine around the buried penis can cause chronic infections and the maceration of the genital and pubic skin. Ultimately, the chronic maceration of the skin and the chronic infections can lead to degenerative changes of the skin and the mucosa such as Lichen Sclerosus (LS) and squamous cell carcionoma of the penis (SCC). Surgical treatment becomes necessary to restore normal sexual and urinary function and to prevent the recurrent infections and almost inevitable skin changes. Surgery consists in freeing the penile shaft from the surrounding tissues in order to expose it and repairing the lack of skin with a split thickness skin graft harvested from a non-genital area, as genital skin may be affected by LS (Figure 2). Generally, this procedure is carried out in combination with an apronectomy or with prepubic lipectomy.

5. *Apronectomy or suprapubic fat pad excision*

Prepubic lipectomy can be achieved either with liposuction or through a transverse suprapubic incision. Patients with redundant abdominal skin can be offered an apronectomy, which consists in the excision of all the excess skin and the prepubic fat in order to expose the penile shaft (Figure 3).

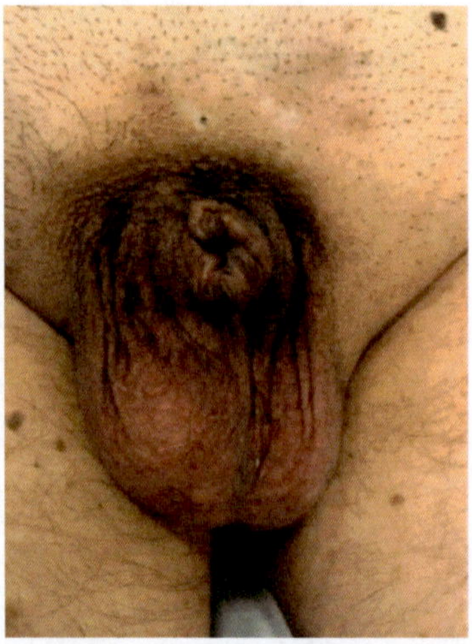

Figure 1. Patient with excessive prepubic adiposity and buried penis after partial penectomy and excessive circumcision.

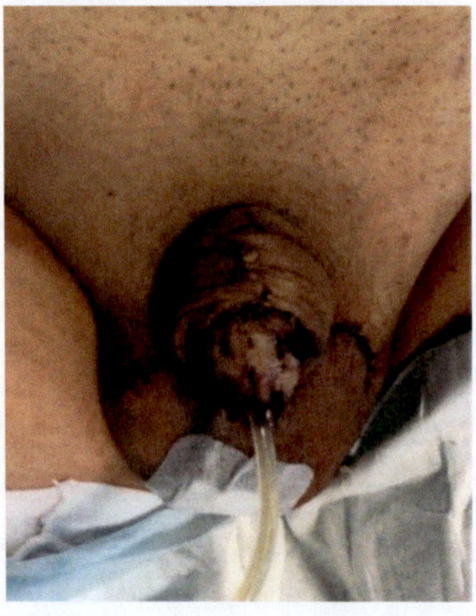

Figure 2. Same patient after freeing the penile shaft from the surrounding tissues for better exposure and use of a split-thickness skin graft harvested from non-genital area. This procedure is performed in combination with apronectomy or prepubic lipectomy.

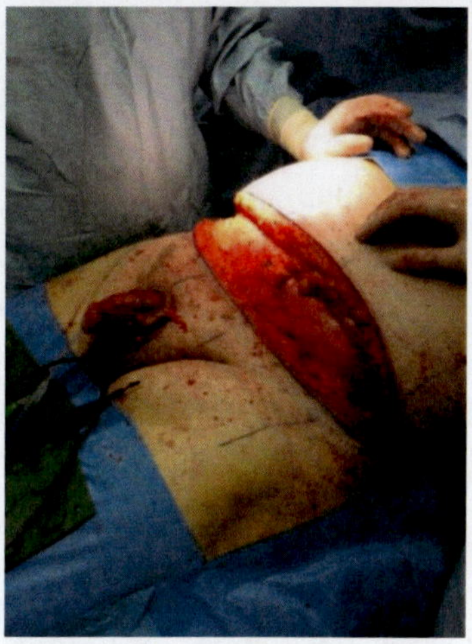

Figure 3. Apronectomy and prepubic lipectomy for exposure of penile shaft.

In properly selected cases these procedures can lead to satisfactory results; in the remainder a TPR should be contemplated.

The Total Phallic Reconstruction Following Penile Amputation for Penile Cancer

A TPR aiming to create a cosmetically acceptable sensate phallus that allows to restore both sexual and urinary function is the only way to improve confidence in patients who have undergone demolitive surgery for a penile cancer. The fact that so many techniques of TPR have been described in the literature so far confirm that an ideal technique still does not exist. The choice of reconstructive technique should be agreed between the patient and the surgeon and take into consideration anatomical factors, pre-existent medical conditions and patient's expectations.

Historical Considerations

Due to the unique anatomy of the male genitalia and to the lack of tissue that may adequately replace the cavernosal bodies and the spongiosum, TPR still represents a challenge for the reconstructive surgeon. The main goals of phallic reconstruction are the creation of a cosmetically acceptable phallus with both tactile and erogenous sensation. Ideally, the phallus should have an incorporated neourethra, to allow the patient to void and ejaculate from the tip of the neoglans, and adequate bulk to allow the insertion of a penile prosthesis to guarantee the rigidity necessary for successful penetrative sexual intercourse.

The first historical attempts aiming to reconstruct a phallus were based on abdominal flaps. The first total phallic reconstruction was described in 1936 by Bogoras [11], who used a random pedicled oblique abdominal flap. Phallic rigidity was obtained by the insertion of a rib cartilage inside the flap.

Subsequently, Matz and Gillies [12], imported the idea to incorporate a neo-urethra in the phallus in a "tube within a tube" fashion to restore urinary and ejaculatory function. These procedures were multi staged, resulted in extensive scarring and disfigurement of the donor area and produced a phallus with no sensation. Therefore, to date, these techniques should be considered only in the case of salvage phalloplasty in patients where the original phalloplasty has failed or who are extremely poor candidates for free flaps.

Infraumbilical and groin skin flaps have been described to minimize donor site disfigurement and to reduce the number of surgical stages [13]. However, the main limitation of these techniques was the formation of a non-sensate wedge-shaped phallus.

Musculocutaneous thigh flaps, used when infraumbilical flaps are contraindicated due to extensive abdominal scarring from previous surgery or radiotherapy, have been abandoned due to poor results, as the muscle tends to scar down and contract [14].

In the 80's, the advent of microsurgical techniques and their application in plastic surgery revolutioned the concept of total phallic reconstruction. In 1982, Song and Chang [15, 16] were the first Authors to describe the use of a sensate radial artery based free flap (RAFF) for phallic reconstruction in patients that had suffered traumatic amputation of the penis. The reconstructive procedure involved the creation of a phallus according to the 'a tube within a tube' concept using a fascio-cutaneous flap harvested from the non-dominant forearm. To minimize complications, the urethra was fashioned from the relatively hairless bearing ulnar area of the flap. The vascular supply of the flap is based on the radial artery, on the venae comitantes of the radial artery and on 1 to 2 main veins.

Following the success of this primary report, many other authors have described personal modifications in flap design in order to improve the cosmesis of the neophallus and to minimize the overall complication rate and donor site morbidity. In particular, the shape of the forearm flap has been modified in order to improve the blood supply to the skin edges in an attempt to reduce the risk of meatal stenosis. Also, an ulnar artery-based flap has been described, aiming to reduce the amount of hair bearing skin incorporated in the neourethra, as the medial aspect of the forearm tends to be less hairy.

Patients' satisfaction following penile amputation for carcinoma with regards to their sexual life is extremely low and therefore they represent the ideal candidates for total phallic reconstruction.

The types of phalloplasty available in this group of patients are:

1. The radial artery-based forearm free flap phalloplasty (RAP)
2. The pedicled infraubilical phalloplasty also known as pubic phalloplasty (PP)

3. The anterolateral thigh flap (ALT)
4. The latissimus dorsi flap (LD)

The Radial Artery Forearm Free Flap Phalloplasty (Figures 4-5)

This is often considered the gold standard technique as it guarantees superior cosmetic and functional results allowing the formation of a cylindrical and sensate phallus with an incorporated neourethra, which reaches the tip of the neoglans. This technique has been demonstrated as a valuable option in patients following penile amputation for carcinoma or trauma, in patients with penile inadequacy and in female to male transsexuals [17–20].

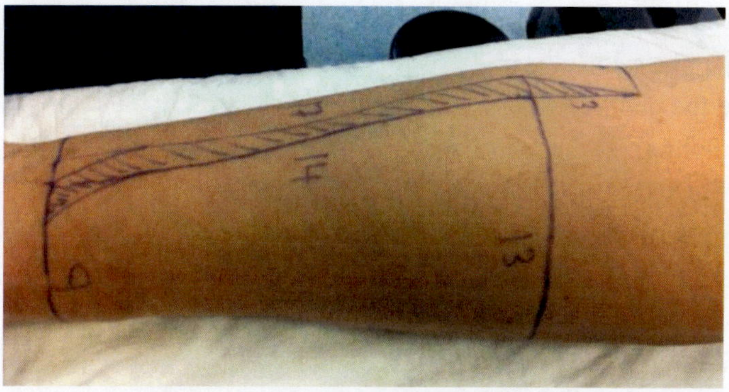

Figure 4. Radial artery forearm free flap phalloplasty.

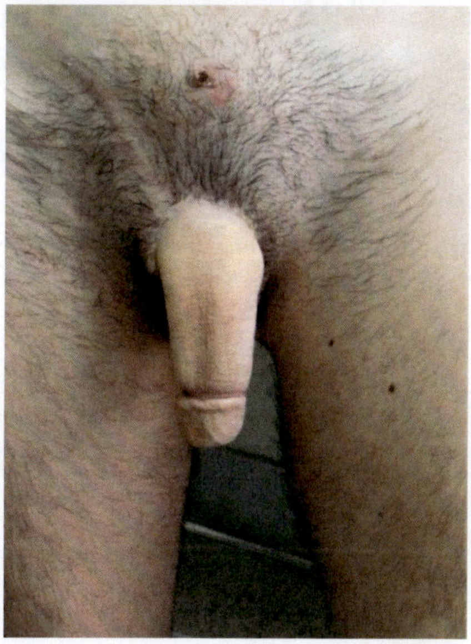

Figure 5. Post-operative appearance after RAFF phalloplasty with excellent cosmetic result.

Although the main limitation of this approach is the visible scar left at the level of the donor site on the non-dominant forearm, functional limitation and sensory changes are virtually absent, as confirmed by various large series published in the literature [21, 22].

Surgery is performed only after the competency of the superficial and deep palmar arteries has been tested with an Allen test. Duplex sonography is reserved to these patients who had a negative Allen test. Laser or electrolysis-based hair removal from the forearm can represent a valuable tool to improve the cosmesis and minimize hair growth in the neourethra, which ultimately may lead to stone formation, recurrent urinary tract infections and voiding dysfunction.

Typically, the total phallic reconstruction with a modified Chang flap is carried out in the following 3 stages, which are carried out at an average of 6 months' intervals:

1. Creation of the phallus with competent neourethra and its' microvascular transfer to the recipient site. Unless the native urethra has been amputated very posteriorly, a primary urethral anastomosis between the native urethra and the neourethra is always performed.
2. Sculpture of the glans and creation of a pseudo-corona according to the Norfolk technique with the use of a full thickness skin graft to fashion the groove of the neoglans. In case the native urethra has been amputated very posteriorly, the anastomosis between the native urethra and the phallic one is carried out at this stage.
3. Insertion of a three-piece inflatable penile prosthesis into the phallus to guarantee the rigidity necessary to engage in penetrative sexual intercourse.

Since its original description by Song and Chang, penile reconstruction with the use of the forearm free flap has proven superior to all other techniques since it:

1. Guarantees a superior cosmetic result by forming a cylindrical phallus rather than the wedge-shaped PP and groin flap phalloplasty and is less prone to postoperative contracture when compared to musculo-cutaneous flaps phalloplasties.
2. Allows the creation of a neourethra that reaches the tip of the phallus, which is significantly less prone to complications than skin graft urethroplasty. Urethral complications with other types of phalloplasties occur in up to 65% of cases and often require multiple revisions. This is the main advantage of this technique when compared to the LD flap, where the only way to fashion a neo-urethra is with a prelaminated buccal mucosa graft applied directly on the muscular portion of the flap.

3. Allows the creation of a sensate phallus whereas in other phalloplasties the sensation is minimal (ALT and LD flap) or absent (Gillies flap and distal 2/3 of PP flap).

Donor site morbidity can be dramatically reduced by adequate preparation of the donor site for grafting. This involves adequate hemostasis and the advancement of the edges of the intact forearm skin to reduce the area that requires grafting and to minimize the step between normal skin and the grafted muscle. With regards to the type of skin graft, thick grafts have proven to be superior to thin grafts as they heal with less scarring and discoloration. Alternatively, excellent results can be achieved with the interposition of a porous matrix of cross-linked bovine tendon collagen between the recipient bed and a split thickness skin graft in order to recreate the appearance of subcutaneous tissue.

In the past, bone and cartilage grafts have been widely used and incorporated in the neophallus in the attempt to guarantee the rigidity necessary to engage in penetrative sexual intercourse. Unfortunately, both these materials create a constant erection difficult to conceal and eventually tend to get reabsorbed and fracture in time.

So far, the best results in terms of rigidity, capacity to conceal and reliability are achieved with the insertion of an inflatable penile prosthesis. In one of the largest series published so far, 247 phalloplasty patients have undergone implantation of a penile prosthesis, after a median follow up of 20 months, the original implant remained in place in 88% of patients were satisfied with the result and 77% were engaging in penetrative sexual intercourse [23].

Infraumbilical Phalloplasty (Figure 6)

This technique, most commonly used for total phallic construction in female to male transsexuals, can be modified for use in penile cancer patients, although no published data is available for this group [13]. The advantages of this technique are that it is more reproducible, technically easier to perform and that the operating time is shorter. Another advantage of this technique is that the donor site scarring is limited to the abdomen, which is more easily concealable than the forearm. The main drawbacks of the technique are the creation of a wedge shaped, hairy phallus, which lacks a neourethra and is insensate for the distal two thirds of its length.

The phallus is fashioned from a cutaneous flap that is raised from the inferior aspect of the abdominal wall. Usually the dimensions of the flap are 12 cm in width and 12- 14 cm in length, which is measured from the base of the penile stump. Where possible, the superficial external pudendal vessels are incorporated into the base of the pedicle. The anterior abdominal wall skin is then dissected off the rectus fascia and mobilized caudally to enable a primary closure of the donor site defect avoiding the need for skin grafting.

The subsequent steps of glans sculpture and prosthetics are similar to the ones previously described for the forearm flap phalloplasty.

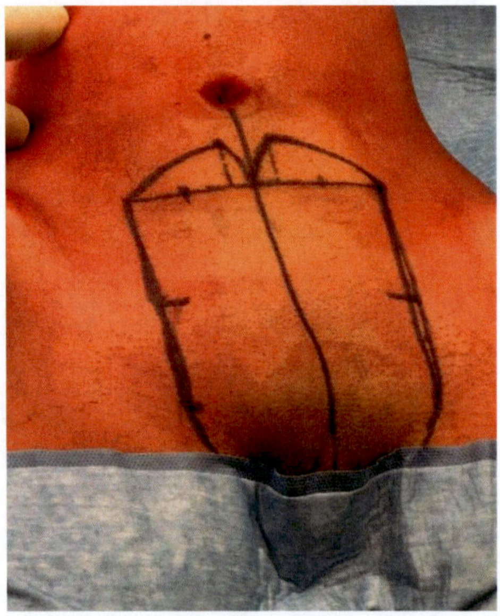

Figure 6. Infraumbilical phalloplasty. A cutaneous flap raised from the inferior aspect of the abdominal wall is used for creation of the neophallus.

Since urethral complications associated with 2 stage skin graft urethroplasty are high in terms of contracture and fistula formation, patients can be offered the delayed incorporation of a radial artery based neourethra into the neophallus (radial artery urethroplasty). The procedure involves the microsurgical transfer of a radial artery based 4 cm wide flap harvested from the inner aspect of the non-dominant forearm. Once tubularized around a 16 Fr catheter, the flap is fitted in a previously fashioned pubic phalloplasty. In expert hands, this procedure is associated with low complication rates, in terms of stricture and fistula formations and it is not prone to sacculation.

Antero-Lateral Thigh Flap Phalloplasty

ALT flap is another reasonable option in patients requiring total phallic reconstruction [24]. This is a fascio-cutaneous flap based on the perforator vessels through the vastus lateralis and rectus femoris from the descending branch of the anterior circumflex femoral artery. The ALT flap is very reliable from a vascular point of view and is commonly used in reconstructive surgery. For total phallic reconstruction purposes, a 16 x 16cm (16 x 20cm if incorporating a neo-urethra) flap needs to be raised. The dissection is a little more difficult than for the radial forearm flap because the perforator vessels need to be released from the surrounding rectus muscle. Frequently there is a long enough pedicle to reach the pubic area after tunneling under the rectus femoris tendon, which then obviates the need for a microsurgical vascular anastomosis. However, the ALT flap has a thick subcutaneous layer and is much hairier than the forearm. These characteristics render simultaneous neo-urethral construction using the "tube within tube" technique difficult. Often the phalloplasty is made from the ALT flap and the neo-urethra is then formed from a 4 cm wide radial forearm flap, with a principle similar to the one previously described for infraumbilical phalloplasty and radial artery urethroplasty. There is only one cutaneous nerve with the ALT flap, so the potential sensation is not as good as in case of radial artery phalloplasty. Careful patient selection is therefore particularly important to achieve good cosmetic results. Because of the large size of the donor site defect, a split skin graft is used to cover the donor site. Although donor site scarring tends to be poor, the area can be easily hidden even if the patient is wearing short trousers.

Latissimus Dorsi Flap

LD flap represents another valid alternative for total penile reconstruction. It is a myocutaneous flap based on the thoracodorsal artery, which is a descending branch of the subscapular artery [25].

Usually a large skin flap, up to 15 cm wide and 20 cm long can be raised on a 3-4 cm strip of latissimus dorsi muscle, as there are many reliable perforators around the anterior intramuscular branch. This technique allows the creation of a sensate phallus, as the thoracodorsal nerve, which runs alongside the thoracodorsal artery and vein, guarantees the innervation of the flap.

The main advantage of LD flap phalloplasty is the limited donor site morbidity as the defect can be primarily repaired without the use of a skin graft and with minimal scarring.

Total phallic reconstruction with the use of LD requires multiple stages. The first is phallus formation with microsurgical tissue transfer techniques to the recipient area. At this stage, the neophallus does not contain a neo-urethra as the flap is too thick to allow the creation of a neourethra with a "tube within a tube" technique. A "prelaminated" urethra can therefore fashioned in 2 stages using buccal mucosa grafts, which are applied on the muscular aspect of the flap. Using this technique urethral strictures and fistulae are rather common. Penile prosthesis implantation is performed using the same technique described for the RAP phalloplasty once sensation has been achieved and flap/urethral complications dealt with.

Conclusion

Reconstructive surgery for penile cancer survivor still represents a real challenge. A special care should be dedicated to minimizing, when oncologically safe, the genital disfiguration. Penile lengthening strategies should be preferred when an adequate residual stump is present. A total phallic reconstruction should be reserved to selected patients and it must be performed in high-volume tertiary referral centers.

Key Points

- The extent of the demolitive surgery for penile cancer should be minimized as much as possible without jeopardizing the clearance rates of the disease.
- Various lengthening procedures may be considered to maximize a residual penile stump after a demolitive surgery for penile cancer.
- Total phallic reconstruction represents the only reconstructive option allowing patients underwent a total/subtotal penectomy to regain both sexual and urinary function.
- Total phallic reconstruction represents a real surgical challenge for the reconstructive surgeon.
- The main goals of a total phallic reconstruction are to create a cosmetically acceptable phallus with both tactile and erogenous sensation, to allow the patient to void and ejaculate from the tip of the neoglans and to have an adequate bulk to allow the insertion of a penile prosthesis.
- The main types of phalloplasty to date are as follows: a) The radial artery phalloplasty, which is a free flap phalloplasty b) The infraubilical phalloplasty also known as pubic phalloplasty c) The anterolateral thigh flap d) The latissimus dorsi flap.
- Total phallic reconstruction, despite the burden of a high incidence of postoperative complications and the possible need for multiple operations, yields to excellent surgical and functional results.

References

[1] Misra S, Chaturvedi A, Misra NC. Penile carcinoma: a challenge for the developing world. *Lancet Oncol* 2004;5:240–7. doi:10.1016/S1470-2045(04) 01427-5.

[2] Barnholtz-Sloan JS, Maldonado JL, Pow-sang J, Giuliano AR, Guiliano AR. Incidence trends in primary malignant penile cancer. *Urol Oncol* 2007;25:361–7. doi:10.1016/j.urolonc.2006.08.029.

[3] Hoffman MA, Renshaw AA, Loughlin KR. Squamous cell carcinoma of the penis and microscopic pathologic margins: how much margin is needed for local cure? *Cancer* 1999;85:1565–8.

[4] Philippou P, Shabbir M, Malone P, Nigam R, Muneer A, Ralph DJ, et al. Conservative surgery for squamous cell carcinoma of the penis: resection margins and long-term oncological control. *J Urol* 2012;188:803–8. doi:10.1016/j.juro.2012.05.012.

[5] Minhas S, Kayes O, Hegarty P, Kumar P, Freeman A, Ralph D. What surgical resection margins are required to achieve oncological control in men with primary penile cancer? BJU Int 2005;96:1040–3. doi:10.1111/j.1464-410X.2005.05769.x.

[6] Hegarty PK, Shabbir M, Hughes B, Minhas S, Perry M, Watkin N, et al. Penile preserving surgery and surgical strategies to maximize penile form and function in penile cancer: recommendations from the United Kingdom experience. *World J Urol* 2009;27:179–87. doi:10.1007/s00345-008-0312-x.

[7] Sedigh O, Falcone M, Ceruti C, Timpano M, Preto M, Oderda M, et al. Sexual function after surgical treatment for penile cancer: which organ sparing approach gives the best results? *Can Urol Assoc J* 2015;9:E423-7. doi:10.5489/cuaj.2801.

[8] Kieffer JM, Djajadiningrat RS, van Muilekom EAM, Graafland NM, Horenblas S, Aaronson NK. Quality of Life for Patients Treated for Penile Cancer. *J Urol* 2014;192:1105–10. doi:10.1016/j.juro.2014.04.014.

[9] Palminteri E, Berdondini E, Lazzeri M, Mirri F, Barbagli G. Resurfacing and Reconstruction of the Glans Penis. *Eur Urol* 2007;52:893–900. doi:10.1016/j.eururo.2007.01.047.

[10] Garaffa G, Raheem AA, Christopher NA, Ralph DJ. Total phallic reconstruction after penile amputation for carcinoma. *BJU Int* 2009;104:852–6. doi:10.1111/j.1464-410X.2009.08424.x.

[11] Bogoras N. Uber die volle plastische wiederherstellung eines zum {Koitus} fahigen {Penis} (peniplastica totalis). *Zentralbl Chir* 1936;63:1271.

[12] Gillies H. Congenital absence of the penis. *Br J Plast Surg* 1948;1:8–28.

[13] Bettocchi C, Ralph DJ, Pryor JP. Pedicled pubic phalloplasty in females with gender dysphoria. *BJU Int* 2005;95:120–4. doi:10.1111/j.1464-410X.2004.05262.x.

[14] Silfen R, Hudson DA, McCulley S. Penile lengthening for traumatic penile amputation due to ritual circumcision: a case report. *Ann Plast Surg* 2000; 44:311–6.

[15] Song R, Gao Y, Song Y, Yu Y, Song Y. The forearm flap. *Clin Plast Surg* 1982;9:21–6.

[16] Chang TS, Hwang WY. Forearm flap in one-stage reconstruction of the penis. *Plast Reconstr Surg* 1984;74:251–8.

[17] Garaffa G, Spilotros M, Christopher NA, Ralph DJ. Total Phallic Reconstruction Using Radial Artery Based Forearm Free Flap Phalloplasty in Patients with Epispadias-Exstrophy Complex. *J Urol* 2014;192:814–20. doi:10.1016/j.juro.2014.03.105.

[18] Garaffa G, Ralph DJ. Free Flap Phalloplasty For Female To Male Gender Dysphoria. *J Sex Med* 2016;13:1942–7. doi:10.1016/j.jsxm.2016.10.004.

[19] Falcone M, Garaffa G, Raheem A, Christopher NA, Ralph DJ. Total Phallic Reconstruction Using the Radial Artery Based Forearm Free Flap After Traumatic Penile Amputation. *J Sex Med* 2016;13. doi:10.1016/j.jsxm.2016.05.003.

[20] Garaffa G, Christopher NA, Ralph DJ. Total Phallic Reconstruction in Female-to-Male Transsexuals. *Eur Urol* 2010;57:715–22. doi:10.1016/j.eururo.2009.05.018.

[21] Selvaggi G, Monstrey S, Hoebeke P, Ceulemans P, Van Landuyt K, Hamdi M, et al. Donor-site morbidity of the radial forearm free flap after 125 phalloplasties in gender identity disorder. *Plast Reconstr Surg* 2006;118:1171–7. doi:10.1097/01.prs.0000221110.43002.a0.

[22] Van Caenegem E, Verhaeghe E, Taes Y, Wierckx K, Toye K, Goemaere S, et al. Long-term evaluation of donor-site morbidity after radial forearm flap phalloplasty for transsexual men. *J Sex Med* 2013;10:1644–51. doi:10.1111/jsm.12121.

[23] Falcone M, Garaffa G, Gillo A, Dente D, Christopher ANAN, Ralph DJDJ. Outcomes of inflatable penile prosthesis insertion in 247 patients completing female to male gender reassignment surgery. *BJU Int* 2018;121:139–44. doi:10.1111/bju.14027.

[24] Felici N, Felici A. A new phalloplasty technique: the free anterolateral thigh flap phalloplasty. *J Plast Reconstr Aesthet Surg* 2006;59:153–7.

[25] Perovic S V., Djinovic R, Bumbasirevic M, Djordjevic M, Vukovic P. Total phalloplasty using a musculocutaneous latissimus dorsi flap. *BJU Int* 2007;100:899–905; discussion 905. doi:10.1111/j.1464-410X.2007.07084.x.

In: Penile Cancer: Challenges and Controversies
Editors: F. E. Martins and M. L. Djordjevic
ISBN: 978-1-53615-950-9

Chapter 21

FUTURE DIRECTIONS AND GOALS

Francisco E. Martins[1,*], MD and
Philippe E. Spiess[2], MD, MS, FACS, FRCS(C)
[1]Department of Urology, University of Lisbon, School of Medicine, Santa Maria University Hospital, CHULN, Lisbon, Portugal
[2]Departments of Genitourinary Oncology and Tumor Biology, Moffitt Cancer Center, Tampa, Florida, US

Penile cancer is an uncommon but often aggressive tumor which is potentially curable particularly if diagnosed and treated at an early stage of progression. Its rarity has prohibited large cooperative randomized controlled trials and the available trials and series are so heterogeneous that meta- or pooled analyses are challenging to conduct. Significant advances have been made in imaging techniques enabling more accurate diagnosis and staging. Recent therapeutic advances have led to a paradigm shift from historically highly mutilating surgery to penile-preserving approaches where indicated. These therapeutic approaches, including penile-sparing surgery, brachytherapy, or radiotherapy should be considered for localized disease. Organ preservation has become the standard approach to low-stage penile cancer, whereas in the setting of lymphatic metastasis particularly bulky disease (> 4cm), multimodal treatment with radical inguinal node surgery and neoadjuvant/adjuvant chemotherapy have been believed to improve outcome based on limited mostly single center peer reviewed data. The currently open multicenter prospective International Penile Cancer Advanced Trial (InPACT) will hopefully define the true benefit of such a multimodal approach to managing locally advanced disease. Efforts to predict accurately nodal involvement in clinically negative

* Corresponding Author's E-mail: faemartins@gmail.com.

node (cN0) patients is essential to better select those patients requiring surgical resection and spare the morbidity of a groin dissection in such patients. Therefore, the goals would be to maximize the chance for cure, while minimizing unnecessary lymphadenectomy-associated morbidity.

Despite excellent oncological outcomes in penile cancer patients with localized disease, metastatic disease remains a therapeutic conundrum. Important research questions remain, such as the role of chemoradiation, and role of targeted and/or immunotherapy. Unfortunately, in view of the disease rarity and little interest among pharmaceutical industry, few clinical trials have been designed and carried out to answer such critical therapeutic dilemmas. Because of the histological and pathophysiological similarities between penile and head and neck squamous cell carcinomas (HNSCC) a further exploration of established systemic agents for HNSCC such as EGFR (epidermal growth factor receptor) targeting therapies should be encouraged. Patients who do not respond to neoadjuvant chemoradiotherapy may in certain instances benefit from undergoing palliative surgery particularly if the endpoint of treatment is locoregional control and/or managing a symptomatic tumor site (either primary penile tumor or inguinal metastasis). It would also be important in the future to identify other predictors of response to systemic therapy, particularly accounting for HPV status, as seen in other cancers. Therefore, the development of new effective systemic therapies for this rare but often devastating disease is critical and we urge the scientific community to embrace this challenge as our patients deserve a more promising fate through the deployment of a more effective therapeutic armamentarium accounting for tumor heterogeneity based on two distinct clinical pathways based on HPV status.

The inclusion of molecular panels may improve available prognostic and therapeutic capabilities. It is explicit that penile cancer possesses distinct molecular pathways with diverse genetic and epigenetic modifications with potential therapeutic implications. Better and additional translational research and collaboration is critical to further develop novel diagnostic biomarkers and effective therapeutic protocols for patients with penile cancer. An improved understanding of the basic biology of penile cancer would be important in the design of future prospective trials including potential precision medicine approaches for this rare disease. Moreover, the cooperation and partnership of regulatory bodies is critical in the early stages of drug development. It is important to incentivize industry, implement a plausible program for disease advocacy and venture philanthropy. Collaborative multi-institutional studies are also encouraged. Being a relatively uncommon disease, the creation of national expert advisory groups for the management of penile cancer with development of proposed nationwide guidelines as has been conducted by the National Comprehensive Cancer Network in the US and the European Urological Association to improve patient care through evidence based diagnostic and treatment strategies is imperative and should be recognized and supported by national governments.

Lastly, and most importantly, prevention and early detection play a vital role and should be the first steps against cancer, in general, and penile cancer, in particular. Because penile cancer is a preventable disease, primary prevention measures including avoidance of HPV risk factors, smoking cessation, patient awareness and self-examination are essential and should be implemented. Neonatal circumcision, smoking cessation and HPV vaccination may substantially reduce the incidence of PC. Indeed, HPV vaccination is already approved in the US for males aged 9 – 26 years for preventing genital warts and anal cancer. Global collaboration is urgently necessary to make these advances in the decrease of penile cancer incidence and improve quality of life. The psychosocial impact of penile cancer is of utmost importance and should not be forgotten; patient survivorship programs should include psychosocial support which have shown proven benefit.

About the Editors

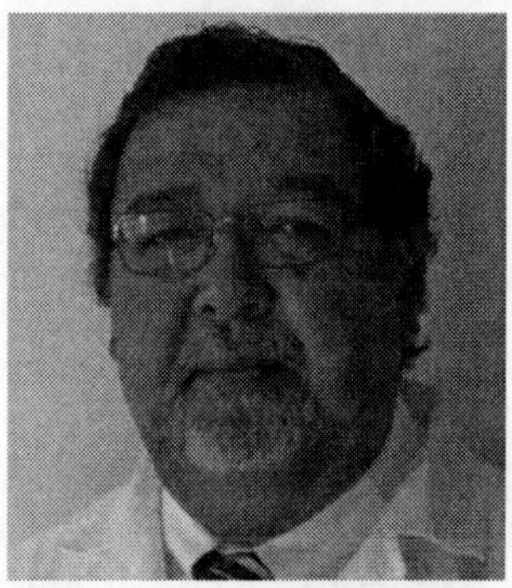

Francisco E. Martins, MD

Consultant Urological Surgeon, Department of Urology, University of Lisbon, School of Medicine, Santa Maria University Hospital, Lisbon, Portugal

Francisco Martins obtained his Medical Degree at the Faculty of Medicine, University of Lisbon in 1983. He earned his title as Specialist in Urology by the Portuguese Medical Association, College of Urology, in 1993. He has been engaged in several humanitarian outreach clinical visits in Ethiopia, Angola and Tanzania. His areas of major clinical and research interest are: Genito-urethral and Pelvic Trauma and Reconstruction, Vesicovaginal and Rectovaginal Fistula, Female Pelvic Medicine, Erectile Dysfunction, Urinary Diversion, and Penile Cancer. He has been Consultant Urological Surgeon at Santa Maria University Hospital (2008-present date). In May 2017, he was elected to the GURS Board of Directors (Genitourinary Reconstructive Surgeons) and in October 2917 and September 2018 was granted Honorary Membership of the Hungarian Urological Association (HUA) and South African Urological

Association (SAUA), respectively. He is member of several national and international societies and associations. He is member of the first EAU (European Association of Urology) Guidelines Panel for Urethral Strictures. He is peer reviewer for several journals, including, Acta Urológica Portuguesa, Actas Urológicas Españolas, Advances in Urology, Biomed Research International, British Journal of Medicine and Medical Research, European Urology, International Urology and Nephrology, Journal of Men's Health, Journal of Surgery, World Journal of Urology and Journal of Urology. He has presented and lectured at numerous national and international meetings, conferences and congresses and has published and co-authored over 60 articles in peer review journals, 7 book chapters and edited 3 books on erectile dysfunction, penile cancer and male genitourethral reconstruction as well as 2 Special Issues for Advances in Urology and Biomed Research International.

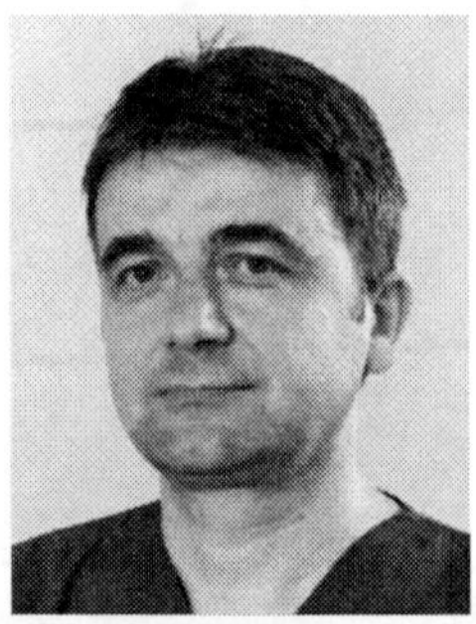

Miroslav L. Djordjevic

Professor of Urology, School of Medicine, University of Belgrade, Serbia

Dr. Miroslav L. Djordjevic is a Professor of Urology and Surgery at the School of Medicine, University of Belgrade, Serbia. The main field of his multidisciplinary work is urogenital reconstructive surgery, encompassing treatment of all anomalies of the genital system, regardless of gender or age. Professor Djordjevic has been multiply awarded for his comprehensive scientific work. He is the Editor of many leading journals and books, and a member of all relevant international associations in the field of urology and genital reconstructive surgery. He has recently been elected as the President of Society of Genitourinary Reconstructive Surgeons (GURS). Professor Djordjevic has been invited lecturer and Visiting Professor on many universities all around the world. As a member of humanitarian societies he actively participated in humanitarian missions over the world. Last but not least, he is the founder and leader of Belgrade Center for Genital Reconstructive Surgery, which is chosen as a fellowship program center by 15-20 foreign colleagues every year.

INDEX

A

B

C

D

E

F

G

H

I

L

M

N

O

P

Q

R

S

T

U

V

W